T0362444

Health Disparities and Health Equity in Critical Care

Editors

CRYSTAL E. BROWN
ELIZABETH J. CHUANG
JORDAN A. KEMPKER

CRITICAL CARE CLINICS

www.criticalcare.theclinics.com

Consulting Editor
GREGORY S. MARTIN

October 2024 • Volume 40 • Number 4

ELSEVIER

1600 John F. Kennedy Boulevard • Suite 1800 • Philadelphia, Pennsylvania, 19103-2899

http://www.theclinics.com

CRITICAL CARE CLINICS Volume 40, Number 4
October 2024 ISSN 0749-0704, ISBN-13: 978-0-443-29384-9

Editor: Joanna Gascoine
Developmental Editor: Saswoti Nath

Critical Care Clinics (ISSN: 0749-0704) is published quarterly by Elsevier Inc., 360 Park Avenue South, New York, NY 10010-1710. Months of issue are January, April, July, and October. Business and Editorial Offices: 1600 John F. Kennedy Blvd., Suite 1800, Philadelphia, PA 19103-2899. Customer Service Office: 6277 Sea Harbor Drive, Orlando, FL 32887-4800. Periodicals postage paid at New York, NY and additional mailing offices. Subscription prices are $279.00 per year for US individuals, $100.00 per year for US students and residents, $317.00 per year for Canadian individuals, $362.00 per year for international individuals, $100.00 per year for Canadian students/residents, and $150.00 per year for foreign students/residents. For institutional access pricing please contact Customer Service via the contact information below. To receive student/resident rate, orders must be accompanied by name of affiliated institution, date of term, and the signature of program/residency coordinator on institution letterhead. Orders will be billed at individual rate until proof of status is received. Foreign air speed delivery is included in all *Clinics* subscription prices. All prices are subject to change without notice. Orders, claims, and journal inquiries: Please visit our Support Hub page https://service.elsevier.com for assistance.

Reprints. For copies of 100 or more of articles in this publication, please contact the Commercial Reprints Department, Elsevier Inc., 360 Park Avenue South, New York, NY 10010-1710. Tel.: 212-633-3874; Fax: 212-633-3820; E-mail: reprints@elsevier.com.

Critical Care Clinics is also published in Spanish by Editorial Inter-Medica, Junin 917, 1ᵉʳ A, 1113, Buenos Aires, Argentina.

Critical Care Clinics is covered in *MEDLINE/PubMed (Index Medicus), EMBASE/Excerpta Medica, Current Concepts/Clinical Medicine, ISI/BIOMED,* and *Chemical Abstracts.*

Contributors

CONSULTING EDITOR

GREGORY S. MARTIN, MD, Msc
Professor, Division of Pulmonary, Allergy, Critical Care and Sleep Medicine, Research Director, Emory Critical Care Center, Director, Emory/Georgia Tech Predictive Health Institute, Co-Director, Atlanta Center for Microsystems Engineered Point-of-Care, Technologies (ACME POCT), President, Society of Critical Care Medicine, Atlanta, Georgia, USA

EDITORS

CRYSTAL E. BROWN, MD, MA
Assistant Professor, Division of Pulmonary, Critical Care, and Sleep Medicine, Adjunct Assistant Professor, Department of Bioethics and Humanities, University of Washington, Seattle, Washington, USA

ELIZABETH J. CHUANG, MD, MPH
Director, Montefiore Einstein Center for Bioethics, Associate Professor of Medicine, Division of Critical Care, Albert Einstein College of Medicine, New Rochelle, New York, USA

JORDAN A. KEMPKER, MD, MSc
Associate Professor of Medicine, Division of Pulmonary, Critical Care, Allergy and Sleep Medicine, Emory School of Medicine, Atlanta, Georgia, USA

AUTHORS

JINNETTE DAWN ABBOTT, MD
Professor, Division of Cardiology, Department of Medicine, Warren Alpert Medical School of Brown University, Professor, Brown Medical School, Lifespan Cardiovascular Institute, Providence, Rhode Island, USA

MANZILAT Y. AKANDE, MD, MPH, MS
Associate Professor, Section of Critical Care, Department of Pediatrics, Oklahoma University Health Sciences Center, Oklahoma City, Oklahoma, USA

DEEPSHIKHA CHARAN ASHANA, MD, MBA, MS
Core Faculty Member, Duke-Margolis Center for Health Policy, Assistant Professor, Department of Population Health Sciences, Duke University, Durham, North Carolina, USA

REBECCA A. ASP, MD, MS
Clinical Fellow, Division of Critical Care Medicine, Cincinnati Children's Hospital Medical Center, University of Cincinnati School of Medicine, Cincinnati, Ohio, USA

MRIDUL BANSAL, MD
Resident, Department of Medicine, East Carolina University Brody School of Medicine, Greenville, North Carolina, USA

TASCE BONGIOVANNI, MD, MPP
Assistant Professor, Department of Surgery, University of California San Francisco School of Medicine, San Francisco, California, USA

HENRY BREMS, MD
Fellow, Division of Pulmonary and Critical Care Medicine, Department of Medicine, Johns Hopkins School of Medicine, Baltimore, Maryland, USA

KARA CALHOUN, MD, MPH
Assistant Professor, Division of Pulmonary Sciences and Critical Care Medicine, University of Colorado, Aurora, Colorado, USA

LEO ANTHONY CELI, MD, MS, MPH
Senior Research Scientist, Laboratory for Computational Physiology, Institute for Medical Engineering and Science, Massachusetts Institute of Technology, Cambridge, Massachusetts, USA; Instructor, Department of Biostatistics, Harvard T.H. Chan School of Public Health, Massachusetts, USA; Associate Program Director, Department of Medicine, Beth Israel Deaconess Medical Center, Boston, Massachusetts, USA

MARIE-LAURE CHARPIGNON, MS
PhD Candidate, Institute for Data, Systems, and Society (IDSS), Massachusetts Institute of Technology, Cambridge, Massachusetts, USA

CHRISTOPHER F. CHESLEY, MD, MSCE
Instructor, Department of Medicine, University of Pennsylvania Perelman School of Medicine, Philadelphia, Pennsylvania, USA; Assistant Professor of Medicine, Division of Pulmonary and Critical Care, Palliative and Advanced Illness Research (PAIR) Center, University of Pennsylvania Perelman School of Medicine, Philadelphia, Pennsylvania, USA; Leonard Davis Institute of Health Economics, University of Pennsylvania, Philadelphia, Pennsylvania, USA

ANAND CHOWDHURY, MD, MMCI
Assistant Professor, Division of Pulmonary, Allergy, and Critical Care Medicine, Department of Medicine, Duke University, Durham, North Carolina, USA

CAITLIN COLLINS, MD
Trauma and Critical Care Fellow, Department of Surgery, University of California San Francisco School of Medicine, San Francisco, California, USA

DANIEL COLON HIDALGO, MD, MPH
Instructor, Division of Pulmonary Sciences and Critical Care Medicine, University of Colorado, Aurora, Colorado, USA

NICOLETA ECONOMOU-ZAVLANOS, PhD
Director, Duke Health, AI Health, Durham, North Carolina, USA

JESSICA FOWLER, MD, MPH
Attending Physician, Division of Critical Care, Department of Anesthesiology and Critical Care Medicine, Children's Hospital of Philadelphia, The University of Pennsylvania Perelman School of Medicine, Philadelphia, Pennsylvania, USA

PANAGIS GALIATSATOS, MD, MHS
Associate Professor, Division of Pulmonary and Critical Care Medicine, Department of Medicine, Johns Hopkins School of Medicine, SDOH and Health Equity SME, Office of Diversity, Inclusion, and Health Equity, Johns Hopkins Health System, Baltimore, Maryland, USA

JACK GALLIFANT, MBBS, MSc
Honorary Researcher, Laboratory for Computational Physiology, Institute for Medical Engineering and Science, Massachusetts Institute of Technology, Cambridge, Massachusetts, USA; Department of Critical Care, Guy's and St Thomas' NHS Trust, London, United Kingdom

CODY-AARON GATHERS, MD, MSHP
Associate Fellow, Leonard Davis Institute of Health Economics, University of Pennsylvania, Fellow, Division of Critical Care, Department of Anesthesiology and Critical Care Medicine, Children's Hospital of Philadelphia, Philadelphia, Pennsylvania, USA

SHERIE A. GAUSE, MD
Assistant Professor, Division of Pulmonary, Allergy, and Critical Care Medicine, Department of Medicine, Oregon Health & Science University, Portland, Oregon, USA

JUDY GICHOYA, MD
Associate Professor, Department of Radiology, Emory University, Atlanta, Georgia, USA

JOCELYN R. GRUNWELL, MD, PhD, MSCR
Associate Professor, Department of Pediatrics, Children's Healthcare of Atlanta, Emory University School of Medicine, Atlanta, Georgia, USA

KATRINA E. HAUSCHILDT, PhD
Faculty Research Associate, Department of Medicine, Johns Hopkins University School of Medicine, Baltimore, Maryland, USA

HEATHER KING, PhD
Research Health Scientist, Health Services Research and Development, Center of Innovation to Accelerate Discovery and Practice Transformation (ADAPT), Durham VA Health Care System, Assistant Professor, Department of Population Health Sciences, Division of General Internal Medicine, Duke University School of Medicine, Durham, North Carolina, USA

MARC KOWALKOWSKI, PhD
Associate Professor, Hospital Medicine, Department of Internal Medicine, Associate Director, Center for Health System Sciences, Wake Forest University School of Medicine, Winston Salem, North Carolina, USA

AKSHAY MACHANAHALLI BALAKRISHNA, MD
Fellow, Section of Cardiovascular Medicine, Department of Medicine, Creighton University School of Medicine, Omaha, Nebraska, USA

PAULA M. MAGEE, MD, MPH
Attending Physician, Division of Pediatric Critical Care Medicine, Department of Anesthesiology and Critical Care Medicine, Children's Hospital of Philadelphia, Philadelphia, Pennsylvania, USA

JOÃO MATOS, MSc
Associate Researcher, Faculty of Engineering, University of Porto (FEUP), Institute for Systems and Computer Engineering, Technology and Science (INESC TEC), Porto, Portugal; Laboratory for Computational Physiology, Institute for Medical Engineering and Science, Massachusetts Institute of Technology, Cambridge, Massachusetts, USA

ARYAN MEHTA, MD
Resident Physician, Department of Medicine, University of Connecticut School of Medicine, Farmington, Connecticut, USA

KRISTINA MONTEMAYOR, MD
Assistant Professor, Division of Pulmonary and Critical Care Medicine, Department of Medicine, Johns Hopkins School of Medicine, Baltimore, Maryland, USA

NICHOLAS MORRIS, MD
Associate Professor, Neurocritical Care Division, Department of Neurology, University of Maryland, Baltimore, Maryland, USA

DARIA C. MUROSKO, MD, MPH
Attending Physician, Division of Neonatology, Department of Pediatrics, Children's Hospital of Philadelphia, Philadelphia, Pennsylvania, USA

CARLIE N. MYERS, MD, MS
Assistant Professor, Division of Critical Care Medicine, Cincinnati Children's Hospital Medical Center, University of Cincinnati School of Medicine, Cincinnati, Ohio, USA

MARYAM Y. NAIM, MD, MSCE
Associate Professor, Department of Anesthesiology and Critical Care, The University of Pennsylvania Perelman School of Medicine, Associate Chief, Division of Cardiac Critical Care Medicine, Children's Hospital of Philadelphia, Philadelphia, Pennsylvania, USA

LAMA NAZER, PharmD
Head, Pharmacy Research and Staff Development, Department of Pharmacy, King Hussein Cancer Center, Amman, Jordan

ANNA NEUMEIER, MD
Assistant Professor, Division of Pulmonary Sciences and Critical Care Medicine, University of Colorado, Denver Health, Pulmonary, Critical Care and Sleep Medicine Division, Denver, Colorado, USA

FADAR OLIVER OTITE, MD, SM
Assistant Professor, Cerebrovascular Division, Upstate Neurological Institute, Syracuse, New York, USA

JESSICA PALAKSHAPPA, MD, MSc
Associate Professor, Division of Pulmonary, Critical Care, Allergy, and Immunologic Diseases, Wake Forest University School of Medicine, Winston-Salem, North Carolina, USA

ERIN PAQUETTE, MD, JD, MBE
Associate Professor, Division of Critical Care Medicine, Ann & Robert H. Lurie Children's Hospital, Northwestern University Feinberg School of Medicine, Assistant Professor (by courtesy), Department of Pediatrics, Northwestern University Pritzker School of Law, Chicago, Illinois, USA

ATHENA POPPAS, MD
Professor, Division of Cardiology, Department of Medicine, Warren Alpert Medical School of Brown University, Chief, Cardiology Division; Director, Lifespan Cardiovascular Institute, Providence, Rhode Island, USA

TYLER RAINER, MD, MSHP
Fellow, Division of Pediatric Emergency Medicine, Department of Pediatrics, Children's Hospital of Philadelphia, Philadelphia, Pennsylvania, USA

ANIREDDY R. REDDY, MD, MSHP
Attending Physician, Division of Critical Care, Department of Anesthesiology and Critical Care Medicine, Children's Hospital of Philadelphia, Leonard Davis Institute of Health Economics, University of Pennsylvania, Department of Anesthesiology and Critical Care, The University of Pennsylvania Perelman School of Medicine, Philadelphia, Pennsylvania, USA

ROBERT O. ROSWELL, MD
Associate Professor, Department of Cardiology, Zucker School of Medicine at Hofstra/ Northwell, Hempstead, New York, USA

MARWAN SAAD, MD, PhD
Assistant Professor, Division of Cardiology, Department of Medicine, Warren Alpert Medical School of Brown University, Director, Interventional Structural Heart Research, Lifespan Cardiovascular Institute, Providence, Rhode Island, USA

YHENNEKO J. TAYLOR, PhD
Co-Director, Center for Health System Sciences, Atrium Health, Charlotte, North Carolina, USA; Adjunct Professor, Department of Sciences and Health Policy, Wake Forest University School of Medicine, Winston Salem, North Carolina, USA

SARASCHANDRA VALLABHAJOSYULA, MD, MSc
Assistant Professor, Division of Cardiology, Department of Medicine, Warren Alpert Medical School of Brown University, Interventional and critical care cardiologist, Lifespan Cardiovascular Institute, Providence, Rhode Island, USA

COREY E. VENTETUOLO, MD, MS
Associate Professor, Division of Pulmonary, Critical Care and Sleep Medicine, Department of Medicine, Warren Alpert Medical School of Brown University, Department of Health Services, Policy and Practice, Brown University, Providence, Rhode Island, USA

JUDITH B. VICK, MD, MPH
Durham VA Health Care System, Consulting Associate, Department of Medicine, Duke University School of Medicine; National Clinician Scholars Program, Duke Clinical and Translational Science Institute, Durham, North Carolina, USA

KELLY C. VRANAS, MD, MCR
Associate Professor, Division of Pulmonary, Allergy, and Critical Care Medicine, Department of Medicine, Oregon Health & Science University, Core Investigator, Center to Improve Veteran Involvement in Care (CIVIC), VA Portland Health Care System, Portland, Oregon, USA

AN-KWOK IAN WONG, MD, PhD
Assistant Professor, Division of Pulmonary, Allergy, and Critical Care Medicine, Department of Biostatistics and Bioinformatics, Division of Translational Biomedical Informatics, Duke University, Durham, North Carolina, USA

Contents

A growing body of literature has identified social determinants of health (SDoH) as potential contributors to health disparities in pediatric critical illness. Pediatric critical care providers should use validated screening tools to identify unmet social needs and ensure appropriate referral through multisector partnerships. Pediatric critical care researchers should consider factors outside of race and insurance status and explore the association between neighborhood-level factors and disparate health outcomes during critical illness. Measuring and addressing the SDoH at the individual and neighborhood level are important next steps in mitigating health disparities for critically ill pediatric patients.

To date, health disparities in critically ill children have largely been studied within, not across, specific intensive care unit (ICU) settings, thus impeding collaboration which may help advance the care of critically ill children. The aim of this scoping review is to summarize the literature intentionally designed to examine health disparities, across 3 primary ICU settings (neonatal ICU, pediatric ICU, and cardiac ICU) in the United States. We included over 50 studies which describe health disparities across race and/or ethnicity, area-level indices, insurance status, socioeconomic position, language, and distance.

Despite legal protections guaranteeing care for patients with trauma, disparities exist in patient outcomes. We review disparities in patient management and outcomes related to insurance status, race and ethnicity, and gender for patients with trauma in the preadmission, in-hospital, and post-discharge settings. We highlight groups understudied and either underrepresented or unrepresented in national trauma databases—including American Indians/Alaska Natives, non-English preferred patients, and patients with disabilities. We call for more study of these groups and of upstream factors affecting the reviewed demographics to measure and improve outcomes for these vulnerable populations.

This article reviews the current evidence base for racial and ethnic disparities related to acute respiratory failure. It discusses the prevailing and most studied mechanisms that underlay these disparities, analytical challenges that face the field, and then uses this discussion to frame future directions to outline next steps for developing disparities-mitigating solutions.

Cardiovascular disease continues to be the leading cause of morbidity and mortality in the United States. Despite advancements in medical care, there remain persistent racial, ethnic, and gender disparity in the diagnosis, treatment, and prognosis of individuals with cardiovascular disease. In this review we seek to discuss differences in pathophysiology, clinical course, and risk profiles in the management and outcomes of acute myocardial infarction and related high-risk states. We also seek to highlight the demographic and psychosocial inequities that cause disparities in acute cardiovascular care.

Racial, ethnicity and sex disparities are pervasive in the evaluation and acute care of ischemic stroke patients. Administration of intravenous thrombolysis and mechanical thrombectomy are the most critical steps in ischemic stroke treatment but compared to White patients, ischemic stroke patients from minority racial and ethnic groups are less likely to receive these potentially life-saving interventions. Sex and racial disparities in intracerebral hemorrhage or subarachnoid hemorrhage treatment have not been well studied.

Critical care pathologies are not immune to potential social challenges in both health equity and health disparities. Over the last century, as sepsis physiology and interventions have continued to improve clinical outcomes, recognition that such improvements are not seen in all diverse populations warrants an understanding of this disproportionate success. In this review, the authors evaluate sepsis incidence and outcomes across ethnicity,

race, and sex and gender, taking into account social and biological categorization and the association of sepsis-related mortality and morbidity.
Further, the authors review how such issues transcend across age groups,
with vulnerability to sepsis.

Patients from groups that are racially/ethnically minoritized or of low socioeconomic status receive more intensive care near the end of life, endorse
preferences for more life-sustaining treatments, experience lower quality
communication from clinicians, and report worse quality of dying than
other patients. There are many contributory factors, including system
(eg, lack of intensive outpatient symptom management resources), clinician (eg, low-quality serious illness communication), and patient (eg, cultural norms) factors. System and clinician factors contribute to
disparities and ought to be remedied, while patient factors simply reflect
differences in care and may not be appropriate targets for intervention.

Health disparities persist among minoritized populations. A diverse clinician workforce may help address these disparities and improve patient
outcomes; however, diversity in the critical are workforce (particularly
among women and those historically underrepresented in medicine
(URiM)) is lacking. This review describes factors contributing to low respre-
sentation of women and URiM in critical care medicine, and proposes
strategies to overcome those barriers.

Pulmonary and Critical Care Medicine (PCCM) fellowship training faces increasing competition but lacks diversity, hindering health care excellence.
Despite a growing interest in the field, programs lack diverse representation. Addressing this issue is crucial to combat health disparities and bias,
benefiting trainees, practitioners, and patients. Sustainable solutions are
vital for achieving diversity, equity, and inclusion in PCCM. Strategies for
achieving equity among training programs include adopting inclusive recruitment practices, recognizing differential attainment, addressing bias,
fostering an equitable academic climate, and implementing multifaceted
strategic processes to enhance diversity in mentorship including recognition and compensation for diversity and equity work.

Yhenneko J. Taylor, Marc Kowalkowski, and Jessica Palakshappa

The coronavirus disease 2019 (COVID-19) pandemic raised new considerations for social disparities in critical illness including hospital capacity and access to personal protective equipment, access to evolving therapies, vaccinations, virtual care, and restrictions on family visitation. This narrative review aims to explore evidence about racial/ethnic and socioeconomic differences in critical illness during the COVID-19 pandemic, factors driving those differences and promising solutions for mitigating inequities in the future. We apply a patient journey framework to identify social disparities at various stages before, during, and after patient interactions with critical care services and discuss recommendations for policy and practice.

João Matos, Jack Gallifant, Anand Chowdhury, Nicoleta Economou-Zavlanos, Marie-Laure Charpignon, Judy Gichoya, Leo Anthony Celi, Lama Nazer, Heather King, and An-Kwok Ian Wong

This narrative review focuses on the role of clinical prediction models in supporting informed decision-making in critical care, emphasizing their 2 forms: traditional scores and artificial intelligence (AI)-based models. Acknowledging the potential for both types to embed biases, the authors underscore the importance of critical appraisal to increase our trust in models. The authors outline recommendations and critical care examples to manage risk of bias in AI models. The authors advocate for enhanced interdisciplinary training for clinicians, who are encouraged to explore various resources (books, journals, news Web sites, and social media) and events (Datathons) to deepen their understanding of risk of bias.

CRITICAL CARE CLINICS

SERIES OF RELATED INTEREST

Emergency Medicine Clinics
https://www.emed.theclinics.com/
Clinics in Chest Medicine
https://www.chestmed.theclinics.com/

THE CLINICS ARE AVAILABLE ONLINE!
Access your subscription at:
www.theclinics.com

Preface

Toward an Equitable Future in Critical Care Medicine

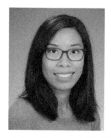
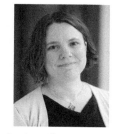
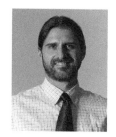

Crystal E. Brown, MD, MA   Elizabeth J. Chuang, MD, MPH   Jordan A. Kempker, MD, MSc

Editors

We are pleased to introduce this issue of *Critical Care Clinics* focused on the stark inequities in access, treatment, and outcomes for critically ill patients, which demand our ongoing attention. The US Department of Health and Human Services' Healthy People 2030 defines health disparity as a "health difference…closely linked with social, economic, and/or environmental disadvantage" and health equity as "the attainment of the highest level of health for all people." They state that "achieving health equity requires valuing everyone equally with focused and ongoing societal efforts to address avoidable inequalities, historical and contemporary injustices, and the elimination of health and health care disparities." In this issue of *Critical Care Clinics*, we present a multifaceted description of disparity and inequity within critical illness, the field of critical care itself, and broader societal structures. This issue contains a series of articles that describe the prevalence, context, characteristics, and effects of health care disparities among the most common conditions and scenarios encountered by critical care practitioners. In addition to disparate patient health and health care outcomes, we look inward and address disparities and inequities in training programs, workforce development, risk assessment tools, and the considerations for rationing scarce critical care resources. Our objective in this multifaceted approach rests on the need to address the underlying societal causes for disparities and inequities in our patients and our own field that are inextricably interrelated.

The articles in this special issue underscore a grim reality of the American health care system: even early in life, geography is destiny. Neighborhood-level social determinants of health, including air quality, access to food, quality housing, transportation, and education, affect the incidence of and recovery from critical illness in children. The existence of "trauma deserts," racial and ethnic minorities and rural populations, decreases the likelihood of timely access to life-saving trauma care. Differences in

Crit Care Clin 40 (2024) xv–xvii
https://doi.org/10.1016/j.ccc.2024.07.001
0749-0704/24/© 2024 Published by Elsevier Inc.

management that result in disparate outcomes in critically ill children and adults with acute respiratory failure and sepsis underscore the need to address the intersectionality of race and ethnicity and other sociodemographic exposures. Adequately addressing and eliminating these inequities, such as those experienced by marginalized populations during the COVID-19 pandemic, requires using best practices for measuring social determinants of health while concurrently addressing the interpersonal, structural, and institutional racism that perpetuates them.

This issue maps a path forward to improve the utility of health disparities research in critical care, including forward-thinking ways to avoid replicating bias, as we advance new technologies and moving beyond mere documentation of disparities and toward concrete actional hypotheses. The use of community-based participatory research, a social justice methodology with proven efficacy in reducing disparities, is described as one effective means of achieving this. Indeed, Hauschildt and colleagues highlight the importance of including community perspectives, reminding us that "when we measure quality of, and disparities in, preference-sensitive outcomes by majority preference, we are most likely to devalue preferences held by marginalized groups."

While we try to present a comprehensive address of disparities and inequities in critical care medicine, we acknowledge that we inevitably fall short. This issue places an emphasis on the population of the United States and its health care system and contains limited discussions around advanced practice providers. In addition, the disparities experienced by LGBTQ+ populations and particular racial and ethnic groups like Native Americans are underdescribed. While we hope this issue inspires greater awareness, empowerment, and action within the topics addressed, we also hope that the issue's limitations encourage additional work in this field, addressing other populations, health care systems, provider groups, and other social domains.

DISCLOSURES

C.E. Brown receives funding from the National Institute of Minority Health and Health Disparities and the Robert Wood Johnson Foundation and has no commercial or financial conflicts of interest. J.A. Kempker has no commercial or financial conflicts of interest to disclose and was not funded during the duration of work for this issue. E.J. Chuang receives funding from the National Institute of Minority Health and Health Disparities and has no commercial or financial conflicts of interest.

Crystal E. Brown, MD, MA
Division of Pulmonary, Critical Care
and Sleep Medicine
Department of Bioethics and Humanities
University of Washington
325 Ninth Avenue
Box 359762
Seattle, WA 98103, USA

Elizabeth J. Chuang, MD, MPH
Montefiore Einstein Center for Bioethics
Division of Critical Care
Albert Einstein College of Medicine
142 Bon Air Avenue
New Rochelle, NY 10804, USA

Jordan A. Kempker, MD, MSc
Division of Pulmonary, Critical Care, Allergy and Sleep Medicine
Emory School of Medicine
89 Jesse Hill Jr Dr SE
Atlanta, GA 30303, USA

E-mail addresses:
crysb@uw.edu (C.E. Brown)
echuang@montefiore.org (E.J. Chuang)
jkempke@emory.edu (J.A. Kempker)

Assessing Social Determinants of Health During Critical Illness
Implications and Methodologies

Paula M. Magee, MD, MPH[a],*, Rebecca A. Asp, MD, MS[b],
Carlie N. Myers, MD, MS[b], Jocelyn R. Grunwell, MD, PhD, MSCR[c],
Erin Paquette, MD, JD, MBe[d], Manzilat Y. Akande, MD, MPH, MS[e]

KEYWORDS

- SDoH • Disparities • Screening • Neighborhood disadvantage • Equity • Pediatrics
- Intensive care unit • Social determinants of health

KEY POINTS

- Social determinants of health (SDoH) have been widely acknowledged as fundamental factors that contribute to a person's overall health and health outcomes.
- Research in pediatrics and pediatric critical care has identified racial/ethnic and socioeconomic disparities in health outcomes for a variety of pediatric conditions.
- The pediatric intensive care unit is an optimal place to identify and address unmet social needs that contribute to health disparities in critical illness using a concerted, multisector approach.
- SDoH screening should occur at the individual level using validated screening tools and the neighborhood level using validated composite measures for research.

[a] Division of Pediatric Critical Care Medicine, Department of Anesthesiology and Critical Care Medicine, Children's Hospital of Philadelphia, 3401 Civic Center Boulevard, 9 Main Suite 9NW45, Philadelphia, PA 19104, USA; [b] Division of Critical Care Medicine, Cincinnati Children's Hospital Medical Center, University of Cincinnati School of Medicine, 3333 Burnet Avenue, ML 2005, Cincinnati, OH 45229, USA; [c] Department of Pediatrics, Children's Healthcare of Atlanta, Emory University School of Medicine, 1405 Clifton Road Northeast, Tower 1, 4th Floor, PCCM Offices, Atlanta GA 30322, USA; [d] Division of Critical Care Medicine, Ann & Robert H. Lurie Children's Hospital, Northwestern University Feinberg School of Medicine, 225 East Chicago Avenue, Chicago, IL 60611, USA; [e] Section of Critical Care, Department of Pediatrics, Oklahoma University Health Sciences Center, 1100 North Lindsay Avenue, Oklahoma City, OK 73104, USA
* Corresponding author.
E-mail address: mageep@chop.edu
Twitter: @GrunwellJocelyn (J.R.G.)

Crit Care Clin 40 (2024) 623–640
https://doi.org/10.1016/j.ccc.2024.05.001
criticalcare.theclinics.com
0749-0704/24/© 2024 Elsevier Inc. All rights are reserved, including those for text and data mining, AI training, and similar technologies.

INTRODUCTION

Addressing social determinants of health (SDoH) has emerged as a key approach to achieving health equity in the United States.[1] SDoH are fundamental social and structural factors in a person's environment that affect a wide range of health, functioning, and quality-of-life outcomes.[2] Categorized into 5 domains by the Center for Disease Control (economic stability, education access and quality, neighborhoods and the built environment, health care access and quality, and social and community), SDoH account for about 80% to 90% of modifiable factors contributing to health outcomes and have been extensively linked to health disparities.[3] SDoH can both directly influence disease onset, progression, and outcomes and indirectly affect health through their effect on health care access.[4] On an individual level, inequitable allocation of resources related to the SDoH yields unmet health-related social needs and poses a significant challenge to achieving good physical health, behavioral health, and well-being.[2] However, there is growing evidence that interventions that address individual-level social needs such as housing or food insecurity result in the downstream effect of improved health outcomes.[5] As such, multiple regulatory bodies and initiatives in the United States have recognized the increasing need to invest in social health as a critical approach to improving individual- and population-level health.[6,7] This has led to many calls for action to address SDoH across the health care continuum through social needs screening and interventions such as linkage with resources and a variety of hospital–community partnerships.[8]

Systemic injustices, rooted in structural racism, are the primary drivers of SDoH, and racism plays a fundamental role in a person's SDoH, such that race and ethnicity are strongly predictive of one's access to SDoH, such as housing, income, and education.[8] Racial/ethnic, gender, and socioeconomic disparities have been identified in adult and pediatric patients across organ-specific diseases. Racial and ethnic minoritized patients, individuals who live in rural communities, people with disabilities, and those who identify as lesbian, gay, bisexual, transgender, queer or questioning, intersex, asexual, and more (LGBTQIA+) are noted to have worse outcomes when compared to White, heterosexual, and urban-living individuals.[2] In adult critical illness, Black patients have a higher incidence of conditions necessitating intensive care unit (ICU) care, a higher incidence of sepsis, acute lung injury and acute respiratory failure, and higher age-adjusted rates of cardiac arrest when compared to White individuals. Similarly, racial and ethnic minoritized patients who live in areas with higher rates of poverty have a higher incidence of sepsis and acute critical illness.[9] There are also notable disparities in clinical management for Black adults compared to their White adult counterparts. Black patients have longer wait times when admitted to the ICU from the emergency department, are less likely to be admitted to cardiac care unit, and receive interventions such as tracheostomy, central venous access, and pulmonary artery catheterizations less often after adjusting for severity of illness.[9]

Decades' worth of research has also identified significant racial/ethnic and socioeconomic disparities across a variety of pediatric conditions. The overall risk of admission, length of stay, hospital costs, and outcomes during hospitalization have been shown to vary by socioeconomic status and race/ethnicity.[10] Researchers have demonstrated the association between SDoH and asthma-related hospitalizations,[11–14] poor glycemic control for children with diabetes mellitus,[15,16] and cancer outcomes, including overall survival, incidence, and prevalence.[17,18] More recently, there is increasing awareness that these disparities extend into pediatric critical illness, with the untoward effect of adverse outcomes during and even after critical illness. Health disparities have been documented during the entire course of critical illness and along the care continuum, from increased risk among certain sociodemographic groups to increased illness severity at ICU admission, worse ICU-based outcomes, and increased risk for adverse outcomes after ICU discharge. However, unlike other pediatric studies, there is limited research on how SDoH contribute to disparities in the risk and outcomes of critical illness in children. Nonetheless, the few studies that exist suggest that social factors, such as poverty, are mediators to health disparities in pediatric critical care outcomes by increasing the risk of worse severity of illness on presentation to the pediatric ICU[19] and overall exposure to the pediatric ICU, which can lead to a diminished quality of life and lower functioning.[20] A more comprehensive understanding of how SDoH impact the risk and outcomes of critical illness across different conditions and among different sociodemographic groups is important and foundational to promoting equity in pediatric critical care. In addition, understanding and addressing the SDoH is a necessary first step in the approach to tackling health disparities in pediatric critical care outcomes. In this article, we discuss the implications of assessing SDoH and provide a methodological approach to screening and addressing SDoH during critical illness.

DISPARITIES IN PEDIATRIC CRITICAL ILLNESS: REVIEW OF LITERATURE
Individual-Level Disparities

Differences in SDoH contribute to persistent health disparities among racial, ethnic, and socioeconomic groups of children. These disparities are potentiated by inequitable distribution of societal resources and exclusionary public policies.[21] Several studies highlight racial and socioeconomic disparities in risk and outcomes of critical illness in children. Observed socioeconomic disparities include higher disease severity,[19] higher mechanical ventilator use,[22,23] and higher mortality in the pediatric ICU (PICU) among critically ill children without health insurance.[22,24] Disparities by race and ethnicity vary. Some studies describe higher disease severity[23] and more in-hospital arrests[25–27] for Latino and Black children compared to White children, while other studies describe no difference in disease severity or mortality between races and ethnicities.[28] Regarding disease-specific outcomes, several studies have shown differences in admission, length of stay, and mechanical ventilation for Black children with asthma,[29,30] differences in mortality and length of stay for minority children with sepsis,[31,32] and greater severity of injury, morbidity, and mortality for Black and Hispanic children with critical injury.[33,34] Racial and ethnic disparities have also been demonstrated in pediatric patients with oncologic disease and patients with other illnesses who interface with the PICU.[35]

Despite this growing body of literature on disparities in critical illness, only few have examined the relationship between specific SDoH and the spectrum of critical illness as an approach to understanding why the observed disparities exist[36] and identifying targets for interventions. In a single-center observational study of critically ill children, Black families reported a higher prevalence of food insecurity than White families.[37] In another study, 60% of families screened in the PICU reported at least one unmet social need, among which difficulty with utilities and living costs, housing instability, and food insecurity were the most identified needs.[38] These findings suggest that critically ill children are at significant risk of exposure to negative outcomes related to SDoH. Therefore, pediatric critical care researchers should include other social factors beyond race and insurance status in their assessment of the impact of SDoH on outcomes in critical illness.

Neighborhood-Level Disparities

Although individual risk factors clearly contribute to the condition of one's health, the contextual factors within one's environment or neighborhood contribute significantly to health status at the individual level and ultimately at the population level.[39] Disadvantaged neighborhoods have a higher proportion of uninsured individuals, lower literacy levels, higher rates of household poverty, and higher rates of minority children living in poverty.[40–42] Area-level socioeconomic factors, which are shaped by structural and political factors such as discriminatory housing policies, residential segregation, and neighborhood disinvestment, affect health through restriction of education and employment opportunities, disruption of neighborhood and housing quality, reinforcement of unhealthy behaviors, and limited access to higher opportunity areas for low-income families due to the higher housing costs in those neighborhoods.[42,43] These area-level factors have been found to be associated with inequities in pediatric preventive care, which is essential for ensuring healthy child development and early intervention to improve outcomes for several diseases and conditions.[44,45] The lack of public transportation, employment and educational opportunities, healthy foods, green space, and exposure to violence, crime, and pollutants are neighborhood factors potentially placing children at risk for higher severity of illness and need for intensive care services.[38,39]

In pediatric critical illness, studies have consistently shown that children living in under-resourced neighborhoods are geographically disadvantaged with limited access to PICUs, which are concentrated in urban areas[46], and have increased risk for critical illness and worse PICU outcomes.[9,32,40] Higher PICU admission rates and severity of illness scores have been observed in neighborhoods with higher rates of persons living in poverty.[19] Children living in disadvantaged neighborhoods have higher risk for post-PICU morbidity, such as decreased health-related quality of life and PICU readmissions.[47,48] Furthermore, children residing in lower socioeconomic areas appear to be at higher risk of critical illness and traumatic injury, and Black children residing in these areas have lower rates of bystander out-of-hospital resuscitation for cardiac arrests, compared to children living in more socioeconomically advantaged areas.[41,49] Neighborhoods with high rates of PICU readmissions for asthma have high social vulnerability and higher exposure to environmental toxins such as industrial pollutants, airborne microparticles, and higher ozone concentrations.[42] Disadvantaged neighborhoods may lack resources needed to make the physical and built environment conducive for optimal health. This leaves families underequipped to support children recovering from critical illness or children with chronic conditions who are at high risk for acute exacerbations and critical care hospitalizations. As such, there is an urgent need for clinicians, administrators, researchers, community leaders, and policy makers to understand the mechanisms of how the neighborhood environment may prevent or attenuate the risk of critical illness and injury.

SCREENING FOR SOCIAL DETERMINANTS OF HEALTH IN PEDIATRIC CRITICAL CARE SETTINGS

Given the association between SDoH and health disparities in pediatrics, several organizations, including the American Academy of Pediatrics and the Center for Medicare and Medicaid Services (CMS), recommend screening for the SDoH.[50,51] *Screening* has several implications and extends beyond the assessment of individual factors experienced by patients interfacing with the PICU to neighborhood-level factors that influence health outcomes during critical illness. To better understand the interplay and causal pathways between social factors and disparate health outcomes during critical illness, providers and researchers need to measure the burden of unmet social needs.[52] We focus the remaining discussion on screening for the SDoH during pediatric critical illness.

SCREENING AT THE INDIVIDUAL LEVEL

Appropriateness of Screening for Social Determinants of Health in the Pediatric Intensive Care Unit

A PICU admission provides a feasible and important opportunity for screening for SDoH.[37,52] Implementation of a stakeholder-informed social risks screening tool could be paradigm shifting for the field of critical care where attention to social risks and relationship to health inequities is increasing. However, there remains a lack of universal screening. Furthermore, screening for traumatic experiences/adverse childhood experiences and relationships to critical illness is underexplored. Having a validated instrument with high acceptability among parents who complete it will have high impact for future research to study critical illness in the context of individual- and neighborhood-level social risk indicators.

Existing Screening Tools

Numerous validated screening tools assessing SDoH have been developed for use in the pediatric population.[53–60] These screening tools have been predominantly developed for the primary care setting with very few targeting the inpatient environment. No published screening tools have been created specifically for the pediatric critical care setting. Most of the published screening tools focus on parents of young children (<5 years of age) and are designed to be incorporated into well-child or routine clinic appointments. Available screening tools are markedly heterogeneous in screening domains and methodologies, including in-person and remote screening options. Further, there is significant variability in response to screening, connection to referral networks, presence of targeted interventions, or follow-up. Last, only a few of the published screening tools incorporate psychometric testing in the development and assessment of the screening tool; these tools include the Safe Environment for Every Kid Parent Questionnaire[61]; Income, Housing, Education, Legal Status, Literacy, Personal Safety Questionnaire[62]; and Well Child Care, Evaluation, Community Resources, Advocacy, Referral, Education[63] screening tools (**Table 1**).

Development of a Validated Screening Tool

A validated SDoH screening tool designed for critically ill children and their families does not currently exist. Screening in the PICU should be guided by several factors including (1) provider education on the impact of SDoH and the relevance of screening; (2) universality of screening; (3) utilization of a strength-based approach; (4) training to screen; (5) pairing of identified needs with appropriate resource referrals; (6) using existing systems to build upon; and (7) development of valid and reliable screening tools.[52] To address the last factor, Asp and colleagues sought to create a validated screen to broadly assess for unmet social needs and risks in a PICU-sensitive approach, recognizing the unique context and challenges of a critical care hospitalization. A primary goal in the development of the screening tool was to draw on the strengths of relevant stakeholders to ensure that the tool captured the voice of patients, their families, and their community in addition to health care professionals. Community stakeholders and families engaged in focus group sessions to elicit input on screening for SDoH. Parents reflected on their experiences with SDoH screening in various health care settings and provided recommendations for future screening initiatives. Community stakeholders and leaders shared suggestions for hospital-based screenings, drawing on personal experiences with pitfalls and successes in screening. After broadly assessing parent and stakeholder perspectives on screening, parents of children who have had critical care hospitalizations participated in one-on-one guided

Table 1 Screening tools and domains	
Individual-Level Screening Tools	
Validated Screening Tools and Indices	**Included Domains and Constructs**
Safe Environment for Every Kid Parent Questionnaire (SEEK PQ-R)	• Parental depression • Parental substance use • Major parental stress • Intimate partner (or domestic) violence • Food insecurity • Harsh punishment
Safe Environment for Every Kid Parent Questionnaire extended (SEEK PQ-Re)	• Home safety • Child behavior • Parental wellness • Food insecurity • Other needs (transportation, utility company, housing, childcare, immigration, employment, education, health care access, public benefits)
Income, Housing, Education, Legal Status, Literacy, Personal Safety (IHELP/IHELLP) Questionnaire	• Employment • Financial strain • Health insurance • Early childhood education and development • Language • Immigration/refugee status • Safety, crime, and violence • Housing quality and stability • Food security
Well Child Care, Evaluation, Community Resources, Advocacy, Referral, Education (WE CARE)	• Parental education • Employment • Child care • Housing security • Food security • Household utilities (heat and electricity)
The Hunger Vital Sign	• Food security
Adverse Childhood Experiences	• Child abuse • Neglect • Trauma

interviews to understand perspectives on screening for social needs specifically in the PICU.[64]

Following input from PICU parents, Asp and colleagues constructed a screening tool building on an extensive literature review of published social needs screening assessments and by engaging with content experts to identify priority domains to include in a PICU-specific screening tool. An expert panel was assembled to review and refined the screening tool through a modified 3 part Delphi method.[65] The developers are currently assessing the face validity of the proposed screening tool through cognitive interviews with parents of children with recent critical care admissions, following which the tool will be assessed for feasibility and acceptability across multiple PICUs. The goal is to create a validated screening tool, developed in concert with relevant stakeholders and rigorously tested, that will result in the identification and support of unmet social needs for critically ill children and their families. However, while this tool is being developed and tested, pediatric critical care providers can assess the unmet social needs of patients and their families using available screening tools guided by the factors mentioned earlier (see **Table 1**).

SCREENING AT THE NEIGHBORHOOD LEVEL TO EVALUATE HEALTH OUTCOMES IN PEDIATRIC CRITICAL CARE

As highlighted earlier, neighborhood disparities in the risk and outcomes of critical illness in children are prevalent. Assessing the SDoH at the neighborhood-level acknowledges the systemic injustices in the United States that have contributed to disparities across health outcomes and identifies modifiable factors that can be intervened upon. To investigate neighborhood-level associations with health outcomes, a geospatial analysis must be performed. Geospatial analysis includes the creation of maps to visualize local trends in clinical data where children experiencing certain health conditions or requiring certain medical interventions reside. Utilizing geospatial analysis can advance the study of geographic disparities in pediatric intensive care by evaluating the association between an area's given attribute (percentage of high school graduates, concentration of environmental air pollutants, and access to green recreational spaces) and health outcomes in pediatric critical illness. Furthermore, geospatial analysis aids in the overlaying of multiple factors such as census tract properties (eg, median income, percentage of single-parent households) and patient residence onto a single map for efficient visualization of patient clusters by census tract.[20,66–69] In this way, geomapping and geospatial analysis can be used to augment understanding of the cultural, socioeconomic, and built environments that contribute to the SDoH.

The impact of the neighborhood environment on health is mediated through the multiple, yet inter-related physical and social characteristics of a given neighborhood. Because of this complexity, the use of multidimensional, validated measures of neighborhood-level SDoH allows for a more nuanced evaluation of the role contextual factors in one's environment play in critical illness.[70–72] Composite measures of the SDoH consist of several key indicators that reflect different SDoH domains such as an area's educational composition, housing conditions, income, or toxic environmental exposures (**Table 2**). Many of these measures are also publicly available for use and can be used in geomapping and geospatial analysis. Brief descriptions of the area deprivation index (ADI),[73] social vulnerability index (SVI),[74] the child opportunity index (COI) 2.0,[75] and the environmental justice index social vulnerability and environmental burden rank (EJI SER) are discussed in the following sections.[76,77]

The Area Deprivation Index

The ADI was created by the Health Resources and Services Administration as a measure of socioeconomic disadvantage in 4 domains, including income, education, employment, and housing quality.[73] The ADI defines a neighborhood as a census block group and ranks neighborhoods by socioeconomic disadvantage at the state or national level using US Census American Community Survey five year estimates as its data source. The ADI ranks each census block from 1 to 100 at the national or state level and then groups each census block into bins representing 1% of the ADI. Group 1 with a ranking of 1 indicates the lowest ADI and the lowest level of disadvantage and group 100 with a ranking of 100 indicates the highest ADI and highest level of disadvantage.[73] The ADI has been used to assess the relationship between poverty and distance to pediatric critical care services[46] and the association between neighborhood-level disadvantage and PICU admission.[78]

The Social Vulnerability Index

Social vulnerability refers to the potential negative effects on communities caused by external stresses on human health. External stresses include natural disasters

Table 2	
Screening tools and indices	
Neighborhood-Level Indices	
Validated Screening Tools and Indices	**Included Domains and Constructs**
Area Deprivation Index (ADI)	• Income • Education • Employment • Housing quality
Social Vulnerability Index (SVI)	• Socioeconomic status • Household composition • Minority status • Housing type • Transportation
Child Opportunity Index (COI)	• Child education • Health and environment • Social and economic opportunity

Environmental Justice Index (EJI)	• Environmental burden
	  ○ Air pollution
	  ○ Potentially hazardous and toxic sites
	  ○ Built environment
	  ○ Transportation infrastructure
	  ○ Water pollution
	• Social vulnerability
	  ○ Poverty
	  ○ Employment
	  ○ Education
	  ○ Minority status
	  ○ Housing quality, type, and security
	  ○ Health insurance status
	  ○ Internet access
	  ○ Household composition
	  ○ Disability
	  ○ Language
	• Health vulnerability
	  ○ Prevalence of asthma
	  ○ Prevalence of cancer
	  ○ Prevalence of high blood pressure
	  ○ Prevalence of diabetes
	  ○ Prevalence of poor mental health

(eg, storm damage from tornadoes or flooding from hurricanes), human-caused disasters (eg, toxin release into the environment), and disease outbreaks (eg, influenza, SARS-CoV-2 pandemics, measles epidemics). Socially vulnerable populations are characterized by socioeconomic status, household composition, minority status, housing type, and transportation.[79] The Centers for Disease Control (CDC)/Agency for Toxic Substances and Disease Registry uses 16 US census variables to determine an SVI of every census tract.[80] The purpose of the SVI is to help local health departments and officials identify communities that may need support before, during, and after a public health emergency.[74,79] In response to the disproportionate impact of the COVID-19 pandemic on racial and ethnic minority communities, the CDC/ATDSR SVI was expanded to create a new social vulnerability metric, the Minority Health SVI.[81] Aggregated data that result from combining information about 2 or more minority groups can obscure local-level social risk factors and prevent the identification of communities at highest risk for unequitable health outcomes during public health emergencies. The Minority Health SVI includes the same socioeconomic status, household composition and disability metrics, and housing type and transportation measures as the SVI; however, it disaggregates minority status into 6 distinct groups (American Indian/Alaska Native, Asian, African American, Native Hawaiian/Pacific Islander, Hispanic or Latinx, and Some Other Race) and expands the native language spoken into 5 separate languages (Spanish, Chinese, Vietnamese, Korean, and Russian). Two additional domains were included: (1) health care infrastructure and access, composed of hospitals, urgent care clinics, pharmacies, primary care physicians, and health insurance and (2) medical vulnerability, composed of cardiovascular disease, chronic respiratory disease, obesity, diabetes, and Internet access.[81] The Minority Health SVI has not been used to study health disparities in children.

The Child Opportunity Index 2.0

The COI is a relative, composite, multidimensional measure of neighborhood (census tract) factors that promote childhood opportunity and healthy development through many causal pathways.[82] It is composed of 29 direct, contemporary indicators within 3 domains of child education, health and environment, and social and economic opportunity.[82] The COI 2.0 has been used to determine the association of SDoH with the use of heath care services and outcomes.[68,69,71,83–85] The COI 2.0 describes and quantifies neighborhood conditions for US children and provides a ranking on a scale from 1 (lowest opportunity) to 100 (highest opportunity). In the United States, the COI 2.0 ranges from the lowest value of 20 (Fresno, CA) to the highest value of 83 (Madison, WI).[42,86] While there is a wide range of child opportunity scores throughout the United States, there is even wider variation in neighborhood opportunity within a metropolitan area.[42] Along with raw and z-score normalized values and levels for each neighborhood-level indicator, the COI 2.0 domain score rankings are available at the national, state, and metropolitan statistical area child opportunity levels to use in an analysis. Child opportunity levels are divided into 5 categories of neighborhood opportunity, including very low, low, moderate, high, and very high opportunity.[87] There are approximately 72,000 census tracts with data available from 2010 and 2015 across all 3 opportunity domains in the United States. These data can be stratified by race/ethnicity, if desired, to assess changes over time and to determine race/ethnicity opportunity gaps within a metro region. What sets the COI 2.0 apart from the SVI is that it does not include race or ethnicity composition as part of neighborhood opportunity measures. Race and ethnicity are associated with both lack of opportunity and structural racism in the United States; therefore, race and ethnicity were not included as COI factors, but should be considered when stratifying the effects of neighborhood opportunity on health outcomes. In pediatric critical care, the COI has been used to explore disparities in health outcomes. Studies have assessed the relationship between neighborhood opportunity and PICU utilization for patients with traumatic brain injury[88] and have explored the association between neighborhood opportunity and emergent readmissions for patients who survived pediatric critical illness in the preceding year.[48] In addition, the COI has been considered in studies seeking to identify neighborhood hot spots associated with life-threatening asthma[66] and acute respiratory failure requiring mechanical ventilation in critically ill pediatric patients.[67]

The Environmental Justice Index

The CDC recently developed a new composite measure called the environmental justice index (EJI) to quantify and rank the cumulative health effects of air and water pollution at the neighborhood level using data from the US Census Bureau, the Environmental Protective Agency, the US Mine Safety and Health Administration, and the CDC. The EJI is composed of 3 modules including environmental burden, social vulnerability, and health vulnerability.[76,77] The health vulnerability module is composed of one domain and indicates high levels of 5 preexisting conditions: asthma, high blood pressure, cancer, diabetes, and poor mental health. The full EJI is not intended for use in secondary analyses where a specific disease is the outcome of interest; however, the EJI SER is designed for this purpose.[76] The EJI SER is composed of 2 distinct modules that are the summed percentile ranks of the individual components of the social vulnerability module (4 thematic domains, 14 items) and environmental burden module (5 thematic domains, 17 items).[12] The percentile rank sum of the EJI SER is ordered from a summed score range of 0 to 2, reranked and converted into a final score ranging between 0 and 1 based on this percentile rank.[12] These modules inform an individual participant's exposure to social vulnerability and environmental pollution at the census tract level. The EJI relies on historical census and government-collected environmental data with varying time scales and is intended to be used as a tool to identify and prioritize areas that may require special attention or additional action to improve health and health equity. The EJI SER can help analyze the unique, local factors driving cumulative impacts on health to inform policy and establish meaningful goals to measure progress toward environmental justice and health equity.[13]

Beyond utilizing these tools to measure the association between neighborhood factors and health outcomes, pediatric critical care providers should begin to consider how and when these tools can be incorporated into the electronic medical record and integrated into patient treatment and management plans to help mitigate health disparities.[51]

COUPLING SCREENING WITH REFERRALS AND RESOURCES

Measuring the social factors experienced by children with critical illness and injury is necessary to evaluate their association with health outcomes. However, it is important to acknowledge that screening for SDoH is only one element in the work toward achieving health equity and improving outcomes for children, especially those with a disproportionately high burden of need. Implementing screening tools focused on assessing unmet social needs may cause unintended harm to families given the sensitive nature of certain topics.[89] In addition, inadequate training and expertise on how to appropriately elicit and address social needs, time restraints, and insufficient knowledge of available resources may cause providers to feel uncomfortable addressing the identified family needs, leaving families and physicians frustrated.[3,89,90] As such, screening for the SDoH without coupling it with referrals to the appropriate resources has been described as ineffective and unethical.[90] Screening for SDoH must take place in an environment that is equipped to respond to identified needs while also championing the strengths and desires of families. In addition, the screening environment should be safe, unbiased, and include recognition that unmet needs were created by systemic structures that are out of the control of the patients or families.

All clinicians have a role in promoting health equity and eliminating health disparities, including those working in intensive care settings. Pediatric critical care divisions and departments are tasked with building infrastructure that supports referral before SDoH screening is implemented. Building the capacity to ensure linkage to "treatment" for unmet social needs requires a multidisciplinary and multisector concerted approach that includes both institutional and community partnerships.[3] In addition, screening should seek to identify social assets that strengthen families, including social connectivity, resiliency, and potential social and built neighborhood-level factors, which have been associated with positive outcomes.[91] Providers should focus on highlighting and strengthening these factors as a part of the treatment plan for unmet social needs. While there are several benefits to screening for the SDoH, it is imperative that all these aspects are included in the approach to screening and referral.

SOCIAL DETERMINANTS OF HEALTH AND RESOURCE ACCESS, ALLOCATION, AND PROVISION

As described earlier, the health care system is wrought with racial, ethnic, and socioeconomic disparities in the access, allocation, and provision of health care, health care resources, and social resources to at-risk populations. Access to health care, specifically health insurance[92,93] and health care resources (eg, physicians, clinics, and pharmacies),[92,94] is imperative for the health of pediatric patients and is dependent on the SDoH. The association between pediatric critical illness and race, ethnicity, poverty, and rurality further highlights the interconnectedness of SDoH, access to care, and pediatric critical care health outcomes.[20,46,78] To achieve health equity, the health system's focus must shift to include the perspective of equity in access to health care and societal resources that are crucial for health and well-being.[95] The lack of access to health care for pediatric patients and their families is perpetuated by health systems built on the foundation of structural racism and the exclusion of the minoritized, marginalized, and the socioeconomically deprived.[95] While the lack of equitable access to health care is a key driver to inequity within pediatric health, the allocation and provision of health care resources are critical components of access to care. Federal and public health programs, supported by the current administration, have rededicated efforts to collecting SDoH data and improving "whole-of-government" collaborations to minimize health care inequities. Targeted government-sponsored efforts to improve geographic (rural vs urban) allocation of workforce resources and physical resources across geographic domains can minimize health care inequities.[96]

Multilevel efforts ranging from federal-, state-, institutional-, and community-level collaborations are needed to assess the health needs of the pediatric population based on the SDoH, to fund and allocate resources equitably, and to ensure equitable provision to patients/families. This extends to the PICU. Partnerships with federal and state government agencies, such as the CMS Innovation Center, can provide funding for initiatives aimed at addressing unmet social needs.[97] Community organizations may already address unmet social needs and can provide patients with access to nontraditional health-related resources such as housing and food; therefore, creating hospital–community partnerships is imperative. Creating effective and sustainable relationships with community organizations requires a stepwise approach. The Health Research & Educational Trust, supported by the Robert Wood Johnson Foundation, provides a guide to creating new community partnerships focused on (1) identifying the community health needs and common goals, (2) identifying community partners, their assets, and their roles; (3) creating a measurable action plan; and (4) assessing the partnership effectiveness and interventions.[98]

As a health care system, we cannot create targeted interventions without adequate measurement of SDoH, their subsequent inequities, and their impact on pediatric health. Therefore, it is the provider's role to examine the influence of the SDoH on access to and the equitable allocation and delivery of health care and social resources to pediatric critically ill patients. We implore providers to use sound methodology to examine and measure the impact of SDoH on pediatric critical illness with tested individual-, neighborhood-, and system-level interventions.

SUMMARY

SDoH have been identified as key drivers of health disparities in pediatric critical illness. As such, the field of Pediatric Critical Care Medicine is now tasked with identifying and addressing unmet social needs that are inextricably linked to worse outcomes for critically ill children. To accomplish this, pediatric critical care providers need to screen for individual unmet social needs, explore the implications of neighborhood factors and disparities through research, employ a multisector approach to ensure equitable provision of resources, and make family referrals to community organizations to address unmet social needs. With this approach, screening for the SDoH can potentially help mitigate health disparities for critically ill children.

CLINICS CARE POINTS

- SDoH account for about 80% to 90% of modifiable factors contributing to health outcomes and have been linked to health disparities.
- In pediatric critical care, social factors, such as poverty, are mediators to health disparities in outcome.
- Providers and researchers need to measure the burden of unmet social needs to better understand the interplay between social factors and disparate health outcomes during critical illness.
- Screening should be coupled with referrals to the appropriate resources and must occur in an environment equipped to respond to identified needs whil championing the strengths of families.

DISCLOSURE

The authors have nothing to disclose.

REFERENCES

1. U.S. Department of health and human services, office of disease prevention and health promotion. Social determinants of health. Social Determinants of Health - Healthy People 2030. Available at: https://health.gov/healthypeople/priority-areas/social-determinants-health. [Accessed 1 November 2023].
2. Whitman A, De Lew N, Aysola V, et al. Addressing social determinants of health: examples of successful evidence-based strategies and current federal efforts. 2022. Available at: https://aspe.hhs.gov/sites/default/files/documents/e2b650 cd64cf84aae8ff0fae7474af82/SDOH-Evidence-Review.pdf.
3. Magnan S. Social determinants of health 101 for health care: five plus five. NAM Perspectives 2017;7(10). https://doi.org/10.31478/201710c.
4. Gillespie C, Wilhite JA, Hanley K, et al. Addressing social determinants of health in primary care: a quasi-experimental study using unannounced standardised patients to evaluate the impact of audit/feedback on physicians' rates of identifying and responding to social needs. BMJ Qual Saf 2022;32(11):632–43.

5. Lipson D. Medicaid's role in improving the social determinants of health: opportunities for states. 2017. Available at: https://www.nasi.org/wp-content/uploads/2017/06/Opportunities-for-States_web.pdf. [Accessed 31 October 2023].

6. Burgard SA, Seefeldt KS, Zelner S. Housing instability and health: findings from the Michigan recession and recovery study. Soc Sci Med 2012;75(12):2215–24.

7. Leventhal T, Brooks-Gunn J. Moving to opportunity: an experimental study of neighborhood effects on mental health. Am J Publ Health 2003;93(9):1576–82.

8. Beck AF, Cohen AJ, Colvin JD, et al. Perspectives from the Society for Pediatric Research: interventions targeting social needs in pediatric clinical care. Pediatr Res 2018;84(1):10–21.

9. Soto GJ, Martin GS, Gong MN. Healthcare disparities in critical illness. Crit Care Med 2013;41(12):2784–93.

10. McKay S, Parente V. Health disparities in the hospitalized child. Hosp Pediatr 2019;9(5):317–25.

11. Sullivan K, Thakur N. Structural and social determinants of health in asthma in developed economies: a scoping review of literature published between 2014 and 2019. Curr Allergy Asthma Rep 2020;20(2). https://doi.org/10.1007/s11882-020-0899-6.

12. Puvvula J, Poole JA, Gwon Y, et al. Role of social determinants of health in differential respiratory exposure and health outcomes among children. BMC Publ Health 2023;23(1). https://doi.org/10.1186/s12889-022-14964-2.

13. Federico MJ, McFarlane AE, Szefler SJ, et al. The impact of social determinants of health on children with asthma. J Allergy Clin Immunol Pract 2020;8(6). https://doi.org/10.1016/j.jaip.2020.03.028.

14. Tyris J, Gourishankar A, Ward M, et al. Social determinants of health and at-risk rates for pediatric asthma morbidity. Pediatrics 2022;150(2). https://doi.org/10.1542/peds.2021-055570.

15. Hershey JA, Morone J, Lipman TH, et al. Social determinants of health, goals and outcomes in high-risk children with type 1 diabetes. Can J Diabetes 2021;45(5):444–50.

16. Lipman TH, Hawkes CP. Racial and socioeconomic disparities in pediatric type 1 diabetes: time for a paradigm shift in approach. Diabetes Care 2020;44(1):14–6.

17. Tran YH, Coven SL, Park S, et al. Social determinants of health and pediatric cancer survival: a systematic review. Pediatr Blood Cancer 2022;69(5). https://doi.org/10.1002/pbc.29546.

18. Aristizabal P, Winestone LE, Umaretiya P, et al. Disparities in pediatric oncology: the 21st century opportunity to improve outcomes for children and adolescents with cancer. American Society of Clinical Oncology Educational Book 2021;41:e315–26.

19. Epstein D, Reibel M, Unger JB, et al. The effect of neighborhood and individual characteristics on pediatric critical illness. J Community Health 2014;39(4):753–9. https://doi.org/10.1007/s10900-014-9823-0.

20. Andrist E, Riley CL, Brokamp C, et al. Neighborhood poverty and pediatric intensive care use. Pediatrics 2019;144(6). https://doi.org/10.1542/peds.2019-0748.

21. McGinnis JM, Williams-Russo P, Knickman JR. The case for more active policy attention to health promotion. Health Aff 2002;21(2):78–93.

22. Lopez AS, Tilford JM, Anand S, et al. Variation in pediatric intensive care therapies and outcomes by race, gender, and insurance status. Pediatr Crit Care Med 2006;7(1):2–6.

23. Sakai-Bizmark R, Chang RKR, Mena LA, et al. Asthma hospitalizations among homeless children in New York state. Pediatrics 2019;144(2):e20182769. https://doi.org/10.1542/peds.2018-2769.

24. Hakmeh W, Barker J, Szpunar SM, et al. Effect of race and insurance on outcome of pediatric trauma. Acad Emerg Med 2010;17(8):809–12.

25. Martinez PA, Totapally BR. The epidemiology and outcomes of pediatric in-hospital cardiopulmonary arrest in the United States during 1997 to 2012. Resuscitation 2016;105:177–81.

26. Meert KL, Donaldson A, Nadkarni V, et al. Multicenter cohort study of in-hospital pediatric cardiac arrest. Pediatr Crit Care Med 2009;10(5):544–53. https://doi.org/10.1097/PCC.0b013e3181a7045c.

27. Berens RJ, Cassidy LD, Matchey J, et al. Probability of survival based on etiology of cardiopulmonary arrest in pediatric patients. Paediatr Anaesth 2011;21(8):834–40.

28. Epstein D, Wong CF, Khemani RG, et al. Race/ethnicity is not associated with mortality in the PICU. Pediatrics 2011;127(3):e588–97.

29. Grunwell JR, Travers C, Fitzpatrick AM. Inflammatory and comorbid features of children admitted to a PICU for status asthmaticus. Pediatr Crit Care Med 2018;19(11):e585–94.

30. Silber JH, Rosenbaum PR, Calhoun SR, et al. Racial disparities in Medicaid asthma hospitalizations. Pediatrics 2016;139(1):e20161221.

31. Mitchell HK, Reddy A, Montoya-Williams D, et al. Hospital outcomes for children with severe sepsis in the USA by race or ethnicity and insurance status: a population-based, retrospective cohort study. The Lancet Child & Adolescent Health 2021;5(2):103–12.

32. Reddy AR, Badolato GM, Chamberlain JM, et al. Disparities associated with sepsis mortality in critically ill children. J Pediatr Intensive Care 2020;11(2). https://doi.org/10.1055/s-0040-1721730.

33. Cassidy LD, Lambropoulos D, Enters J, et al. Health disparities analysis of critically ill pediatric trauma patients in Milwaukee, Wisconsin. J Am Coll Surg 2013; 217(2):233–9.

34. Haider AH, Efron DT, Haut ER, et al. Black children experience worse clinical and functional outcomes after traumatic brain injury: an analysis of the national pediatric trauma Registry. J Trauma Inj Infect Crit Care 2007;62(5):1259–63.

35. Mitchell HK, Reddy A, Perry MA, et al. Racial, ethnic, and socioeconomic disparities in paediatric critical care in the USA. The Lancet Child & Adolescent Health 2021;5(10):739–50.

36. Huang E, Albrecht L, Menon K. 262: reporting of social determinants of health in PICU randomized controlled trials. Crit Care Med 2023;51(1):116.

37. La Count S, McClusky C, Morrow SE, et al. Food insecurity in families with critically ill children: a single-center observational study in pittsburgh. Pediatr Crit Care Med 2021;22(4):e275–7.

38. Maholtz DE, Riley CL. Screening for social needs in critically ill patients: addressing more than health conditions. Pediatr Crit Care Med 2022;23(11):e541–2.

39. Diez Roux AV, Mair C. Neighborhoods and health. Ann N Y Acad Sci 2010; 1186(1):125–45.

40. Diez Roux AV. Neighborhoods and health: what do we know? What should we do? Am J Publ Health 2016;106(3):430–1.

41. Kirby JB, Kaneda T. Neighborhood socioeconomic disadvantage and access to health care. J Health Soc Behav 2005;46(1):15–31.

42. Acevedo-Garcia D, Noelke C, McArdle N, et al. Racial and ethnic inequities in children's neighborhoods: evidence from the new child opportunity Index 2.0. Health Aff 2020;39(10):1693–701.
43. Williams DR, Collins C. Racial residential segregation: a fundamental cause of racial disparities in health. Publ Health Rep 2001;116(5):404–16. Available at: https://www.ncbi.nlm.nih.gov/pmc/articles/PMC1497358/.
44. Hambidge SJ, Emsermann CB, Federico S, et al. Disparities in pediatric preventive care in the United States, 1993-2002. Arch Pediatr Adolesc Med 2007; 161(1):30.
45. Jones MN, Brown CM, Widener MJ, et al. Area-level socioeconomic factors are associated with noncompletion of pediatric preventive services. Journal of Primary Care & Community Health 2016;7(3):143–8.
46. Brown LE, França UL, McManus ML. Socioeconomic disadvantage and distance to pediatric critical care. Pediatr Crit Care Med 2021;22(12):1033–41.
47. Kachmar AG, Watson RS, Wypij D, et al. For the randomized evaluation of sedation titration for respiratory failure (RESTORE) investigative team. Association of socioeconomic status with postdischarge pediatric resource use and quality of life. Crit Care Med 2022;50(2):e117–28.
48. Akande MY, Ramgopal S, Graham RJ, et al. Child opportunity Index and emergent PICU readmissions: a retrospective, cross-sectional study of 43 U.S. Hospitals. Pediatr Crit Care Med 2023;24(5):e213.
49. Javed Z, Haisum Maqsood M, Yahya T, et al. Race, racism, and cardiovascular health: applying a social determinants of health framework to racial/ethnic disparities in cardiovascular disease. Circulation: Cardiovascular Quality and Outcomes 2022;15(1). https://doi.org/10.1161/circoutcomes.121.007917.
50. Council on Community Pediatrics. Poverty and child health in the United States. Pediatrics 2016;137(4):e20160339. https://doi.org/10.1542/peds.2016-0339.
51. Committee on the recommended social and behavioral domains and measures for electronic health records, board on population health and public health practice, institute of medicine. Capturing social and behavioral domains and measures in electronic health records: phase 2. National Academies Press (US); 2015. Available at: https://www.ncbi.nlm.nih.gov/books/NBK268995/. [Accessed 30 October 2022].
52. Akande M, Paquette ET, Magee P, et al. Screening for social determinants of health in the pediatric intensive care unit: recommendations for clinicians. Crit Care Clin 2023;39(2):341–55.
53. Ye M, Hessler D, Ford DC, et al. Pediatric ACEs and related life event screener (PEARLS) latent domains and child health in a safety-net primary care practice. BMC Pediatr 2023;23(1). https://doi.org/10.1186/s12887-023-04163-2.
54. Billioux A, Verlander K, Anthony S, et al. Standardized screening for health-related social needs in clinical settings the accountable health communities screening tool. National Academy of Medicine; 2017. Available at: https://nam.edu/wp-content/uploads/2017/05/Standardized-Screening-for-Health-Related-Social-Needs-in-Clinical-Settings.pdf. [Accessed 3 October 2023].
55. Children's health watch. Available at: https://childrenshealthwatch.org/wp-content/uploads/Full-CHW-Survey-English.pdf. [Accessed 3 October 2023].
56. Health Leads. Social needs screening toolkit. 2016. Available at: https://healthleadsusa.org/resources/the-health-leads-screening-toolkit/. [Accessed 3 October 2023].
57. Kenyon C, Sandel M, Silverstein M, et al. Revisiting the social history for child health. Pediatrics 2007;120(3):e734–8. PMID: 17766513.

58. Safe Environment for Every Kid (SEEK). Parent Questionnaire. Available at: https://seekwellbeing.org/wp-content/uploads/2022/10/SEEK-PQ-R-English-9-22.pdf. [Accessed 3 October 2023].

59. Garg A, Toy S, Tripodis Y, et al. Addressing social determinants of health at well child care visits: a cluster RCT. Pediatrics 2015;135:e296–304.

60. National Association of Community Health Centers Inc. Association of asian pacific community health organizations, Oregon primary care association. PRAPARE: Protocol for Responding to and Assessing Patient Assets, Risks, and Experiences 2016. [Accessed 27 June 2019].

61. The SEEK Project. SEEK materials. SEEK - safe environment for every Kid. Available at: https://seekwellbeing.org/seek-materials/. [Accessed 19 October 2023].

62. Kaiser permanente social interventions research & evaluation network. iHELP/iHELLP. sdh-tools-review.kpwashingtonresearch.org. 2020. Available at: https://sdh-tools-review.kpwashingtonresearch.org/screening-tools/ihellp-questionnaire. [Accessed 1 November 2023].

63. Child Health Equity Center. WE CARE. child health equity center. Available at: https://childhealthequitycenter.org/we-care/. [Accessed 19 October 2023].

64. Asp R and Paquette E. Feasibility and acceptability of screening for social determinants of health in the PICU, American Academy of pediatrics national conference & exhibition 2022; Anaheim, CA.

65. Nasa P, Jain R, Juneja D. Delphi methodology in healthcare research: how to decide its appropriateness. World J Methodol 2021;11(4):116–29.

66. Grunwell JR, Opolka C, Mason C, et al. Geospatial analysis of social determinants of health identifies neighborhood hot spots associated with pediatric intensive care use for life-threatening asthma. J Allergy Clin Immunol Pract 2021. https://doi.org/10.1016/j.jaip.2021.10.065.

67. Najjar N, Opolka C, Fitzpatrick AM, et al. Geospatial analysis of social determinants of health identifies neighborhood hot spots associated with pediatric intensive care use for acute respiratory failure requiring mechanical ventilation. Pediatr Crit Care Med 2022;23(8):606–17.

68. Beck AF, Huang B, Wheeler K, et al. The child opportunity Index and disparities in pediatric asthma hospitalizations across one Ohio metropolitan area, 2011-2013. J Pediatr 2017;190:200–206 e1.

69. Krager MK, Puls HT, Bettenhausen JL, et al. The child opportunity Index 2.0 and hospitalizations for ambulatory care sensitive conditions. Pediatrics 2021;148(2). https://doi.org/10.1542/peds.2020-032755.

70. Singh GK, Wilkinson AV, Song FF, et al. Health and social factors in Kansas: a data and chartbook, 1997–98. Lawrence, Kan: Allen Press; 1998.

71. Singh GK, Miller BA, Hankey BF, et al. Changing area socioeconomic patterns in US cancer mortality, 1950–1998: part I—all cancers among men. J Natl Cancer Inst 2002;94:904–15.

72. Singh GK, Siahpush M. Increasing inequalities in all-cause and cardiovascular mortality among US adults aged 25–64 years by area socioeconomic status, 1969–1998. Int J Epidemiol 2002;31:600–13.

73. Kind AJH, Buckingham WR. Making neighborhood-disadvantage metrics accessible - the neighborhood atlas. N Engl J Med 2018;378(26):2456–8.

74. Centers for Disease Control and Prevention/Agency for Toxic Substances and Disease Registry/Geospatial Research A, and Services Program. Social vulnerability Index data documentation. Available at: https://www.atsdr.cdc.gov/placeandhealth/svi/data_documentation_download.html. [Accessed 25 August 2021].

75. Noelke C, McArdle N, Baek M, et al. Child opportunity Index 2.0 technical documentation. 2020. Available at: http://new.diversitydatakids.org/research-library/research-brief/how-we-built-it. [Accessed 20 October 2021].

76. Registry CfDCaPaAfTSD. Environmental justice Index. Available at: https://www.atsdr.cdc.gov/placeandhealth/eji/index.html. [Accessed 18 August 2023].

77. Stephenson J. Federal agencies launch tool to measure health effects of environmental hazards for communities. JAMA Health Forum 2022;3(8):e223527.

78. Myers CN, Chandran A, Psoter KJ, et al. Indicators of neighborhood-level socioeconomic position and pediatric critical illness. Chest 2023;S0012-3692(23):01037–1041.

79. Centers for Disease Control and Prevention/Agency for Toxic Substances and Disease Registry/Geospatial Research A, and Services Program. Social vulnerability Index. Available at: https://www.atsdr.cdc.gov/placeandhealth/svi/index.html. [Accessed 10 March 2021].

80. Centers for disease control and prevention/agency for toxic Substances and disease Registry/geospatial research A, and services program. CDC social vulnerability Index 2018 database Georgia. 2021. Available at: https://www.atsdr.cdc.gov/placeandhealth/svi/data_documentation_download.html.

81. Index MHSV. Available at: https://www.minorityhealth.hhs.gov/minority-health-svi/. [Accessed 28 November 2022].

82. Diversity Data Kids. Childhood opportunity Index 2.0. Available at: https://data.diversitydatakids.org/dataset/coi20-child-opportunity-index-2-0-database. [Accessed 25 August 2021].

83. Javalkar K, Robson VK, Gaffney L, et al. Socioeconomic and racial and/or ethnic disparities in multisystem inflammatory syndrome. Pediatrics 2021;147(5). https://doi.org/10.1542/peds.2020-039933.

84. Givens M, Teal EN, Patel V, et al. Preterm birth among pregnant women living in areas with high social vulnerability. Am J Obstet Gynecol MFM 2021;3(5):100414.

85. Paro A, Hyer JM, Diaz A, et al. Profiles in social vulnerability: the association of social determinants of health with postoperative surgical outcomes. Surgery 2021. https://doi.org/10.1016/j.surg.2021.06.001.

86. Diversity Data Kids. Data visualization childhood opportunity Index by metropolitan statistical area. Available at: https://www.diversitydatakids.org/research-library/data-visualization/snapshot-child-opportunity-across-us. [Accessed 25 August 2021].

87. Diversity Data Kids. What is child opportunity?. Available at: https://www.diversitydatakids.org/research-library/research-brief/what-child-opportunity#Child-Opportunity-Levels. [Accessed 1 August 2023].

88. Gray MM, Malay S, Kleinman LC, et al. Child opportunity Index and hospital utilization in children with traumatic brain injury admitted to the PICU. Critical Care Explorations 2023;5(2):e0840.

89. Andermann A. Taking action on the social determinants of health in clinical practice: a framework for health professionals. Canadian Medical Association Journal 2019;188(17–18):474–83.

90. Garg A, Boynton-Jarrett R, Dworkin PH. Avoiding the unintended consequences of screening for social determinants of health. JAMA 2016;316(8):813.

91. Kawachi I. Social capital and community effects on population and individual health. Ann N Y Acad Sci 1999;896(1):120–30.

92. Institute of Medicine (US). Committee on monitoring access to personal health care services. In: Millman M, editor. Access to health care in America. National Academies Press (US); 1993. Available at: https://www.ncbi.nlm.nih.gov/books/NBK235882/.

93. Musumeci M. Medicaid's role for children with special health care needs. J Law Med Ethics 2018;46(4):897–905.

94. Douthit N, Kiv S, Dwolatzky T, et al. Exposing some important barriers to health care access in the rural USA. Publ Health 2015;129(6):611–20.

95. Yearby R, Clark B, Figueroa JF. Structural racism in historical and modern US health care policy. Health Aff 2022;41(2):187–94.

96. Dong E, Xu J, Sun X, et al. Differences in regional distribution and inequality in health-resource allocation on institutions, beds, and workforce: a longitudinal study in China. Arch Publ Health 2021;79(1). https://doi.org/10.1186/s13690-021-00597-1.

97. Centers for Medicare and Medicaid Services. Health care innovation awards | CMS. Available at: www.cms.gov. [Accessed 30 October 2023] https://www.cms.gov/priorities/innovation/innovation-models/health-care-innovation-awards.

98. American Hospital Association. A playbook for fostering hospital-community partnerships to build a culture of health, AHA. Available at: www.aha.org. [Accessed 30 October 2023] https://www.aha.org/ahahret-guides/2017-07-27-playbook-fostering-hospital-community-partnerships-build-culture-health.

Health Disparities in the Management and Outcomes of Critically Ill Children and Neonates: A Scoping Review

Anireddy R. Reddy, MD, MSHP[a,b,c,*],
Cody-Aaron Gathers, MD, MSHP[b,d], Daria C. Murosko, MD, MPH[e],
Tyler Rainer, MD, MSHP[f,g], Maryam Y. Naim, MD, MSCE[c,h],
Jessica Fowler, MD, MPH[a,c]

KEYWORDS

• Health disparities • Pediatric critical care • Cardiac intensive care • Neonatology

KEY POINTS

• Health disparities are present in the three primary settings (neonatal intensive care unit [NICU], pediatric intensive care unit [PICU], and cardiac intensive care unit [CICU]) that care for critically ill children in the United States.

• We describe over 50 studies which were designed to evaluate health disparities based on sociodemographic exposures. All of the included studies were published after 2010; the majority of studies describe NICU and PICU populations, with emerging CICU literature.

Continued

[a] Division of Critical Care, Department of Anesthesiology and Critical Care Medicine, Children's Hospital of Philadelphia, 3401 Civic Center Boulevard, Main Hospital, Ninth Floor, Room 9NW102, Philadelphia, PA 19104, USA; [b] Leonard Davis Institute of Health Economics, University of Pennsylvania, Philadelphia, PA, USA; [c] Department of Anesthesiology and Critical Care, The University of Pennsylvania Perelman School of Medicine, Philadelphia, PA, USA; [d] Division of Critical Care, Department of Anesthesiology and Critical Care Medicine, Children's Hospital of Philadelphia, 3401 Civic Center Boulevard, Main Hospital, Ninth Floor, Suite 9NW45, Philadelphia, PA 19104, USA; [e] Division of Neonatology, Department of Pediatrics, Children's Hospital of Philadelphia, 3401 Civic Center Boulevard, 2-Main, Philadelphia, PA 19104, USA; [f] Division of Pediatric Emergency Medicine, Department of Pediatrics, Children's Hospital of Philadelphia, Philadelphia, PA, USA; [g] Division of Emergency Medicine, Children's Hospital of Philadelphia, 3501 Civic Center Boulevard, 2nd Floor, Philadelphia, PA 19104, USA; [h] Division of Cardiac Critical Care, Department of Anesthesiology and Critical Care Medicine, Children's Hospital of Philadelphia, 3401 Civic Center Boulevard, Main Hospital, Eighth Floor 8555, Philadelphia, PA 19104, USA
* Corresponding author. Division of Critical Care, Department of Anesthesiology and Critical Care Medicine, Children's Hospital of Philadelphia, 3401 Civic Center Boulevard, Main Hospital, Ninth Floor, Room 9NW102, Philadelphia, PA 19104.
E-mail address: Reddya2@chop.edu

Crit Care Clin 40 (2024) 641–657
https://doi.org/10.1016/j.ccc.2024.05.002
0749-0704/24/© 2024 Elsevier Inc. All rights reserved, including those for text and data mining, AI training, and similar technologies.

criticalcare.theclinics.com

Continued

- Race and ethnicity were the most common exposures among the included studies, followed by area-level indices, insurance status, socioeconomic position, language, and distance to ICU.
- Future observational studies should improve collection and reporting of social determinants of health and acknowledge intersectionality of sociodemographic exposures.
- There are few interventional studies, though there is potential for individual-, institution-, neighborhood-, and policy-level solutions to reduce health disparities.

BACKGROUND

Health disparities are defined as differences in health care quality and outcomes that do not arise from differences in clinical appropriateness or patient preferences, but rather from structural or interpersonal discrimination.[1] Health disparities are widely prevalent and have persisted despite a national call to action to address inequities over 2 decades ago in the seminal publications *Health Disparities: Bridging the Gap*[2] and *Unequal Treatment: Confronting Racial and Ethnic Disparities in Health Care*.[1] Understanding and eliminating health disparities are crucial to providing high-quality and equitable care. In the past 20 years, the field has slowly shifted from *incidentally* describing significantly worse outcomes for poor individuals and racial and ethnic minorities to *intentionally* seeking to understand the drivers of structural inequities. Structural inequities are systems (policies, laws, cultural norms) and institutional processes that systematically disadvantage some groups compared to others[3] and influence personally held biases that together create inequitable outcomes. Recently, the COVID-19 pandemic illuminated racial inequities and created new urgency for health care systems to confront health disparities.[4]

Health disparities are pervasive and present in the care of neonates, infants, and children in the intensive care unit (ICU) setting. Critically ill children are primarily cared for in three settings: the neonatal ICU (NICU), pediatric ICU (PICU), and cardiac ICU (CICU). To date, health disparities in critically ill children have largely been studied within, not across, specific ICU settings, thus impeding collaboration that may help advance the care of critically ill children. The aim of this scoping review is to summarize the literature intentionally designed to examine health disparities, across 3 primary ICU settings in the United States, with the goal of describing cross-cutting themes and identifying priorities for future investigation.

METHODS

We searched MEDLINE and Embase databases for full-text articles published in English from January 1, 2000 to August 22, 2023. In consultation with a medical librarian, we used the search terms "pediatric," "child*," "neonat*," "infant" AND "health disparit*," "*equit*," AND "critically ill," "critical care," "intensive care" found in titles or abstracts. We used the Preferred Reporting Items for Systematic Reviews and Meta-Analysis (PRISMA)[5] to report the study search, screening, and selection process. The studies identified in these databases were then assessed for duplicates, which were removed. The remaining studies were screened by 2 authors (ARR and CAG) for inclusion; items flagged for inclusion by either reviewer subsequently underwent full article screening. The authors ARR, CAG, DCM, and TR participated in full article screening and discussion of final studies to include. We excluded review articles, abstracts, poster presentations, and articles published in languages other than English. We also excluded studies outside of the United States, as the structural determinants that influence health disparities are tied to the unique demographics, history, and political context of each country. To focus on inequities in ICU care, we excluded studies in which the outcome was measured prior to ICU admission. Articles were assessed for quality, design, size, and explicit aim of studying health disparities; we therefore excluded studies that were designed for another purpose and incidentally found disparate health outcomes based on sociodemographic factors. We acknowledge that structural inequities are pervasive and likely to be found in any study; thus, we chose to focus on studies which were designed and powered to detect health disparities. Citations included in key publications were manually reviewed to supplement literature search. Last, we described the study design, setting, sample, outcomes, and results of the final included studies.

RESULTS

Our search yielded 872 studies (Medline 608, EMBASE 264), of which 125 were duplicates (**Fig. 1**). The subsequent 746 studies were screened for inclusion criteria, yielding 96 studies for which full article screening was completed. Subsequently, 47 studies were excluded due to wrong population (24), wrong outcome (7), wrong setting (6), wrong publication type (5), or wrong exposure (5). Studies which analyzed data collected prior to 2000 but were published after 2000 were classified as "wrong setting." Studies which incidentally found disparities but were not designed with the intent of investigating disparities were classified as "wrong exposure." Citations included in key publications were manually reviewed to supplement the literature search, yielding 7 additional studies. In total, 56 studies were included in the final version of this review, for which we categorized by ICU setting (NICU, PICU, or CICU) and described study design, setting, population, sample size, and results.

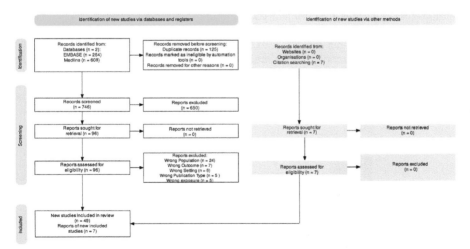

Fig. 1. PRISMA flow diagram of study identification, screening, and selection. Identification of 872 studies via databases (*left*) was completed using Embase and Medline, from which 125 duplicate studies were removed prior to screening. A total of 746 records were screened and 650 did not meet initial inclusion criteria. The remaining 96 reports were fully reviewed and assessed for eligibility, ultimately yielding 49 eligible studies. There were 7 studies included via other manual citation search (*right*). A total of 56 studies were included.

There were 43 retrospective cohort studies, 6 prospective cohort studies, 3 geospatial analyses, 3 interventional studies, and one secondary analysis of a randomized control trial. Studies were further categorized by NICU, PICU, and CICU as study populations are pragmatically divided into these groups based on practice setting. Of 56 total studies, the majority were NICU (24) and PICU (21) followed by CICU (9) with 2 PICU/CICU studies (**Fig. 2**).

Race and ethnicity were the most common exposures among the included studies (33), followed by composite area-level indices (12), insurance status (10), socioeconomic position (8), language (7), distance (3), telemedicine (1), and segregation (1; **Table 1**). Exposures such as race and ethnicity are reported here as they were originally published, noting that language and best practices for reporting race have evolved over time.[6] Last, we depicted studies by publication year (**Fig. 3**); all were published after 2010, with an overall increase in the number of publications in the last 5 years.

DISCUSSION

Our scoping review of studies investigating health disparities in critically ill children across multiple ICU settings yielded over 50 studies, all of which were published after 2010 with an overall surge in publications in the last 5 years. The majority of studies were retrospective cohort studies, with much fewer prospective cohort studies, and only 3 interventional studies. The paucity of prospective and interventional studies may reflect the need to characterize the existence of health disparities in multiple care and patient population settings prior to intervention. It likely also signifies the feasibility and effort with which retrospective studies can be completed in comparison to prospective and interventional work, which is needed in this space. We present the findings and themes within and across, ICU settings.

Not All Enter the Intensive Care Unit Equitably

Prior to interpreting the included studies, it is important to acknowledge the wealth of literature that illustrates that not everyone enters the ICU equitably. Prehospital care presents an important element of the care continuum not represented in our review. Children from geographic regions with the lowest child opportunity index (COI)—an area-based index describing resources and conditions which contribute to child health[7]—comprised a higher proportion of hospital admissions, critical care utilization,

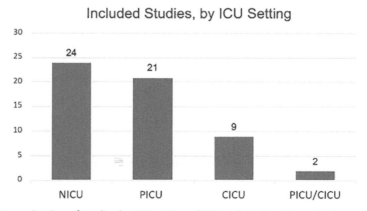

Fig. 2. Categorization of studies by ICU setting of 56 total studies: the majority are NICU (24) and PICU (21) followed by CICU (9) and PICU/CICU (2) studies.

Table 1	
Categorization of primary exposures within included studies	
Exposure	**Number of Studies**
Race and/or Ethnicity	33
Area-level Index	12
Childhood opportunity index	5
Social vulnerability index	4
Area deprivation index	2
Diez-Roux score	1
Insurance Status	10
Socioeconomic Position	8
Median household income by zip code	4
Child poverty rate	1
Self-reported household income	1
WIC eligibility	1
Composite SES index	1
Language	7
Distance	3
Access to Telemedicine	1
Segregation	1

As some studies assessed more than one exposure, the total number of exposures is greater than the number of included studies.

Abbreviation: WIC, special supplemental nutrition program for women, infants, and children.

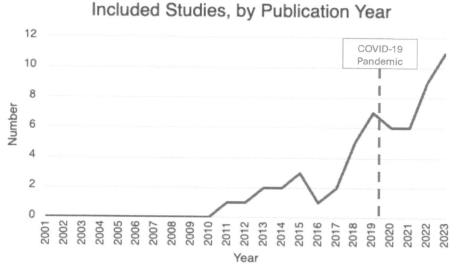

Fig. 3. Categorization of included studies by publication year in this review: all were published after 2010, with an overall increase in the number of publications in the last 5 years. The COVID-19 pandemic is denoted with red dashed line.

and mortality.[8] Emergency medical services research has also demonstrated disparities for patients with limited English proficiency (LEP), including longer time to dispatch, higher rates of unnecessary intubation,[9] more frequent hospitalization, higher critical care utilization, and delayed transport to the hospital.[10–12] Geography poses another area of health disparities for critically ill patients, as further travel for definitive care among rural populations and variation in clinical practice between urban and rural/suburban centers can impact outcomes.[8]

Care within the hospital emergency department prior to the critical care setting often reflects inequities in health care access, and utilization is disproportionately higher for children from regions with lower COI,[13] who identify as racial and ethnic minorities[14] and those with LEP.[15] Black pediatric patients with asthma are shown to have increased ICU utilization,[6] possibly reflecting delayed or more severe presentation to the emergency department related to limited access to care. Conversely, Black children requiring pediatric trauma team activation at a Level 1 trauma center were less likely to be admitted to the PICU[16]—a practice which may reflect bias in determining patient disposition. Further research in prehospital and emergency department care of critically ill patients is needed to better understand the drivers of pediatric critical care health disparities.

Disparities in the Neonatal Intensive Care Unit

Inequities in outcomes for infants have been rigorously documented, with many studies noting disparities in birth weight and prematurity, characteristics that are observable at birth and typically reflect maternal health and pregnancy-related exposures.[17] Because this review sought to describe inequities in the intensive care medicine, we focus on clinical outcomes that evolve during an infant's NICU admission, finding disparities across a broad range of clinical outcomes. Compared to infants born to non-Hispanic White (NHW) mothers, infants born to non-Hispanic Black (NHB) mothers are at greater risk of experiencing complications of prematurity,[18] including retinopathy of prematurity (ROP),[19,20] necrotizing enterocolitis (NEC),[19,21] and tracheostomy for treatment of bronchopulmonary dysplasia (BPD)[22] though some of these differences are at least partially attributable to higher rates of premature birth in NHB women. Inequities were less clear for infants born to Hispanic mothers, with some studies finding that Hispanic ethnicity was protective against requiring tracheostomy for BPD,[23] while others found increased risk of NEC[21] and ROP.[20] Analyses for other racial groups were extremely limited,[19] though one study examined a single NICU in Hawaii and found that infants born to mothers who were Pacific Islanders had greater rates of intraventricular hemorrhage (IVH) and NEC compared to Asian infants.[24] Only 2 NICU studies investigated other exposures: one found that residential racial segregation increased the risk of IVH in infants[25] and another documented increased risk of mortality for uninsured infants.[26]

Many studies examined disparities in parental engagement during the NICU hospitalization. Measures of parental engagement, including time spent at bedside,[27] participating in kangaroo mother care,[28] and remote viewing of infant[29] differed by parental language preference and socioeconomic status (SES). Barriers such as limited time away from work or the need for financial and/or personnel resources to care for other children may limit parental engagement. Preferred language other than English was associated with a significant decrease in parental understanding of medical care,[30] as shown in a powerful qualitative piece by Palau and colleagues. Preferred language other than English was also associated with increased provision of mother's own milk (MOM) at discharge.[31] Taken together, these findings suggest that language concordant care can be a powerful opportunity to foster resilience and increase parental engagement. As parental engagement is increasingly recognized as a driver of NICU outcomes, the effects of such interventions on infant health inequities must be examined.

Unique among the ICU settings analyzed, many NICU studies revealed a growing recognition that hospital-level differences in care quality may contribute to broad disparities in outcomes. The definition of "high quality care" remains the subject of ongoing debate, though racial and ethnic inequities were noted across multiple measures, including composite measures such as Baby MONITOR[32,33] or care processes including antenatal steroids,[19] hospital-acquired infections,[34,35] and provision of MOM.[24,36,37] Two studies suggested that nursing staffing and practice environment[35,38,39] might mediate the association between care quality and specific disparities. An exploration of provider strain, individual biases, and institutional culture at each NICU is needed to guide interventions that can improve and standardize quality of care for all infants. A quality improvement approach may be a potential solution to address disparities, as suggested by Parker and colleagues showing the impact of quality improvement (QI) methodology in improving in process measures related to MOM.[36] However, the population-level effect of such interventions is limited, as NHB and Hispanic infants are more likely to receive care at hospitals with lower quality scores[40,41] compared to NHW infants, Asian infants,[33,41] or those from more affluent neighborhoods.[33] Thus, eliminating racial and ethnic inequities in NICU outcomes will require both unit-specific interventions and addressing population-level NICU distribution.

Disparities in the Pediatric Intensive Care Unit

The included PICU studies described differences from prevalence/severity of illness on presentation to in-hospital management to ICU utilization and mortality. For example, incidence of penetrating trauma was higher for Black populations[42] and those residing in areas with higher social vulnerability index (SVI).[43] There were also higher rates of asthma,[44] bronchiolitis,[45] and respiratory failure requiring mechanical ventilation[46] in lower resourced neighborhoods. Studies additionally described the association of neighborhood deprivation with higher severity of illness on presentation,[47] increased likelihood of admission,[48] and increased risk of emergent readmission.[49] With regard to mortality, racial minority groups with cancer admitted to the PICU experienced higher mortality,[50] as did pediatric sepsis patients who were poor, uninsured, or publicly insured.[51]

While it follows that patients who are sicker on admission subsequently have higher ICU utilization[44–46] and longer length of stay,[44–46,52,53] there were mixed results observed within inpatient management. For example, in a propensity-matched cohort of pediatric patients with traumatic brain injury, private insurance status was associated with increased odds of undergoing invasive intracranial pressure monitoring and having cranial procedures.[54] Another study described single-center racial differences in rapid response team (RRT) activation; RRTs for NHW patients were more often called by attendings compared to Hispanic patients whose RRTs more likely to be called by trainees. In this center, Hispanic patients were observed to have 2.5 greater odds of mortality compared to NHW patients, raising the possibility of provider bias in recognition of clinical deterioration.[55] Distinct from these examples of differential inpatient management was an analysis of a multicenter randomized control trial that found no differences in sedation management by race or ethnicity,[56] suggesting that care standardization and equitable provision of care is plausible and may reduce practice variation between racial and ethnic groups.

In studying mechanisms to mitigate these disparities, there are few interventional studies. Because distance to pediatric critical care increases with poverty, potentially affecting time to care and subsequent severity of illness on presentation, telemedicine is a potential mechanism to reduce time to care. One interventional study found that telemedicine decreased severity of illness on presentation, finding a significant difference in Pediatric Risk of Mortality III score in patients for whom telemedicine was utilized.[57] The use of such services may be increasingly more relevant as we observe the regionalization of pediatric critical care and closures of PICUs across the country.[58,59] Another interventional study described a single center in which, prior to intervention, Latino patients' odds of mortality were 3.7 times that of non-Latino patients. The difference in mortality is supported by caregiver data in other studies wherein LEP families reported they were less likely to understand what was discussed on rounds or that they could rely on their nurses to spend enough time, including for medical updates.[60] After a multilevel intervention including cultural competency training, recruitment of bilingual staff, increased availability of interpreting services, translation of written materials, and community outreach, the mortality differences disappeared.[61] This study is an example of how system-level improvement efforts can have meaningful impact on health disparities.

Disparities in the Cardiac Intensive Care Unit

The CICU literature consists of retrospective cohort studies utilizing race, ethnicity, insurance status, parental income, and composite socioeconomic scores to characterize differences in outcomes. Among infants and children who undergo cardiac surgery for congenital heart disease (CHD), Black patients experience higher mortality,[62,63] have worse postoperative severity of illness,[64] and have an increased risk of death without etracorporeal membrane oxygenation (ECMO).[63] A study utilizing more granular data from the Pediatric Cardiac Critical Care Consortium database found that infants and children who were Black and other races had increased ECMO utilization during surgical hospitalizations and still had higher mortality despite the difference in ECMO use.[65] Infants and children who are Hispanic have worse preoperative severity of illness.[64] When considering SES, lower income was associated with worse mortality, longer length of stay, and higher health care costs.[62] A large single-center study identified a higher risk of early mortality, higher risk of transplant, and longer hospitalizations after Norwood operation for neonates in the lowest SES tertile status.[66] Infants who are uninsured have greater mortality risk,[67] while children with public insurance have higher mortality and an increased risk of death without ECMO.[63] A recent study analyzing race, ethnicity, and COI found that non-Hispanic Black patients, Asian patients, and patients from the lowest COI quintile had higher mortality, and COI only partially mediated the relationship between race/ethnicity and mortality.[68]

Understanding the contributions to racial, ethnic, and socioeconomic disparities in CICU outcomes requires better comprehension of preoperative, intraoperative, and postoperative risk factors. It is reasonable to hypothesize that disparities arise from differences in the prenatal diagnosis of CHD and timing to subspecialty care based on previously observed higher mortality in uninsured patients and those with delayed referral.[67,69] Delayed recognition and care of CHD may contribute to higher preoperative severity of illness and influence mortality or the likelihood of transplant.[70]

Tjoeng and colleagues demonstrated that postoperative severity of illness mediates the relationship between race and mortality after cardiac surgery for CHD.[64] While preoperative severity of illness did not mediate this relationship, postoperative severity of illness represents a contribution of preoperative and intraoperative factors. As such, a deeper analysis of preoperative risk factors including access to care, environmental exposures, economic stressors such as financial toxicity and food insecurity, timing of surgery, and intraoperative factors is warranted. Many of these factors can be difficult to measure on a large scale and may require local analysis of practice patterns to better elucidate this relationship. When explicitly considering the contribution of postoperative risk factors on mortality, Chan and colleagues identified that children who are Black or publicly insured have an increased risk of death without ECMO, suggesting that there may be variations in ECMO use related to race and insurance status.[63] However, Brunetti and colleagues suggest that differences in mortality may be attributed to factors other than ECMO utilization.[65] Moreover, the contribution of additional postoperative factors warrants evaluation in determining the underlying causes for surgical disparities in CHD. Institutional practice patterns, health care provider implicit and explicit biases, and complication rates after surgery may be additional contributors to these disparities.

Themes Across Intensive Care Unit Settings

Disparities across a multitude of exposures were observed across ICU settings, though notable differences emerged. The NICU patient population demonstrates the intergenerational effects of structural inequalities which manifest as differences in risk of prematurity. Prematurity has a major influence on, though is not the only driver of, inequities in clinical outcomes in the NICU. Compared to studies of outcomes in PICUs and CICUs, studies in NICUs have identified hospital-level differences in practice and process metrics such as administration of antenatal steroids, hospital-acquired infections, provision of MOM, and parental engagement, which can serve as potential targets for intervention. The PICU and CICU studies are more descriptive with fewer studies describing process metrics or intervention, though differences in management such as RRT activation (PICU) and ECMO (CICU) could contribute to disparate outcomes. Taken together, no setting is immune from disparities, and yet each setting is in a different stage of understanding and intervening upon these disparities. We therefore subsequently describe limitations to exposure assignment and future directions for research and intervention.

Limitations to Exposure Assignment

A limitation of the included studies is the paradigm of focusing on individual outcomes based on potentially blunt exposures such as individual race, ethnicity, income, language, or insurance status. These classifications can be imperfect proxies for structural inequities such as racism, classism, and discrimination and may introduce misclassification bias. In this review, the majority of studies use race and/or ethnicity as an exposure (which is further complicated by whether or not it is self-reported) and do not capture the impact of racism. Additionally, limited data collection and incomplete category options for many data sets do not allow for meaningful analysis of racial complexity, such as those who identify as biracial or multiracial patients who are often labeled as "other" in studies. There is further intricacy if we acknowledge intersectionality of exposures; poverty, for example, may modify the relationship between race and mortality. One way to overcome this is through joint modeling to account for effect modification between exposure and outcome. Composite area-level indices similarly attempt to address complexity, but it is unclear which index might be most appropriate for child health. In recent years, there have been 15 indices published which incorporate anywhere from 4 to 29 input variables.[71] SVI, for example, is used by the Centers for Disease Control to predict communities which may be vulnerable during disasters but is not specific to child health.[72] The area deprivation index uses American Community Survey data and was created to inform health delivery and policy.[73] Childhood opportunity index has potential for pediatric research in that it incorporates neighborhood resource variables in addition to ACS data, is available at the census level, and weighs factors based on the ability to predict health outcomes.[71] Like any measured variable, these indices are limited by input data and how often inputs are updated. Despite these limitations, these indices shift focus away from individual-level exposures toward investigating the *systems* which create disparate outcomes and, unlike many individual factors, are potentially modifiable.

Gaps in Research and Next Steps

The next stage in health disparities research in pediatric critical care involves embedding a health equity lens to all steps of the research process,[74–76] to consider additional exposures which are understudied, shift toward systems-based exposures, and step into the interventional space. Applying a health equity lens to research includes everything from designing a study with the intent of sampling a purposively stratified and diverse sample, to accurately capturing social determinants of health to inform statistical analysis. Community-based participatory research is an additional tool to integrate diverse stakeholders and patient/family input in academic research and is critical to creating local change that may not be applicable at the population level.[77] In addition to the exposures observed in this review, there are less explored populations relating to gender and sexual identity, education level, health literacy, urban versus rural settings, immigration status, and political context. As we move to more sophisticated data gathering, there are opportunities to better understand the contexts which create unequal outcomes. Contexts that shape policies and practices, and subsequently impact where patients receive care, live, work, and play need to be better understood in order for systemic change to occur. Most importantly, we must move from problem characterization and causal inference to intervention. Interventions must be developed and executed across multiple levels, recognizing that overlapping and intersecting processes will be necessary to counteract the pervasive effects of structural inequities.

At the policy level, paid family leave is associated with decreased postneonatal mortality[78,79] and has the potential to improve ICU outcomes by increasing parental presence at the bedside.[80] In a similar attempt to mitigate financial hardship, unconditional cash transfer programs are being studied, with mixed results thus far.[81–83] At the neighborhood level, opportunities for intervention include modifying resource distribution and improving neighborhoods, and prior studies have shown interventions such as cleaning vacant lots ("greening") can improve mental health[84] and decrease crime and violence.[85] Within institutions, quality improvement efforts can rapidly and effectively narrow health inequities, such as the multilevel linguistic intervention which eliminated the mortality difference between Latino and NHW in a single center.[61] Some institutions are moving toward more comprehensive screening for social determinants of health[86] or implementing quality or equity dashboards to provide real-time monitoring of care outcomes and potential disparities.[87,88] Similarly, interventions such as telemedicine have the potential to support centers which are far from critical care resources in order to reduce the severity of illness on subsequent ICU presentation.[57] Lastly, individuals who provide care to critically ill infants and children must receive education and training on bias recognition and mitigation strategies.[89,90] Health disparities research is replete with opportunities to reduce inequitable outcomes and improve care for all.

SUMMARY

In this scoping review, we summarize literature designed to examine health disparities, across 3 primary ICU settings in the United States. We included over 50 studies which describe health disparities across race and/or ethnicity, area-level indices, insurance status, socioeconomic position, language, and distance (Supplementary Table 1). Future observational studies should improve collection and reporting of social determinants of health and acknowledge intersectionality of sociodemographic exposures. While there are only a few interventional studies, there is potential for individual-, institution-, neighborhood-, and policy-level solutions to reduce health disparities.

CLINICS CARE POINTS

- There is increasing literature describing health disparities observered in the NICU, PICU and CICU, predominately describing racial and/or ethnic differences.
- Data collection and reporting of social determinants of health, including community and system-level determinants, is paramount for future research and intervention.

DISCLOSURE

The work of C-A. Gathers and D.C. Murosko was supported by the NIH, United States-funded training grant T32HL098054.

SUPPLEMENTARY DATA

Supplementary data to this article can be found online at https://doi.org/10.1016/j.ccc.2024.05.002.

REFERENCES

1. Institute of Medicine (US) Committee on. Understanding and Eliminating Racial and Ethnic Disparities in Health Care. Unequal Treatment: Confronting Racial and Ethnic Disparities. In: Smedley BD, Stith AY, Nelson AR, editors. Health Care. Washington, DC: National Academies Press (US); 2003.
2. National Institute of Child Health and Huma Development (US). Health Disparities: Bridging the Gap 2000 The Development.
3. National Academies of Sciences, Engineering, and Medicine; Health and Medicine Division; Board on Population Health and Public Health Practice; Committee on Community-Based Solutions to Promote Health Equity in the United States. Communities in Action: Pathways to Health Equity. Baciu A, Negussie Y, Geller A. Weinstein JN, editors. National Academies Press (US); Washington, DC, 2017.
4. Nana-Sinkam P, Kraschnewski J, Sacco R, et al. Health disparities and equity in the era of COVID-19. Journal of Clinical and Translational Science 2021;5(1). e99. e99.
5. Moher D, Liberati A, Tetzlaff J, et al, PRISMA Group* t. Preferred reporting items for systematic reviews and meta-analyses: the PRISMA statement. Annals of internal medicine 2009;151(4):264–9.
6. Flanagin A, Frey T, Christiansen SL, et al. Updated guidance on the reporting of race and ethnicity in medical and science Journals. JAMA 2021;326(7): 621–7.

7. diversitydatakids.org. Child opportunity index 2.0 ZIP code data. Available at: https://data.diversitydatakids.org/dataset/coi20_zipcodes-child-opportunity-index-2-0-zip-code-data?_external=True. Accessed February 1, 2023.

8. Heneghan JA, Goodman DM, Ramgopal S. Hospitalizations at United States children's hospitals and severity of illness by Neighborhood Child Opportunity Index. J Pediatr 2023;254:83–90. e8.

9. Bard MR, Goettler CE, Schenarts PJ, et al. Language barrier leads to the unnecessary intubation of trauma patients. Am Surg 2004;70(9):783–6.

10. Grow RW, Sztajnkrycer MD, Moore BR. Language barriers as a reported cause of prehospital care delay in Minnesota. Prehosp Emerg Care 2008;12(1):76–9.

11. Perera N, Birnie T, Ngo H, et al. "I'm sorry, my English not very good": Tracking differences between Language-Barrier and Non-Language-Barrier emergency ambulance calls for Out-of-Hospital Cardiac Arrest. Resuscitation 2021;169: 105–12.

12. Lee ED, Rosenberg CR, Sixsmith DM, et al. Does a physician-patient language difference increase the probability of hospital admission? Acad Emerg Med 1998;5(1):86–9.

13. Ramgopal S, Attridge M, Akande M, et al. Distribution of emergency department encounters and subsequent hospital admissions for children by child opportunity index. Academic Pediatrics 2022;22(8):1468–76.

14. Shapiro DJ, Fine AM. Patient ethnicity and pediatric visits to the emergency department for fever. Pediatr Emerg Care 2021;37(11):555–9.

15. Lowe JT, Monteiro KA, Zonfrillo MR. Disparities in pediatric emergency department length of stay and utilization associated with primary language. Pediatr Emerg Care 2022;38(4):e1192–7.

16. Slain KN, Wurtz MA, Rose JA. US children of minority race are less likely to be admitted to the pediatric intensive care unit after traumatic injury, a retrospective analysis of a single pediatric trauma center. Injury epidemiology 2021;8(1):1–10.

17. Singh GK. Trends and social inequalities in maternal mortality in the United States, 1969-2018. Int J MCH AIDS 2021;10(1):29–42.

18. Tanner LD, Chen H-Y, Sibai BM, et al. Racial and ethnic disparities in maternal and neonatal adverse outcomes in college-educated women. Obstet Gynecol 2020;136(1):146–53. Available at: http://elinks.library.upenn.edu/sfx_local?sid=EMBASE&issn=1873233X&id=doi:10.1097%2FAOG.0000000000003887&atitle=Racial+and+Ethnic+Disparities+in+Maternal+and+Neonatal+Adverse+Outcomes+in+College-Educated+Women&stitle=Obstet.+Gynecol.&title=Obstetrics+and+Gynecology&volume=136&issue=1&spage=146&epage=153&aulast=Tanner&aufirst=Lisette+D.&auinit=L.D.&aufull=Tanner+L.D.&coden=OBGNA&isbn=&pages=146-153&date=2020&auinit1=L&auinitm=D.

19. Boghossian NS, Geraci M, Lorch SA, et al. Racial and ethnic differences over time in outcomes of infants born less than 30 weeks' gestation. Pediatrics 2019;144(3). https://doi.org/10.1542/peds.2019-1106.

20. Reer K, Marie A, Tahmieh R, et al. Association between social determinants of health and retinopathy of prematurity outcomes. JAMA ophthalmology 2022; 140(5):496–502.

21. Jammeh ML, Adibe OO, Tracy ET, et al. Racial/ethnic differences in necrotizing enterocolitis incidence and outcomes in premature very low birth weight infants. Article. J Perinatol 2018;38(10):1386–90.

22. Smith MA, Steurer MA, Mahendra M, et al. Sociodemographic factors associated with tracheostomy and mortality in bronchopulmonary dysplasia. Pediatr Pulmonol 2023 2023;58(4):1237–46. Available at: http://elinks.library.upenn.edu/sfx_

local?sid=EMBASE&issn=10990496&id=doi:10.1002%2Fppul.26328&atitle=
Sociodemographic+factors+associated+with+tracheostomy+and+mortality+in+
bronchopulmonary+dysplasia&stitle=Pediatr.+Pulmonol.&title=Pediatric+
Pulmonology&volume=58&issue=4&spage=1237&epage=1246&aulast=Smith&
aufirst=Michael+A.&auinit=M.A.&aufull=Smith+M.A.&coden=PEPUE&isbn=
&pages=1237-1246&date=2023&auinit1=M&auinitm=A.

23. Smith MA, Steurer MA, Mahendra M, et al. Sociodemographic factors associated
    with tracheostomy and mortality in bronchopulmonary dysplasia. Article. Pediatr
    Pulmonol 2023;58(4):1237–46.

24. MeganY K, Chieko K, Kara WR. Racial disparities in breastmilk receipt and
    extremely low gestational age neonatal morbidities in an asian pacific islander
    population. Journal of racial and ethnic health disparities 2023-4 2023;10(2):
    952–60.

25. Murosko D, Passerella M, Lorch S. Racial segregation and intraventricular hem-
    orrhage in preterm infants. Pediatrics 2020;145(6). https://doi.org/10.1542/peds.
    2019-1508.

26. Jr MF. Increased risk of death among uninsured neonates. Health Serv Res
    2013-8 2013;48(4):1232–55.

27. SL B, BW W, MA P, et al. The association of social factors and time spent in the
    NICU for mothers of very preterm infants. Hosp Pediatr 2021-9 2021;11(9):
    988–96.

28. E B-P, M S, HM F, et al. Disparities in Kangaroo care for premature infants in the
    neonatal intensive care unit. Journal of developmental and behavioral pediatrics :
    JDBP (J Dev Behav Pediatr) 2022-6-01 2022;43(5):e304–11.

29. Patel RK, Kreofsky BL, Morgan KM, et al. Sociodemographic factors and family
    use of remote infant viewing in neonatal intensive care. J Perinatol 2023;43(3):
    350–6. Available at: http://elinks.library.upenn.edu/sfx_local?sid=EMBASE&issn=
    14765543&id=doi:10.1038%2Fs41372-022-01506-2&atitle=Sociodemographic+
    factors+and+family+use+of+remote+infant+viewing+in+neonatal+intensive+
    care&stitle=J.+Perinatol.&title=Journal+of+Perinatology&volume=43&issue=3&
    spage=350&epage=356&aulast=Patel&aufirst=Rahul+K.&auinit=R.K.&aufull=
    Patel+R.K.&coden=JOPEE&isbn=&pages=350-356&date=2023&auinit1=R&
    auinitm=K.

30. MA P, MR M, JT B, et al. The impact of parental primary language on communi-
    cation in the neonatal intensive care unit. J Perinatol 2019;39(2):307–13.

31. Kalluri NS, Melvin P, Belfort MB, et al. Maternal language disparities in neonatal
    intensive care unit outcomes. Article. J Perinatol 2022;42(6):723–9.

32. Jochen P, ErikaM E, DaWayne P. Getting to health equity in NICU care in the USA
    and beyond. Arch Dis Child Fetal Neonatal Ed 2023;108(4):326–31.

33. Padula AM, Shariff-Marco S, Yang J, et al. Multilevel social factors and NICU
    quality of care in California. J Perinatol 2021;41(3):404–12.

34. Liu J, Sakarovitch C, Sigurdson K, et al. Disparities in health care-associated in-
    fections in the NICU. Am J Perinatol 2020;37(2):166–73.

35. Lake ET, Staiger D, Horbar J, et al. Disparities in perinatal quality outcomes for
    very low birth weight infants in neonatal intensive care. Health Serv Res 2015;
    50(2):374–97.

36. Parker MG, Gupta M, Melvin P, et al. Racial and ethnic disparities in the use of
    mother's milk feeding for very low birth weight infants in Massachusetts. Article.
    J Pediatr 2019;204:134–41.e1.

37. Patel AL, Schoeny ME, Hoban R, et al. Mediators of racial and ethnic disparity in
    mother's own milk feeding in very low birth weight infants. Pediatr Res 2019;85(5):

662–70. Available at: http://elinks.library.upenn.edu/sfx_local?sid=EMBASE& issn=15300447&id=doi:10.1038%2Fs41390-019-0290-2&atitle=Mediators+of+ racial+and+ethnic+disparity+in+mother%E2%80%99s+own+milk+feeding+ in+very+low+birth+weight+infants&stitle=Pediatr.+Res.&title=Pediatric+Research& volume=85&issue=5&spage=662&epage=670&aulast=Patel&aufirst=Aloka+L. &auinit=A.L.&aufull=Patel+A.L.&coden=PEREB&isbn=&pages=662-670&date= 2019&auinit1=A&auinitm=L.

38. ET L, D S, EM E, et al. Nursing care disparities in neonatal intensive care units. Health Serv Res 2018;53:3007–26.

39. E L, J R, J W. Improving the lives of fragile newborns: what does nursing have to offer? LDI Issue Brief 2016-4 2016;20(1):1–4.

40. JD H, EM E, LT G, et al. Racial segregation and inequality in the neonatal intensive care unit for very low-birth-weight and very preterm infants. JAMA Pediatr 2019;173(5):455–61.

41. J P, JB G, M B, et al. Racial/ethnic disparity in NICU quality of care delivery. Pediatrics 2017-9 2017;140(3). https://doi.org/10.1542/peds.2017-0918.

42. Cassidy LD, Lambropoulos D, Enters J, et al. Health disparities analysis of critically ill pediatric trauma patients in Milwaukee, Wisconsin. J Am Coll Surg 2013; 217(2):233–9.

43. Stevens J, Reppucci ML, Pickett K, et al. Using the social vulnerability index to examine disparities in surgical pediatric trauma patients. Article. J Surg Res 2023;287:55–62.

44. JR G, C O, C M, et al. Geospatial analysis of social determinants of health identifies neighborhood hot spots associated with pediatric intensive care use for life-threatening asthma. J Allergy Clin Immunol Pract 2022-4 2022;10(4):981–91.e1.

45. Slain KN, Shein SL, Stormorken AG, et al. Outcomes of children with critical bronchiolitis living in poor communities. Clin Pediatr (Phila) 2018;57(9):1027–32.

46. N N, C O, AM F, et al. Geospatial analysis of social determinants of health identifies neighborhood hot spots associated with pediatric intensive care use for acute respiratory failure requiring mechanical ventilation. Pediatr Crit Care Med 2022-8-1 2022;23(8):606–17.

47. Epstein D, Reibel M, Unger JB, et al. The effect of neighborhood and individual characteristics on pediatric critical illness. J Community Health 2014;39(4): 753–9.

48. Myers CN, Chandran A, Psoter KJ, et al. Indicators of neighborhood-level socioeconomic position and pediatric critical illness. Chest 2023. https://doi.org/10. 1016/j.chest.2023.07.014.

49. Akande MY, Ramgopal S, Graham RJ, et al. Child opportunity index and emergent PICU readmissions: a retrospective, cross-sectional study of 43 U.S. Hospitals. Pediatr Crit Care Med 2023;24(5):e213–23.

50. Leimanis Laurens M, Snyder K, Davis AT, et al. Racial/ethnic minority children with cancer experience higher mortality on admission to the ICU in the United States. Pediatr Crit Care Med 2020;21(10):859–68.

51. Reddy AR, Badolato GM, Chamberlain JM, et al. Disparities associated with sepsis mortality in critically ill children. Journal of Pediatric Intensive Care 2022;11(2):147–52.

52. Andrist E, Riley CL, Brokamp C, et al. Neighborhood poverty and pediatric intensive care Use. Pediatrics 2019;144(6). https://doi.org/10.1542/peds.2019-0748.

53. Gray MM, Malay S, Kleinman LC, et al. Child opportunity index and hospital utilization in children with traumatic brain injury admitted to the PICU. Crit Care Explor 2023;5(2):e0840. https://doi.org/10.1097/cce.0000000000000840.

54. Porter A, Brown CC, Tilford JM, et al. Association of insurance status with treatment and outcomes in pediatric patients with severe traumatic brain injury. Crit Care Med 2020 2020;48(7):E584–91. Available at: http://elinks.library.upenn. edu/sfx_local?sid=EMBASE&issn=15300293&id=doi:10.1097%2FCCM.000000 0000004398&atitle=Association+of+Insurance+Status+with+Treatment+and+ Outcomes+in+Pediatric+Patients+with+Severe+Traumatic+Brain+Injury&stitle= Crit.+Care+Med.&title=Critical+Care+Medicine&volume=48&issue=7&spage= E584&epage=E591&aulast=Porter&aufirst=Austin&auinit=A.&aufull=Porter+A. &coden=CCMDC&isbn=&pages=E584-E591&date=2020&auinit1=A&auinitm=.

55. Lawson NR, Acorda D, Guffey D, et al. Association of social determinants of health with rapid response events: a retrospective cohort trial in a large pediatric academic hospital system. Frontiers in pediatrics 2022 2022;10:853691.

56. Natale JE, Asaro LA, Joseph JG, et al. Association of race and ethnicity with sedation management in pediatric intensive care. Annals of the American Thoracic Society 2021;18(1):93–102.

57. Parul D, Nayal H, Kissee JL, et al. Impact of telemedicine on severity of illness and outcomes among children transferred from referring emergency departments to a children's hospital PICU. Pediatr Crit Care Med 2016;17:516–21.

58. Mahant S, Guttmann A. Shifts in the hospital care of children in the US—a health equity Challenge. JAMA Netw Open 2023;6(9):e2331763.

59. Cushing AM, Bucholz EM, Chien AT, et al. Availability of pediatric inpatient services in the United States. Pediatrics 2021;148(1). https://doi.org/10.1542/peds. 2020-041723.

60. Zurca AD, Fisher KR, Flor RJ, et al. Communication with limited english-proficient families in the PICU. Hosp Pediatr 2017;7:9–15.

61. Anand KJ, Sepansi RJ, Giles K, et al. Pediatric intensive care unit mortality among Latino children before and after a multilevel health care delivery intervention. JAMA Pediatr 2015-4 2015;169(4):383–90.

62. Anderson BR, Fieldson ES, Newburger JW, et al. Disparities in outcomes and resource use after hospitalization for cardiac surgery by neighborhood income. Pediatrics 2018-3 2018;141(3). https://doi.org/10.1542/peds.2017-2432.

63. Chan T, Barrett CS, Tijeng YL, et al. Racial variations in extracorporeal membrane oxygenation use following congenital heart surgery. J Thorac Cardiovasc Surg 2018;156:306–15.

64. Tjoeng YL, Jenkins K, Deen JF, et al. Association between race/ethnicity, illness severity, and mortality in children undergoing cardiac surgery. Article. J Thorac Cardiovasc Surg 2020;160(6):1570–9.e1.

65. Brunetti Marissa A, Griffis Heather M, O'Byrne Michael L, et al. Racial and ethnic variation in ECMO utilization and outcomes in pediatric cardiac ICU patients. JACC (J Am Coll Cardiol): Advances 2023;2(9):100634.

66. Sengupta A, Bucholz EM, Gauvreau K, et al. Impact of neighborhood socioeconomic status on outcomes following first-stage palliation of single ventricle heart disease. Article. J Am Heart Assoc 2023;12(6). https://doi.org/10.1161/JAHA. 122.026764.

67. JE K, CH C, CJ A, et al. Role of health insurance on the survival of infants with congenital heart defects. Am J Public Health 2014-9 2014;104(9):e62–70.

68. Duong SQ, Elfituri MO, Zaniletti I, et al. Neighborhood childhood opportunity, race/ethnicity, and surgical outcomes in children with congenital heart disease. J Am Coll Cardiol 2023;82(9):801–13.

69. Fixler DE, Xu P, Nembhard WN, et al. Age at referral and mortality from critical congenital heart disease. Pediatrics 2014;134(1):e98–105.

70. Peterson JK, Chen Y, Nguyen DV, et al. Current trends in racial, ethnic, and healthcare disparities associated with pediatric cardiac surgery outcomes. Congenit Heart Dis 2017;12(4):520–32.

71. Trinidad S, Brokamp C, Mor Huertas A, et al. Use of area-based socioeconomic deprivation indices: a scoping review and qualitative analysis. Health Aff 2022; 41(12):1804–11.

72. Flanagan BE, Gregory EW, Hallisey EJ, et al. A social vulnerability index for disaster management. J Homel Secur Emerg Manag 2011;8(1). 0000102202154773551792.

73. Kind AJH, Buckingham WR. Making neighborhood-disadvantage metrics accessible — the neighborhood Atlas. N Engl J Med 2018;378(26):2456–8.

74. AD Z, ML S, TW O. An antiracism approach to conducting, reporting, and evaluating pediatric critical care research. Pediatr Crit Care Med 2022;23(2): 129–32.

75. Montoya-Williams D, Fraiman YS, Peña MM, et al. Antiracism in the field of neonatology: a foundation and concrete approaches. NeoReviews 2022; 23(1):e1–12.

76. Montoya-Williams D, Peña MM, Fuentes-Afflick E. In pursuit of health equity in pediatrics. J Pediatr X 2020. https://doi.org/10.1016/j.ympdx.2020.100045.

77. Wallerstein N, Duran B. Community-based participatory research contributions to intervention research: the intersection of science and practice to improve health equity. Am J Public Health 2010;100(S1):S40–6.

78. Montoya-Williams D, Passarella M, Lorch SA. The impact of paid family leave in the United States on birth outcomes and mortality in the first year of life. Health Serv Res 2020;55:807–14.

79. Burtle A, Bezruchka S. Population health and paid parental leave: what the United States can learn from two decades of research. MDPI; 2016. p. 30.

80. Montez K, Thomson S, Shabo V. An opportunity to promote health equity: national paid family and medical leave. Pediatrics 2020;146(3).

81. Sperber JF, Gennetian LA, Hart ER, et al. Unconditional cash transfers and maternal assessments of children's health, nutrition, and sleep: a randomized clinical trial. JAMA Netw Open 2023;6(9):e2335237.

82. Copeland WE, Tong G, Gaydosh L, et al. Long-term outcomes of childhood family income supplements on adult functioning. JAMA Pediatr 2022;176(10): 1020–6.

83. Flynn EF, Kenyon CC, Vasan A. Cash transfer programs for child health—Elucidating Pathways and Optimizing program design. JAMA Pediatr 2023;177(7): 661–2.

84. South EC, Hohl BC, Kondo MC, et al. Effect of greening vacant land on mental health of community-dwelling adults: a cluster randomized trial. JAMA Netw Open 2018;1(3):e180298.

85. Branas CC, South E, Kondo MC, et al. Citywide cluster randomized trial to restore blighted vacant land and its effects on violence, crime, and fear. Proc Natl Acad Sci USA 2018;115(12):2946–51.

86. Akande M, Paquette ET, Magee P, et al. Screening for social determinants of health in the pediatric intensive care unit: recommendations for clinicians. Crit Care Clin 2023;39(2):341–55.

87. Razdan S, Hedli LC, Sigurdson K, et al. Disparity drivers, potential solutions, and the role of a health equity dashboard in the neonatal intensive care unit: a qualitative study. J Perinatol 2024;44(5):659–64.

88. Menda N, Edwards E. Measuring equity for quality improvement. Clin Perinatol 2023;50(2):531–43.
89. Torr C. Culturally competent care in the neonatal intensive care unit, strategies to address outcome disparities. J Perinatol 2022;42(10):1424–7.
90. Castillo EG, Isom J, DeBonis KL, et al. Reconsidering systems-based practice: advancing structural competency, health equity, and social responsibility in graduate medical education. Acad Med 2020;95(12):1817–22.

Disparities in Access, Management and Outcomes of Critically Ill Adult Patients with Trauma

Caitlin Collins, MD, Tasce Bongiovanni, MD, MPP*

KEYWORDS

- Disparities • Trauma • Patient outcomes • Race and ethnicity • Health equity
- Insurance status

KEY POINTS

- Disparities exist for patients with trauma across the care continuum, from prehospital settings to postdischarge.
- Lacking private insurance, identifying as a racial or ethnic minority, and being women can negatively impact the management and outcomes of patients with trauma at every step of care.
- Certain demographics are understudied and either underrepresented or completely unrepresented in large national trauma databases such as American Indian/Alaska Native patients, patients with a preferred language other than English, and patients with disabilities.
- More data on unrepresented groups and research on upstream factors affecting all patients with trauma are critical to measure and improve outcomes for these vulnerable populations.

INTRODUCTION

Disparities in health and health care exist across multiple dimensions. Greater recognition and understanding of the social determinants of health has led to a considerable amount of research on the ways racism affects health outcomes, socioeconomic status, insurance status, the physical environment, and more. The results of these studies have shown disparities in cancer, infectious disease, and chronic disease outcomes among vulnerable populations.[1] However, it is not a foregone conclusion that the

Department of Surgery, University of California San Francisco School of Medicine, San Francisco, CA, USA
* Corresponding author. 513 Parnassus Avenue, HSW 1601, San Francisco, CA 94143-0790.
E-mail address: Tasce.Bongiovanni@ucsf.edu
Twitter: @TasceB (T.B.)

Crit Care Clin 40 (2024) 659–670
https://doi.org/10.1016/j.ccc.2024.05.003   criticalcare.theclinics.com
0749-0704/24/© 2024 Elsevier Inc. All rights reserved, including those for text and data mining, AI training, and similar technologies.

same disparities in care and outcomes would also affect patients with trauma, because unlike care for chronic or subacute medical problems, the receipt of emergent care for traumatic injuries is a protected right under the Emergency Medical Treatment and Active Labor Act (EMTALA). EMTALA was passed by Congress in 1986 to ensure access to the treatment of medical emergencies regardless of a person's ability to pay. Hospitals are required to provide stabilizing treatment of patients with emergency medical conditions regardless of insurance status. If the hospital cannot provide the necessary level of care, it must stabilize the patient to the best of its ability before transferring the patient to another facility.[2] Consequently, patients with trauma are protected from discrimination and exclusion in ways that are not true for patients suffering from any other nonemergent medical problem. Yet, despite legal protections that guarantee access to care for patients with trauma, research has repeatedly demonstrated health and health care disparities among this population. Since trauma care is a continuum, we aimed to review disparities at each step of the journey for a severely injured patient with trauma, from prehospital care to postdischarge outcomes (**Fig. 1**).[3–6]

BARRIERS TO CARE IN THE PREHOSPITAL SETTING

Time plays a particularly crucial role in outcomes for patients with trauma. Because access to a trauma center is not equally distributed across the US population, the disparity in care and subsequent disparity in outcome after traumatic injury begins the second the patient is injured. Therefore, a discussion of disparities in care and outcomes of critically injured adult patients with trauma must first consider who makes it to the hospital and who does not.

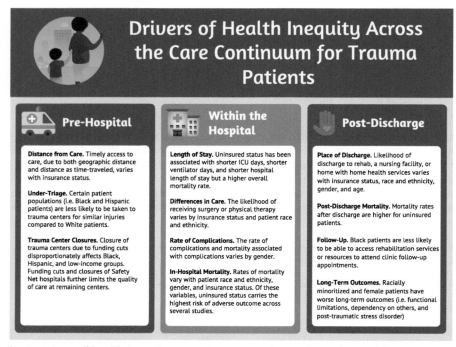

Fig. 1. Drivers of health inequity across the care continuum for patients with trauma.

Much like some hospitals carry certifications for stroke centers, some hospitals have specific designations as trauma centers. Trauma centers are hospitals with specialized personnel and equipment capable of providing care for the unique needs of patients with trauma. Because trauma centers are expensive and the various levels of trauma center designation have specific requirements, not all hospitals can obtain this designation, nor would it be practical. However, patients with trauma who were treated at level I trauma centers had a 20% lower in-hospital mortality than those treated at nontrauma hospitals and a 25% lower 1 year mortality rate.[7] It is similarly well documented that patients suffer worse outcomes when they lack timely access to a trauma center.[8–11] The notable difference in outcome by trauma center designation becomes especially important because the distribution of trauma centers in the United States is not random and often reveals the sinister disparities driven by human design decisions.

Across the United States, nearly 30 million people lack timely access to trauma care.[3,12,13] Census block groups with a high rate of uninsured individuals are over 90% less likely to have access to a level I or level II trauma center.[3] In a similar vein, census block groups with a high proportion of people eligible for Medicare or Medicaid are 31% less likely to have access to a trauma center than census block groups with predominantly insured individuals.[3]

While individuals living in urban areas may be geographically closer to a trauma center, many studies fail to account for significant variability in actual transit times due to vehicular congestion within urban settings. In an investigation of travel times and subsequent mortality rates for individuals suffering gunshot wounds in Chicago, which has one of the country's highest homicide rates from penetrating injury, Crandall and colleagues found that individuals who were shot more than 5 miles from a trauma center had 23% higher odds of death.[14] The authors coined the term "relative trauma desert" to describe these areas within urban settings that suffer from disparate outcomes because of time-based differences in access to definitive care.[14] Building on this study, Tung and colleagues evaluated the racial composition of "relative trauma deserts" in New York City, Chicago, and Los Angeles, demonstrating that US Census tracts containing a majority Black population were more likely to be located in an urban trauma desert.[15] Further compounding this differential access to timely trauma care, another study also found that severely injured Black and Hispanic patients with trauma were more likely to be undertriaged, meaning they were more likely to be sent to a nontrauma center than White patients with trauma with similar injuries.[8] Undertriage following major trauma is associated with a considerable increase in mortality,[16] likely from delays in receipt of time-sensitive, life-saving care.

Although trauma center access in the United States improved significantly in the last 2 decades, in recent years, several trauma centers had to close their doors because of financial constraints stemming from disadvantageous health policy regarding reimbursement for trauma care.[12,17,18] These closures have also disproportionately impacted Black, Hispanic, and low-income groups.[19] Furthermore, safety-net hospital closures and funding restrictions have limited the quality of care the remaining centers can provide. A lack of funding restricts hospital participation in regional quality improvement initiatives, which have been shown to reduce rates of major complications and mortality.[20]

OUTCOME AND MANAGEMENT DISPARITIES WITHIN THE HOSPITAL SETTING

Insurance status may be the most significant driver of disparate outcomes among patients with trauma. According to a study of the National Trauma Data Bank (NTDB), from 2002 to 2006, uninsured status was associated with a higher risk of death (hazard ratio [HR] 1.69) than minoritized ethnicity (HR 1.08) or male gender (HR 1.14). This difference in mortality began on the first day after injury and widened throughout the hospitalization.[21] Further, the inequities in mortality among uninsured patients exist for both penetrating and blunt injuries.[22,23] Another study of NTDB data demonstrated that although penetrating injury carries an overall higher mortality than blunt injury regardless of insurance status, in subset analysis, uninsured patients within the 2 groups had significantly higher mortality.[23] One proposed explanation for this disparity in mortality is that uninsured patients have preexisting poorly managed chronic comorbidities due to the lack of access to health care that drives their subsequent increased mortality when they become victims of trauma. However, these disparities by insurance status are evident even among 18 to 30 year old patients with trauma who presumably have few, if any, comorbidities.[21,23]

The increased mortality for uninsured patients with trauma is recapitulated across populations with differing mechanisms of injury and injury severity scores (ISSs). An NTDB analysis for the years 2013 to 2015 found that uninsured patients suffering penetrating injury had higher odds of death, not only among the severely injured population (odds ratio [OR] 2.68) but also among patients with mild-to-moderate injury (ISS <15), where the odds of death were 56% higher for uninsured patients.[24] A study of 26,404 vehicle-struck pedestrians within the NTDB reported that uninsured patients had 77% greater odds of mortality than privately insured patients.[25]

Several additional studies point to measurable differences in management decisions when stratified by insurance status, which could contribute to the mortality differences.[26,27] An analysis of all adults hospitalized following traumatic injury in Massachusetts in 1990 showed that, compared to privately insured patients, uninsured patients were as likely to be admitted to the intensive care unit (ICU) but less likely to undergo surgery or receive physical therapy. Uninsured patients were also more than twice as likely to die in the hospital (OR 2.15). Medicaid status did mitigate the disparities in access to physical therapy and mortality, but these patients were still less likely to undergo surgery than privately insured patients.[26] A study evaluating predictors of morbidity and mortality after spine trauma found that compared with insured patients, uninsured patients had a lower number of hospital days, ICU days, and ventilator time as well as a higher rate of mortality.[27]

Many studies also highlight the complex interplay between race and ethnicity and insurance status, which produces particularly poor outcomes for already marginalized and excluded populations. A study of NTDB data found that uninsured status compounds the disparate outcomes experienced by Hispanic and Black patients with trauma; the adjusted odds of mortality for Black and Hispanic patients were 1.17 and 1.47, respectively, when compared to White patients.[22] However, when compared to insured White patients with trauma, uninsured Black and Hispanic patients had ORs of 1.78 and 2.30, respectively.[22] The disparate outcomes remain disheartening even in publicly funded hospitals that specialize in trauma care. An analysis of data from a single, publicly funded, level I trauma center in California indicated that although uninsured patients were younger and had lower ISSs than insured patients, they had a significantly higher mortality rate (adjusted OR 3.4). When the analysis was stratified by race and ethnicity, the disparity in mortality by insurance status only existed for Black and Hispanic patients.[28] No mortality difference was found between insured and uninsured patients from White or Asian backgrounds. These results further underscore how overlapping areas of vulnerability have a synergistic effect in worsening outcomes.

The impact of race and ethnicity on mortality after traumatic injury has been the subject of a systematic review and meta-analysis by Haider and colleagues.[4] Their analysis of 35 studies prior to 2012 indicated that Black patients had a significantly higher odds of death (OR 1.19) than White patients. While there was a trend toward higher odds of death in Hispanic patients with trauma compared to White patients, this result was not statistically significant.[4] A study of Black motorcyclists found they were more likely to wear a helmet (OR 1.30) than White motorcyclists, but still suffered substantially higher odds of mortality (1.58) even after controlling for age and injury-related characteristics.[29] A study of vehicle-struck pedestrians showed that Black and Hispanic pedestrians had 22% and 33% higher odds of mortality, respectively, than White pedestrians. Although uninsured status carried the highest odds of mortality (OR 1.77) in that study, Black and Hispanic communities suffer a disproportionately higher burden of pedestrian trauma and were also more likely to be uninsured.[25]

We know of no studies that describe differential access to trauma care based on gender or sex, but differences in mortality have been documented between male and female patients with trauma. Specifically, male patients with trauma have higher mortality rates than female patients with trauma.[21,30] Likely driving the lower adjusted risk of death compared to men (OR 1.79), female patients with trauma were less likely to acquire life-threatening complications, such as pneumonia, pulmonary embolism, acute respiratory distress syndrome, or acute renal failure.[30] However, when female patients with trauma did acquire a life-threatening complication, they suffered a higher risk of dying than their male counterparts.[30]

OUT-OF-HOSPITAL OUTCOMES

Patients who live to discharge after admission for a traumatic incident can still suffer from disparate outcomes, including place of discharge, postdischarge mortality, hospital readmission, and other markers of quality of life. Some aspects of these outcomes have been studied extensively, with specific attention to how outcomes are different for vulnerable communities. Insurance status is often described as affecting disparities in out-of-hospital outcomes. Overall, the uninsured patients tend to have worse outcomes after discharge in all studied domains. As noted earlier, the systematic review and meta-analysis by Haider and colleagues found higher mortality rates for uninsured patients than for insured patients.[4] Yet, another study showed that safety-net hospitals, where the proportion of uninsured patients is higher, do not have increased mortality.[31] Several studies have found that uninsured patients are less likely than insured patients to be transferred to acute rehabilitation or a skilled nursing facility or be discharged with home health after a trauma admission.[32,33] This remained true even among older adults in a study that looked specifically at patients with traumatic brain injury (TBI).[34]

The literature on out-of-hospital outcomes details numerous disparities between groups based on race and ethnicity. One study looking specifically at the difference between Black and White patients found that 5% of deaths at a national level could be attributable specifically to racial disparities.[35] Discharge location is another area in which disparities have been found by race and ethnicity, with racially minoritized patients less likely to be discharged to rehabilitation services.[36] In a national study of 58,792 patients with TBI, Black and Hispanic patients were 15% less likely to be discharged to a rehabilitation center than non-Hispanic White patients, even after the analysis controlled for injury severity and insurance status.[37] An even larger study of 299,205 patients found that Black and Hispanic patients were less likely than non-Hispanic White patients to be discharged to a higher level of rehabilitation (eg, inpatient rehabilitation vs skilled nursing facility), and this held true even when the analysis controlled for uniform insurance coverage in a Medicare group.[38] This disparity was also found in similar studies of older adults with TBI.[34] In a single-center study of patients with TBI followed for 12 months found that racially minoritized patients were more likely to have worse long-term functional outcomes and increased dependency on others for standard of living, leisure, and work/school domains compared to non-Hispanic White patients, even after the analysis controlled for age, gender, injury scores, and head-specific injury scores.[39] We found only one study, from 2007, in which discharge disposition was similar between racially minoritized and non-Hispanic White groups, but the long-term functional outcomes were still worse in racially minoritized groups at 6 and 12 months post-TBI.[40] A study that included subgroup analysis of frail older adults (age $\geq$ 65 years) found that non-Hispanic White patients were more likely than Hispanic or Black patients to be discharged to a skilled nursing facility.[41]

Follow-up is another postdischarge outcome that has been analyzed by race and ethnicity. One study found that Black patients were less likely than White patients to use rehabilitation services, including physical and occupational therapy, and had less clinic follow-up for their traumatic injuries.[6] Black patients were more likely than their White counterparts to have a trauma-injury related visit to the emergency department, but this was not statistically significant in the adjusted model.[6] Only one study examined disparities between American Indian (AI)/Alaska Native (AN) and non-Hispanic Whites, finding that most AI/AN patients were discharged home without services (80% vs 62%) and AI/AN patients were less likely to be discharged to rehabilitation or long-term or skilled nursing facilities.[42]

Some investigators have postulated that many of these disparities are in fact due to a lack of insurance, not race.[43] A study of 87,112 patients with trauma from 2006 to 2014 showed that outcomes disparities among racial and ethnic minorities seem to be mitigated by universal health insurance.[44] Although there was no difference in mortality and readmission at 30 and 90 days, 60% of the study cohort were active duty National Guard and Reserve service members and their dependents; the rest were retirees and dependents who still paid a fee for coverage,[44] limiting generalizability to the rest of the country. While insurance may be one piece contributing to disparities, implicit bias may also be playing a part. In fact, one study of 248 members of a large trauma association found that 74% of participants did have unconscious preference toward White persons in a study using vignettes and responses, despite 79% explicitly stating they had no race preferences.[45]

There are studies of gender-based and sex-based disparities in out-of-hospital outcomes. A study of survivors of TBI who were aged 65 years or older found that, after controlling for age, mechanism of injury, ISS, and length of stay, female patients were 1.3 times more likely to be discharged to a long-term care facility than to home compared with male patients.[46] A more recent study had similar findings, with female patients more likely to be discharged to a skilled nursing facility than their male counterparts.[47] The authors posit that this may be because women, as primary caretakers of the home, are less likely to have the social support to be able to return home. Female patients also have worse outcomes after hospitalization for traumatic injury 6 to 12 months afterward, including having more functional limitations, continuance of pain medication, and a higher rate of posttraumatic stress disorder.[48]

OTHER CONSIDERATIONS

This review would not be complete without a section focused on other groups of patients with trauma that are less likely to be studied due to lack of data or inclusion in national databases and trauma registries. These groups include patients with non-English preferred language, patients with unknown immigration status, patients in rural areas, and patients where even less data are available, such as patients with disabilities or nonbinary or transgender identity (**Box 1**). Few studies feature these specific groups, and they are unrepresented or underrepresented in large databases, which means the literature consists primarily of single-center reports in which investigators pull variables directly from the electronic health record. In fact, a review of 82 studies on motor vehicle collisions found that 28% outright excluded non-English preferred patients and none included preferred language as a variable of analysis.[49] The single-center studies that did examine outcomes for non-English preferred patients varied in group and outcome studied. A study of pain assessment for non-English preferred patients found that they were less likely than English-preferred patients to have their pain assessed, and when assessed, they had lower pain scores.[50] A study of mortality found that non-English preferred patients had higher mortality than English-preferred patients (7% vs 4%), and that in adjusted models, speaking languages other than Spanish and Chinese (Mandarin and Cantonese) was associated with significantly increased mortality compared to English-preferred patients.[51] As for disparities in discharge disposition, one study found that undocumented immigrants were more likely to be discharged home than to be sent to acute rehabilitation.[5] Finally, a study of Latino patients found no difference in documented versus undocumented status with respect to in-hospital outcomes, but it did not assess disposition location.[52]

Living in more rural areas is another source of disparity since location of injury and triage to the correct center is vital. According to a study using the NTDB,[53] level I trauma centers have better outcomes than lower level centers for patients with specific injuries associated with high mortality and poor functional outcomes, and this finding was not affected by volume of major trauma admissions at either type of center.[10] Further, undertriage, or initial transport to a nontrauma center is associated with increased mortality, though neither of these studies examined patient demographics.[10,16] In fact, 16% of the US population lives more than an hour away from a level I or II trauma center,[11] limiting timely access to the trauma system, and leading to the finding that rural patients with trauma have an increased likelihood of undertriage and a decreased likelihood of transportation to a level I or II trauma center as their first stop along their care.[54] Studies looking at older adults who live in rural areas have also found that older adults are undertriaged and suffer worse outcomes.[55]

Box 1
Unstudied and understudied patient demographics

The following groups of patients with trauma are less likely to be studied due to lack of data or lack of inclusion in national databases and trauma registries.
- *Non-English preferred patients*: Less likely to have their pain assessed, lower pain scores, and higher mortality.
- *Patients of unknown immigration status*: Undocumented patients less likely to discharge to rehab.
- *Rural patients*: More likely to be undertriaged or have primary transport to a nontrauma center hospital.
- *Patients with disability*: Insufficient data available.
- Transgender and nonbinary patients: Insufficient data available.
- *AI, AN, Native Hawaiian, and Other Pacific Islanders*: Insufficient data available. Existing data combine these groups with other minorities, impeding the ability to study disparities specific to these identities.

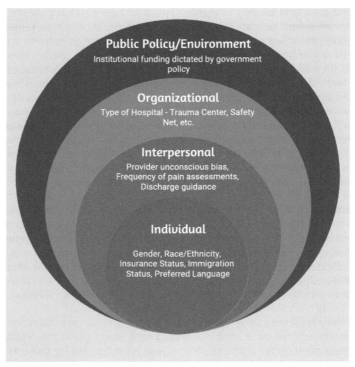

Fig. 2. Factors contributing to care disparities within the social ecological model framework.

Studies have also tried to link geography based on social vulnerability to outcomes. A recent study linking a social vulnerability index to identify vulnerable communities found that a higher index led to a higher likelihood of presenting with penetrating injuries, shock, and higher injury scores, but that risk-adjustment for these clinical characteristics resulted in similar mortality rates.[56]

Finally, there are specific groups of patients who are rarely, if ever, reported on. Particularly understudied groups are AI/AN and Native Hawaiian and Pacific Islander populations. While many of the studies we describe may include these patients, given the larger number of White, Black, and Hispanic patients, the remaining groups are lumped together as "Other," which may negate any effect that might be seen in each group individually.

SUMMARY

Our review highlights numerous disparities along the continuum of trauma care. It should be evident that disparities related to insurance status and race and ethnicity have been investigated the most, whereas other groups—including AI/NA and other smaller racial and ethnic groups, non-English preferred patients, patients with unknown immigration status, patients with disabilities, and patients with nonbinary or transgender identity—are understudied and underrepresented or unrepresented completely in large national trauma databases. There are likely many more disparities that we are simply unable to measure given this lack of data. There is a clear need to improve data collection both locally and nationally. Without clear data on a wide range of social issues, there will be scant ability to measure and improve on outcomes for these vulnerable populations. This will need to be done remembering to build trust with and partner with vulnerable communities who may be directly affected by an increase in data collection.

It is important to remember that race and ethnicity is a social construct, and therefore, any study aiming to find genetic variations or genetic causes based on race and ethnicity for these disparities is unwarranted. However, there are clear associations between race and ethnicity and outcomes across many studies. Finding the root causes of these disparities will be crucial to improving trauma care. Another way to improve care and build trust in the system will be to advocate for and provide trauma-informed care, which accounts for both the mental and physical aspects of trauma, to each patient.[57] As the American College of Surgeons states, "Engaging at-risk communities can help address structural racism and social determinants of health and create a solutions-based narrative."[57]

While several studies look at the effects of both race and ethnicity and insurance status on care and outcomes in critically ill adult patients with trauma, to our knowledge, no studies specifically examine the ways that discriminatory upstream policies and structures permeate our trauma system and dictate the disparities that researchers subsequently describe across a spectrum of dimensions (**Fig. 2**). To this end, improving trauma care including access, in-hospital care, and survival among vulnerable communities will require interventions and policies that target not only in-hospital quality improvement projects and postdischarge follow-up but also social and structural inequities upstream of trauma center admission.

ACKNOWLEDGMENTS

The authors would like to thank Julia Axelrod for support with the figures.

DISCLOSURE

Dr T. Bongiovanni was funded by the National Institute of Aging of the National Institutes of Health under Award Number K23AG073523 and the Robert Wood Johnson Foundation, United States under the Award P0553126. The content is solely the responsibility of the authors and does not necessarily represent the official views of the National Institutes of Health or the Robert Wood Johnson Foundation. The authors have no conflicts of interest.

REFERENCES

1. National Academies of Sciences E, Division H and M, Practice B on PH and PH. The state of health disparities in the United States. In: Communities in action: pathways to health equity. National Academies Press (US); 2017. Available at: https://www.ncbi.nlm.nih.gov/books/NBK425844/. [Accessed 5 November 2023].

2. Emergency medical treatment & labor Act (EMTALA) | CMS. Available at: https://www.cms.gov/medicare/regulations-guidance/legislation/emergency-medical-treatment-labor-act. [Accessed 29 October 2023].

3. Carr BG, Bowman AJ, Wolff CS, et al. Disparities in access to trauma care in the United States: a population-based analysis. Injury 2017;48(2):332–8.

4. Haider AH, Weygandt PL, Bentley JM, et al. Disparities in trauma care and outcomes in the United States: a systematic review and meta-analysis. J Trauma Acute Care Surg 2013;74(5):1195–205.

5. Ram P, Miah FT, Wyrick JM, et al. Outcomes in critically ill patients with traumatic brain injury: ethnicity, documentation, and insurance status. Crit Care Med 2020; 48(1):31.

6. Chun Fat S, Herrera-Escobar JP, Seshadri AJ, et al. Racial disparities in post-discharge healthcare utilization after trauma. Am J Surg 2019;218(5):842–6.

7. MacKenzie EJ, Rivara FP, Jurkovich GJ, et al. A national evaluation of the effect of trauma-center care on mortality. N Engl J Med 2006;354(4):366–78.

8. Alber DA, Dalton MK, Uribe-Leitz T, et al. A multistate study of race and ethnic disparities in access to trauma care. J Surg Res 2021;257:486–92.

9. Champion HR, Sacco WJ, Copes WS. Improvement in outcome from trauma center care. Arch Surg Chic Ill 1960 1992;127(3):333–8, discussion 338.

10. Demetriades D, Martin M, Salim A, et al. The effect of trauma center designation and trauma volume on outcome in specific severe injuries. Ann Surg 2005; 242(4):512.

11. Choi J, Carlos G, Nassar AK, et al. The impact of trauma systems on patient outcomes. Curr Probl Surg 2021;58(1):100849.

12. Choi J, Karr S, Jain A, et al. Access to American College of surgeons committee on trauma–verified trauma centers in the US, 2013-2019. JAMA 2022;328(4): 391–3.

13. Population clock. Available at: https://www.census.gov/popclock/. [Accessed 5 November 2023].

14. Crandall M, Sharp D, Unger E, et al. Trauma deserts: distance from a trauma center, transport times, and mortality from gunshot wounds in chicago. Am J Publ Health 2013;103(6):1103–9.

15. Tung EL, Hampton DA, Kolak M, et al. Race/ethnicity and geographic access to urban trauma care. JAMA Netw Open 2019;2(3):e190138.

16. Haas B, Gomez D, Zagorski B, et al. Survival of the fittest: the hidden cost of undertriage of major trauma. J Am Coll Surg 2010;211(6):804–11.

17. Branas CC, MacKenzie EJ, Williams JC, et al. Access to trauma centers in the United States. JAMA 2005;293(21):2626–33.

18. Shen YC, Hsia RY, Kuzma K. Understanding the risk factors of trauma center closures. Med Care 2009;47(9):968–78.

19. Hsia RY, Shen YC. Changes in geographical access to trauma centers for vulnerable populations in the United States. Health Aff Proj Hope 2011;30(10):1912–20.

20. Hemmila MR, Cain-Nielsen AH, Jakubus JL, et al. Association of hospital participation in a regional trauma quality improvement collaborative with patient outcomes. JAMA Surg 2018;153(8):747–56.

21. Downing SR, Oyetunji TA, Greene WR, et al. The Impact of insurance status on actuarial survival in hospitalized trauma patients: when do they die? J Trauma Acute Care Surg 2011;70(1):130.

22. Haider AH, Chang DC, Efron DT, et al. Race and insurance status as risk factors for trauma mortality. Arch Surg Chic Ill 1960 2008;143(10):945–9.

23. Greene WR, Oyetunji TA, Bowers U, et al. Insurance status is a potent predictor of outcomes in both blunt and penetrating trauma. Am J Surg 2010;199(4):554–7.

24. Alaniz L, Billimek J, Figueroa C, et al. Increased mortality in underinsured penetrating trauma patients. Am Surg 2021;87(10):1594–9.

25. Maybury RS, Bolorunduro OB, Villegas C, et al. Pedestrians struck by motor vehicles further worsen race- and insurance-based disparities in trauma outcomes: the case for inner-city pedestrian injury prevention programs. Surgery 2010; 148(2):202–8.

26. Haas JS, Goldman L. Acutely injured patients with trauma in Massachusetts: differences in care and mortality, by insurance status. Am J Publ Health 1994; 84(10):1605–8.
27. Schoenfeld AJ, Belmont PJ, See AA, et al. Patient demographics, insurance status, race, and ethnicity as predictors of morbidity and mortality after spine trauma: a study using the National Trauma Data Bank. Spine J 2013;13(12): 1766–73.e1.
28. Salim A, Ottochian M, DuBose J, et al. Does insurance status matter at a public, level I trauma center? J Trauma 2010;68(1):211–6.
29. Crompton JG, Pollack KM, Oyetunji T, et al. Racial disparities in motorcycle-related mortality: an analysis of the national trauma data bank. Am J Surg 2010;200(2):191–6.
30. Haider AH, Crompton JG, Oyetunji T, et al. Females have fewer complications and lower mortality following trauma than similarly injured males: a risk adjusted analysis of adults in the National Trauma Data Bank. Surgery 2009;146(2): 308–15.
31. Vettukattil AS, Haider AH, Haut ER, et al. Do trauma safety-net hospitals deliver truly safe trauma care? A multilevel analysis of the national trauma data bank. J Trauma 2011;70(4):978–84.
32. Nirula R, Nirula G, Gentilello LM. Inequity of rehabilitation services after traumatic injury. J Trauma 2009;66(1):255–9.
33. Sacks GD, Hill C, Rogers SO. Insurance status and hospital discharge disposition after trauma: inequities in access to postacute care. J Trauma 2011;71(4): 1011–5.
34. Hosseinpour H, El-Qawaqzeh K, Magnotti LJ, et al. The unexpected paradox of geriatric traumatic brain injury outcomes: uncovering racial and ethnic disparities. Am J Surg 2023. https://doi.org/10.1016/j.amjsurg.2023.05.017.
35. Scott VK, Hashmi ZG, Schneider EB, et al. Counting the lives lost: how many black trauma deaths are attributable to disparities? J Surg Res 2013;184(1): 480–7.
36. Englum BR, Villegas C, Bolorunduro O, et al. Racial, ethnic, and insurance status disparities in use of posthospitalization care after trauma. J Am Coll Surg 2011; 213(6):699–708.
37. Shafi S, de la Plata CM, Diaz-Arrastia R, et al. Ethnic disparities exist in trauma care. J Trauma 2007;63(5):1138–42.
38. Racial and ethnic disparities in discharge to rehabilitation following traumatic brain injury in. J Neurosurg 2015;122(3). Journals. Available at: https://thejns.org/view/journals/j-neurosurg/122/3/article-p595.xml. [Accessed 30 October 2023].
39. Staudenmayer KL, Diaz-Arrastia R, de Oliveira A, et al. Ethnic disparities in long-term functional outcomes after traumatic brain injury. J Trauma 2007;63(6): 1364–9.
40. Shafi S, Marquez de la Plata C, Diaz-Arrastia R, et al. Racial disparities in long-term functional outcome after traumatic brain injury. J Trauma 2007;63(6): 1263–8 ; discussion 1268-1270.
41. Anand T, Khurrum M, Chehab M, et al. Racial and ethnic disparities in frail geriatric trauma patients. World J Surg 2021;45(5):1330–9.
42. Fuentes MM, Moore M, Qiu Q, et al. Differences in injury characteristics and outcomes for american indian/Alaska native people hospitalized with traumatic injuries: an analysis of the national trauma data bank. J Racial Ethn Health Disparities 2019;6(2):335–44.

43. Grenn E, Kutcher M, Hillegass WB, et al. Social determinants of trauma care: associations of race, insurance status, and place on opioid prescriptions, postdischarge referrals, and mortality. J Trauma Acute Care Surg 2022;92(5):897.

44. Chaudhary MA, Sharma M, Scully RE, et al. Universal insurance and an equal access healthcare system eliminate disparities for Black patients after traumatic injury. Surgery 2018;163(4):651–6.

45. Haider AH, Schneider EB, Sriram N, et al. Unconscious race and class bias: its association with decision making by trauma and acute care surgeons. J Trauma Acute Care Surg 2014;77(3):409.

46. Strosberg DS, Housley BC, Vazquez D, et al. Discharge destination and readmission rates in older trauma patients. J Surg Res 2017;207:27–32.

47. Ingram MCE, Nagalla M, Shan Y, et al. Sex-based disparities in timeliness of trauma care and discharge disposition. JAMA Surg 2022;157(7):609–16.

48. Herrera-Escobar JP, El Moheb M, Ranjit A, et al. Sex differences in long-term outcomes after traumatic injury: a mediation analysis. Am J Surg 2021;222(4):842–8.

49. Smith M, Tibbetts C, Agrawal P, et al. Representation of patients with non-English language preferences in motor vehicle collision trauma and emergency medicine research. Inj Prev 2023;29(3):253–8.

50. Schwartz H, Menza R, Lindquist K, et al. Limited English proficiency associated with suboptimal pain assessment in hospitalized trauma patients. J Surg Res 2022;278:169–78.

51. Castro MRH, Schwartz H, Hernandez S, et al. The association of limited English proficiency with morbidity and mortality after trauma. J Surg Res 2022;280: 326–32.

52. Chong VE, Lee WS, Victorino GP. Potential disparities in trauma: the undocumented Latino immigrant. J Surg Res 2014;191(2):251–5.

53. National Trauma Data Bank. ACS. Available at: https://www.facs.org/quality-programs/trauma/quality/national-trauma-data-bank/. [Accessed 2 November 2023].

54. Newgard CD, Fu R, Bulger E, et al. Evaluation of rural vs urban trauma patients served by 9-1-1 emergency medical services. JAMA Surg 2017;152(1):11–8.

55. Staudenmayer K, Lin F, Mackersie R, et al. Variability in California triage from 2005 to 2009: a population-based longitudinal study of severely injured patients. J Trauma Acute Care Surg 2014;76(4):1041–7.

56. Neiman PU, Flaherty MM, Salim A, et al. Evaluating the complex association between Social Vulnerability Index and trauma mortality. J Trauma Acute Care Surg 2022;92(5):821.

57. Trauma informed care can help break the cycle of violence. ACS. Available at: https://www.facs.org/for-medical-professionals/news-publications/news-and-articles/press-releases/2021/isave-073021/. [Accessed 8 November 2023].

Race and Ethnicity Disparities in Management and Outcomes of Critically Ill Adults with Acute Respiratory Failure

Christopher F. Chesley, MD, MSCE[a,b,c,d,*]

KEYWORDS

- Acute respiratory failure • Racial disparities • Ethnic disparities
- Minority serving hospitals

KEY POINTS

- Racial and ethnic minority patients experience higher burden of disease, death, and hospital length of stay from acute respiratory failure.
- Investigations into acute respiratory failure disparities are limited by missingness, data aggregation, and racially biased disease severity scores.
- Conventionally understood mechanisms for racial and ethnic disparities in acute respiratory failure center on presenting disease severity, socioeconomic status, and hospital-level variation in care quality.
- Acute respiratory failure research must move toward identifying actionable mechanisms and work with minority serving hospitals to develop mitigating solutions.

INTRODUCTION

Acute respiratory failure (ARF) describes a life-threatening and abrupt onset of impaired gas exchange of oxygen and/or carbon dioxide.[1] Though ARF's national impact is tremendous, its population-level impact is disproportionate. A common theme in the epidemiology of ARF is that populations who are socially and historically marginalized are also most burdened by ARF-related disease. The objective of this

[a] Division of Pulmonary, Allergy, and Critical Care, University of Pennsylvania Perelman School of Medicine; [b] Palliative and Advanced Illness Research (PAIR) Center, University of Pennsylvania Perelman School of Medicine; [c] Leonard Davis Institute of Health Economics, University of Pennsylvania; [d] Department of Medicine, Hospital of the University of Pennsylvania, 3400 Spruce Street, 839 West Gates Building, Philadelphia, PA 19104, USA
* Corresponding author.
E-mail address: Christopher.Chesley@pennmedicine.upenn.edu

Crit Care Clin 40 (2024) 671–683
https://doi.org/10.1016/j.ccc.2024.05.004   criticalcare.theclinics.com
0749-0704/24/© 2024 Elsevier Inc. All rights reserved, including those for text and data mining, AI training, and similar technologies.

review is to provide an overview of the disproportionate health impacts of ARF on racial and ethnic minority groups, discuss prevailing mechanisms for these disparities, and identify important future directions that will facilitate ARF disparities mitigation. Because the extent of health and health care disparities reflect unique sociohistorical patterns of racialization and discrimination, this review will focus on racial and ethnic disparities as they exist within the United States. While certain general concepts discussed in this review may apply to non-US settings, the pathways through which American systemic racism has culminated in ARF health disparities are expected to be specific to American populations. Indeed, future research that better delineates how these mechanisms apply to racial and ethnic disparities in ARF among non-US populations is needed.

KNOWN SCOPE OF ACUTE RESPIRATORY FAILURE DISPARITIES
Incidence

ARF is the most commonly managed condition in intensive care units (ICUs). In the United States, 1274.4 adults per 100,000 experience ARF every year, with an incidence that has increased over time.[2,3] In general, approximately 40% of those who experience ARF will require mechanical ventilation, accounting for an incidence of 455 per 100,000 adults.[3] Mechanically ventilated patients with ARF accumulate tremendous costs for hospitals, accounting for US$27 billion annually, or 12% of all hospital costs.[4]

While these estimates of overall ARF disease burden are determined from large national administrative datasets, using these data sources to determine racial and ethnic group-specific estimates of ARF disease burden is made challenging by missing data, sampling bias, data representativeness, and data aggregation. To overcome these challenges, one study used imputation to determine race-specific population differences in ARF incidence as well as assess temporal trends.[5] They found that overall ARF incidence for Black patients was nearly double that of White patients (123.6 vs 65.0 per 100,000 adults). Unfortunately, estimates about other racial groups were more complicated. Because this study used the National Hospital Discharge Survey (NHDS) database, standard errors for Asian American, Pacific Islander, American Indian, Alaskan Native, and other racial groups were unfortunately aggregated. As a result, disaggregated analyses for these groups could not be determined, though among the "other" group consisting of patients with these identities, estimated ARF incidence was 108.8 per 100,000 adults. These race-specific estimates differ by several orders of magnitude compared to the previously referenced study[3]; this is most likely due to a more limited case definition of patients requiring mechanical ventilation and the exclusion of several diagnosis codes for patients that experienced trauma, surgery, and chronic respiratory failure. Additionally, data from the present study were also limited by changes in the 2000 US Census, in which self-identification as more than one race was finally possible.[6] This made determining ARF trends in the "other" group particularly unstable; however, all groups tended to demonstrate an overall increasing incidence in ARF over the study period. Unfortunately, data concerning Hispanic ethnicity was not measured by NHDS, and convincing data concerning ethnicity differences in ARF incidence are not available.

Mortality

Evidence suggests that minority patients, particularly Black patients, are at higher independent risk of mortality from ARF compared to nonminority patients. Using the National Inpatient Sample, a database containing discharge information for approximately 20% of all nonfederal inpatient hospitals, researchers found that Black, Hispanic, Asian American, and Pacific Islander patients each had an increased risk of in-hospital mortality relative to White patients (13%, 17%, and 15% increased odds, respectively). These findings were independent of adjustment for patient age, gender, year of admission, comorbidity measures, median income approximated by ZIP code, diagnosis-related group subclass, and select hospital characteristics.[7] Further evidence from acute respiratory distress syndrome (ARDS) supports the signal for increased mortality among minority patients. One study paired death certificate information with diagnosis coding for ARDS to measure independent associations between death and patient race after adjusting for age, gender, rural designation, and Census geographic division. Black patients were found to have 30% increased odds of mortality relative to Asian American or Pacific Islander patients (who were selected as the comparison group due to having the lowest population odds of mortality in this study). White patients were found to have 6% increased odds of mortality relative to Asian American and Pacific Islander patients, but this difference was not statistically significant. In this study, these relationships were most pronounced for patients aged under 65 years. This study also suggested that ARDS mortality did not differ between Hispanic and non-Hispanic patients. Lastly, for all groups, ARDS-related mortality decreased during the study period, with no observed race-specific differences in the rate of decrease.[8]

Hospital Length of Stay

Investigations designed to determine race and ethnicity-specific disparities in hospital length of stay (LOS) have been relatively limited. One retrospective matching study found that among a cohort of severely ill patients with ARF, LOS was on average 1 day longer among Black patients but shorter among Asian American, Pacific Islander, and Hispanic patients compared to White patients. These findings were independent of other study variables, notably including do-not-resuscitate status, which may vary among racial groups.[9] Few other studies have measured LOS disparities related to ARF, though some evidence for prolonged LOS among minority racial and ethnic groups exists for patients who were acutely hospitalized with coronavirus disease 2019 (COVID-19), a sizable proportion of which required respiratory support.[10–12]

Hospital Readmission

At present, no study has specifically investigated readmission disparities among a large, nationally representative cohort of ARF survivors. However, supportive evidence for a signal of increased risk of hospital readmission comes from analyses among related disease syndromes. Among Medicare patients who survived hospital admission for pneumonia in 2006 to 2008, a retrospective cohort study found that Black patients were at 15% to 25% increased risk of hospital readmission compared to non-Black patients. Unfortunately, all non-Black racial groups were aggregated in this study, precluding more granular analysis of other racial groups; additionally, ethnicity was also not studied.[13,14] Similarly, a retrospective cross-sectional analysis of 12 states in 2008 found that Black patients with chronic obstructive pulmonary disease had highest all-cause hospital readmission (23.1%) compared to White (20.5%), Hispanic (20.4%), and Asian American and Pacific Islander (19.1%) patients, though independent risk ratios and population-adjusted rates were not examined.[15]

Other Domains

Disparities related to many other post-ARF survivorship outcomes are currently unstudied. Among them, the disparities in the occurrence of physical and cognitive disability after ARF has yet to be studied in depth. Physical and cognitive disability is increasingly recognized to be common after acute critical illness, complicating the recovery of many critical illness survivors, and is common among survivors of mechanical ventilation. Given the established disproportionate impact of ARF on minority racial and ethnic groups, fundamental research gaps exist in (1) characterizing the impact of population-level racial and ethnic disparities of post-ARF physical and cognitive disability, (2) evaluating the equity of postacute care delivery for rehabilitation, and (3) assessing the equitability of functional outcomes following postacute care rehabilitation for post-ARF disability.

Another important but unstudied qualitative outcome in the context of ARF care concerns patient experiences of racism and other forms of discrimination. In the context of critical or acute respiratory care, no study has determined the incidence of patient-perceived discriminatory experiences resulting from clinical care providers, hospital care workflows, or health system experiences more generally. Some evidence exists that while overt experiences of discrimination may be in decline, as many as 1 in 5 Black patients with chronic illnesses continue to report receiving inferior treatment because of their race.[16] Notably, this survey was performed in a study population that was not acutely ill, and performing similar investigations during the course of ARF care represents a major research priority. During ARF, complex decisions are made in the context of patient and family members' care preferences, treatment goals, and directives. Patient perceived discrimination stands to threaten patient autonomy and respect during medical care and might be particularly noticeable during ARF care delivery and impact patient-centered outcomes. Thus, developing strategies that ensure antiracist patient care for ARF illness is a pressing knowledge gap.

PREVAILING MECHANISMS OF ACUTE RESPIRATORY FAILURE DISPARITIES

Evidence for currently postulated mechanisms of racial and ethnic disparities in ARF outcomes relies on retrospective data from large administrative datasets as well as secondary analyses of prospective registries originally designed to investigate nonequity research questions. In most of these studies, multivariable regression models have been used to determine how measures of association between clinical outcomes and racial and/or ethnic group identities are affected by confounding variables. When confounding variables have been found that sufficiently temper these relationships, researchers have erroneously implied that these confounding variables actually serve as mechanistic determinants of these relationships. The result has left the field with the assumption that 3 main "mechanisms" of ARF disparities exist: presenting disease severity, interhospital variation in care delivery, and socioeconomic determinants.

Presenting Disease Severity

Leveraging data from the ARDS Network randomized controlled trials platform, researchers investigated associations between patient race, ethnicity, and 60 day mortality following ARDS. Among this study population, both Black and Hispanic patients had elevated age-adjusted 60 day mortality compared to White patients (59% and 85% increased odds, respectively). Researchers found that these differences persisted after adjustment for processes of care (including the receipt of lung protective ventilation), degree of lung injury by $Pao_2:Fio_2$ ratio, and presence of select comorbid conditions. However, when adjusting for acute disease severity (operationalized in this study by the acute physiology score [APS]), the association between Black patient identity and mortality was no longer significant, while this association remained significant among Hispanic patients. Researchers concluded that acute disease severity on presentation accounted for mortality differences among Black but not Hispanic patients.[17] This study group also used retrospective data across 35 hospitals in California to determine measures of association between patient race and mortality among a cohort of patients receiving critical care, though the study did not quantify the proportion meeting criteria for ARF. They similarly found that by adjusting for the APS, acute physiology and chronic health evaluation (APACHE) score, admission type, and do-not-resuscitate status, no differences in hospital mortality were found among Black, Hispanic, Asian and Pacific Islander, and White patients. Because Black patients presented with increased physiologic derangement as measured by the APS, researchers again concluded that acute disease severity was a mechanism for mortality-related disparities.[18] Similar conclusions were reached in a different study of ICU admissions[19] and pneumonia hospitalizations.[20] However, the latter study is notable for finding that Black patients had *lower* pneumonia severity index and APACHE score than White patients in their secondary analysis of Genetic and Inflammatory Markers of Sepsis (GenIMS) a prospective inception cohort study examining inflammatory markers in sepsis.

Hospital Care Quality

Between-hospital variation has been implicated as an important mechanism of racial and ethnic disparities related to ARF. In the previously mentioned secondary analysis of GenIMS, researchers also assessed the relative importance of within-hospital and between-hospital variation on provision of guideline-concordant care. In crude analyses, Black patients were less likely than White patients to receive antibiotic care within 4 hours (62% vs 75%). Using both generalized estimating equations and random effects regression models, researchers determined that within-hospital clustering of variation resulted in no significant association between race and guideline concordant care, whereas between-hospital clustering maintained significant differences (16% decreased odds among Black compared to White patients). Notably, within-hospital effects appeared to account for decreased crude likelihood of receiving guideline-adherent antibiotics and increased likelihood of mechanical ventilation observed among Black patients. Researchers concluded that hospital-level variation in adherence to guideline-concordant care accounted for racial disparities in care quality such that within hospitals themselves, care quality tended to be equivalent.[20] Together, these data signal that important determinants of racial ARF disparities relate to factors that impact care delivery and that vary among hospitals; many of these factors may themselves be manifestations of structural inequalities that disproportionately impact certain predominantly minority-serving hospitals than others.

Socioeconomic Status

While no study has specifically characterized the impact of socioeconomic status on clinical outcomes resulting from ARF, a previously mentioned study sought to examine the question in a cohort of critically ill patients.[18] In the cohort of patients who were managed at California hospitals with critical illness, researchers operationalized socioeconomic status using an index validated by the Agency for Health Research and Quality developed from ZIP code and Census block-level measures that included employment, household income, education, and the federal poverty line. This index was also added as an adjustment variable in regression models and as stated previously, researchers found no differences in mortality after full covariate adjustment.[18]

However, which components of the index are relevant to clinical outcomes generally, and to ARF outcomes specifically, were not explored.

LIMITATIONS OF PREVAILING MECHANISMS
Generalizability

At least 3 features threaten the generalizability of the currently available evidence of mechanisms for ARF disparities. First, the studies that established these mechanisms were published between over one to nearly 3 decades ago. In the time since the oldest study, dramatic changes in standards of care for the management of patients with ARF have occurred, including the proven efficacy of lung protective ventilation, changing guidelines governing definitions and management of sepsis (a leading cause of ARF), and numerous public health catastrophes, including the opioid epidemic and ongoing COVID-19 pandemic. The modern landscape of critical care medicine has highlighted the importance of adherence to guideline-established standards of care to save lives and improve outcomes. Simultaneously assessing the equity of care delivery in the context of this dynamic field has been a major challenge to the field to date. While several recent studies have sought to characterize health equity in the context of the COVID-19 pandemic, identifying mechanisms that are proven to be generalizable to care delivery in other contexts of ARF are lacking.

Second, the study populations included in these studies may not be generalizable to many care delivery settings in the United States. As stated previously, several studies were conducted as secondary analyses of prospective studies originally designed for study questions that did not originally focus on health equity.[17,20] While performing well-designed supplementary studies among enriched prospective datasets represents important research efficiency, the validity of conclusions from these studies may be limited due to differences in trial datasets and populations compared to real-life care delivery settings. For example, secondary analyses of the ARDS Net trial indicated that increased disease severity was more common among Black and Hispanic patients as measured by the APS; subsequently, researchers used statistical analyses to demonstrate how this diminished associations among patient race, ethnicity, and mortality.[17] In contrast, secondary analysis of the GenIMS trial found that Black patients had lower acute illness compared to White patients based on pneumonia severity index and APACHE scores.[20] Together, these 2 studies observed acute disease burdens in opposite directions between Black and White patients, yet both concluded that the same mechanism accounted for ARF-related disparities. This difference in covariate balance between studies, likely represents the different enrolled populations between the 2 parent trials. Nevertheless, it also underscores the challenge of generalizing study conclusions to broader populations and highlights that a deep understanding of relationships among presenting disease severity, ARF disease burden, and racial and ethnic disparities have yet to be elucidated.

Third, structural racism in the United States likely threatens the generalizability of these mechanistic studies. Clinical trials randomize care delivery interventions with the intention of achieving balance in population characteristics between study arms. In clinical trials that successfully achieve between-arm balance with respect to patient race and ethnicity, population-level differences in care delivery prescribed by trial protocols (regardless of allocation to study interventions) may limit race-specific and ethnicity-specific variation that leads to disparate care outcomes. In other words, care delivery defined by protocol adherence that minimizes between-hospital variation in care processes and physician variation in delivery of emerging and novel therapies may mask the determinants of implicit and explicit racism that fail to accurately approximate actual care delivery outside of clinical trial settings. These complications are sure to threaten the validity of any study that is not specifically designed to measure health equity. Additionally, inpatient health care delivery is tremendously segregated in the United States. Among all Medicare patients acutely hospitalized, only 5% of nonfederal hospitals manage over 50% of Black patients, and 25% of hospitals care for nearly 90% of elderly Black patients.[21] Hospitals that predominantly manage minority patients are often called minority serving hospitals (MSHs), and how well these hospitals have been represented in the discussed mechanistic studies is unclear. Ensuring appropriate representation from MSHs is critical because of evidence suggesting that race-specific disparities in pneumonia care quality[20,21] and non-ARF clinical outcomes[13,22–25] persist when MSH status is taken into account—though importantly, not across all metrics.[26]

Racial Bias in Disease Severity Scores

Recent investigations into the equitability of crisis standards of care (CSCs) and other resource allocation frameworks have demonstrated severe limitations resulting from racially biased misclassification. One retrospective study demonstrated that CSCs based on the sequential organ failure assessment (SOFA) score consistently underestimated in-patient mortality for White patients and overestimated mortality for Black patients, which culminated in excluding over 80% of Black patients from favorable CSC categories. Additionally, different severity scores varied in their predictive performance, with the Sequential Organ Failure Assessment score performing most poorly despite being the most commonly used.[27] The inequitable performance of SOFA has been observed in several retrospective studies[28,29] and may be related to an increased mortality risk assigned to serum creatinine.

Risk stratification is key in ARF epidemiologic research given high risks of death and morbidity associated with multiple presenting characteristics. Unfortunately, this represents an additional challenge for health equity research in critical care that attempts to account for confounding using these scores. It is rare for any study to measure whether any risk score equitably predicts mortality across different racial and ethnic groups comprising its study population; therefore, given the established and inequitable misclassification bias that exists among commonly used severity scores, the potential for analytical bias introduced by explanatory models using these scores as covariates is potentially tremendous. Together, the potential for bias related to inequitable disease severity scores, along with poor external validity of existing literature, demonstrate that many evidence gaps remain concerning the identification of likely mechanisms of ARF disparities.

Poorly Targetable Mechanisms

Though the proposed mechanisms are clearly associated with some disparities related to ARF, they do not yet represent actionable targets for disparities-mitigating interventions. Patient disease severity on admission and patient socioeconomic status are difficult, if not improbable, targets to modify at the time of hospital admission. Additionally, while clinician adherence to standards of care may be modifiable, current understanding of the specific care processes that directly impact ARF disparities are currently unknown, leaving health systems without evidenced-based targets to safeguard health equity. Additionally, even though hospital characteristics such as teaching, safety net, public ownership, rural designation, and size are all associated with outcomes,[20,30–35] these represent immutable characteristics of care delivery centers. In short, while our current evidence base has identified potential sources of variability related to disparities, our field has yet to identify discreet, directly actionable mechanisms that have relevance to bedside providers, health system administrators, or policy makers. This is likely a major reason for the current lack of evidence-based interventions that mitigate racial and ethnic ARF disparities.

FUTURE DIRECTIONS

Developing solutions that mitigate racial and ethnic ARF disparities is possible. To better position our field toward finding these solutions, future research priorities must identify targetable mechanisms of racial and ethnic ARF disparities; develop a more granular understanding of the impacts of socioeconomic disadvantage (SED) on inequitable ARF outcomes; and establish MSHs as an important setting to effect equitable ARF care delivery.

Targetable Mechanism-Oriented Equity Research

A primary goal of characterizing mechanisms of ARF disparities is to identify modifiable aspects of health care delivery that have the potential to eliminate disparities. Under this framework, our field must seek to move beyond identifying measures of association between patient racial identity, clinical outcomes, and convenience variables that are already captured in established quantitative datasets. Before performing these analyses, the ideal equity-focused research objectives will be able to articulate how quantifying any association might inform hypothetical future interventions, policies, and other actionable initiatives that can be based on the study's findings. If actionable solutions are not likely to culminate from research interventions, future investigators might consider revising study questions. To assist with study question design, conceptual models based on causal inference (eg, directed acyclic graphs and other tools) can be crucial for developing testable hypotheses related to health inequity.

Additionally, investigators must consider whether a study's data structures are designed to fill knowledge gaps, or continue to perpetuate them. A major limitation of the existing evidence base concerns unstudied racial and ethnic populations resulting from missing and inappropriately aggregated data, a common limitation of administrative datasets. Often, these limitations result in the collapsing of distinct racial and ethnic groups into single categories, perpetuating disparities in knowledge through further data aggregation. Such categorization fails to account for population-level differences in disease incidence, care delivery, experiences of discrimination, and patterns of resilience; effectively, this erases the unique health care experiences of aggregated groups and prevents investigators, clinicians, and policy makers from developing solutions. If our field is unable to accurately identify the populations who are experiencing disparities, it will continue to fall short of developing solutions that safeguard their equity. Equitable data collection, quality control, and study design continue to represent the greatest threats of bias for all health equity investigations into critical care and must be overcome for disparity-mitigating interventions to become a reality.

Granular Characterization of Socioeconomic Disadvantage

Current understanding of socioeconomic impacts on critical care outcomes depends on relationships with neighborhood-level socioeconomic deprivation indices.[18,36,37] These studies are important because they demonstrate that ARF outcomes are likely impacted by the effects of poverty and other forms of socioeconomic disenfranchisement. However, relying on neighborhood indices promotes further knowledge gaps through aggregation of multiple measures of SED. SED is defined as low-quality social and economic resources that are available to citizens[36,38] and can exist at the levels of the individual, neighborhoods, and other distinctions. Neighborhood-level deprivation indices are designed to blend measures of neighborhood poverty, income, and unemployment to approximate individual-level SED.[36,37,39-41] While this approach brings us closer to understanding that relationships exist between SED and health outcomes, they fail to identify *how* they relate, and in particular, whether these relationships may be targeted to promote equitable ARF outcomes. Ideally, future studies will move beyond reinforcing that socioeconomic status is associated with ARF outcomes, and toward identifying how the context of a patient's lived SED can inform care delivery and health policy to reduce disparities.

Focus on Minority Serving Hospitals

MSHs represent the predominant care location for a majority of patients who identify as Black. The extent to which racial minority groups predominantly receive ARF care in MSHs is currently unstudied yet is a fundamental knowledge gap. While population imbalances in care received at MSHs may represent a health care manifestation of de facto segregation, the concentration of most minority patient care among a limited number of hospitals may represent opportunity to efficiently target those hospitals to promote equitable care.[21] Therefore, it is crucial that in all future studies designed to mitigate ARF disparities, these MSHs are represented not merely as study sites, but also as partners in study design. MSHs face unique organizational challenges,[24,42-44] and too frequently, policies designed to improve health care quality often result in excessive penalties for these hospitals.[43,45-48] An ideal pathway that might avoid these penalties requires leadership from MSH specialists throughout the process of health services research, intervention strategy, and health policy development.

SUMMARY

Racial and ethnic disparity research related to ARF faces a number of unique methodological challenges. To date, convincing evidence exists for increased disease burden and worse clinical outcomes among racial and ethnic minority patients with ARF. However, the comprehensive characterization of actionable mechanisms for these disparities is still lacking. Some studies have begun to identify presenting disease severity, individual hospital care quality, and socioeconomic status as important factors, and though relevance of their association with disparities in ARF clinical outcomes is relevant, multiple knowledge gaps preclude this evidence from being actionable. To develop disparities mitigating solutions relevant to clinicians and policy makers, future investigations must identify modifiable determinants of ARF disparities, better contextualize ARF care delivery within the lived experience of patient SED, and be developed through partnerships between experts at MSHs as well as the patients that receive care at these institutions to develop novel solutions that will eliminate ARF disparities.

CLINICS CARE POINTS

- Racial and ethnic minority patients experience highest risk of disease, death, and LOS from ARF and related disease.
- Mechanistic relationships regarding ARF disparities that have been inferred are related to presenting disease severity, between-hospital variation in standards of care, and socioeconomic status.

- Many knowledge gaps exist that limit the development of targetable interventions and health policies that might promote health equity for ARF outcomes.
- Challenges that must be overcome to develop disease-mitigating solutions focus on data disaggregation of demographic groupings; comprehensive mapping of causal relationships between SED, race, ethnicity, and clinical outcomes; and partnership with MSHs.

DISCLOSURE

The author has nothing to disclose.

FUNDING

This commentary was funded by NHLBI R01HL146386.

REFERENCES

1. Roussos C, Koutsoukou A. Respiratory failure. Eur Respir J Suppl 2003;47: 3s–14s. https://doi.org/10.1183/09031936.03.00038503.
2. Stefan MS, Shieh MS, Pekow PS, et al. Epidemiology and outcomes of acute respiratory failure in the United States, 2001 to 2009: a national survey. J Hosp Med 2013;8(2):76–82. https://doi.org/10.1002/jhm.2004.
3. Kempker JA, Abril MK, Chen Y, et al. The epidemiology of respiratory failure in the United States 2002-2017: a Serial cross-sectional study. Crit Care Explor 2020; 2(6):e0128. https://doi.org/10.1097/CCE.0000000000000128.
4. Wunsch H, Linde-Zwirble WT, Angus DC, et al. The epidemiology of mechanical ventilation use in the United States. Crit Care Med 2010;38(10):1947–53. https://doi.org/10.1097/CCM.0b013e3181ef4460.
5. Cooke CR, Erickson SE, Eisner MD, et al. Trends in the incidence of noncardiogenic acute respiratory failure: the role of race. Crit Care Med 2012;40(5): 1532–8. https://doi.org/10.1097/CCM.0b013e31824518f2.
6. Citro CF, Cork DL, Norwood JL. *The 2000 Census: Counting Under Adversity. Chapter 8: race and ethnicity measurement.* Washington, DC: National Research Council. The National Academies Press; 2004.
7. Bime C, Poongkunran C, Borgstrom M, et al. Racial differences in mortality from severe acute respiratory failure in the United States, 2008-2012. Ann Am Thorac Soc 2016;13(12):2184–9. https://doi.org/10.1513/AnnalsATS.201605-359OC.
8. Cochi SE, Kempker JA, Annangi S, et al. Mortality trends of acute respiratory distress syndrome in the United States from 1999 to 2013. Ann Am Thorac Soc 2016;13(10):1742–51. https://doi.org/10.1513/AnnalsATS.201512-841OC.
9. Chesley CF, Chowdhury M, Small DS, et al. Racial disparities in length of stay among severely ill patients presenting with sepsis and acute respiratory failure. JAMA Netw Open 2023;6(5):e239739. https://doi.org/10.1001/jamanetworkopen.2023.9739.
10. Qeadan F, VanSant-Webb E, Tingey B, et al. Racial disparities in COVID-19 outcomes exist despite comparable Elixhauser comorbidity indices between Blacks, Hispanics, Native Americans, and Whites. Sci Rep 2021;11(1):8738. https://doi.org/10.1038/s41598-021-88308-2.
11. Vardar U, Ilelaboye A, Murthi M, et al. Racial disparities in patients with COVID-19 infection: a national inpatient Sample analysis. Cureus 2023;15(2):e35039. https://doi.org/10.7759/cureus.35039.

12. Rao A, Alnababteh MH, Avila-Quintero VJ, et al. Association between patient race and ethnicity and outcomes with COVID-19: a retrospective analysis from a large mid-atlantic health system. J Intensive Care Med 2023;38(5):472–8. https://doi.org/10.1177/08850666221149956.

13. Joynt KE, Orav EJ, Jha AK. Thirty-day readmission rates for Medicare beneficiaries by race and site of care. JAMA 2011;305(7):675–81. https://doi.org/10.1001/jama.2011.123.

14. Calvillo-King L, Arnold D, Eubank KJ, et al. Impact of social factors on risk of readmission or mortality in pneumonia and heart failure: systematic review. J Gen Intern Med 2013;28(2):269–82. https://doi.org/10.1007/s11606-012-2235-x.

15. Elixhahuser A, Au D, Podulka J. Readmissions for chronic obstructive pulmonary disease. HCUP Statistical Brief #121. Agency for Health Research and Quality 2008. Available at: http://www.hcup-us.ahrq.gov/reports/statbriefs/sb121.pdf. [Accessed 30 October 2023].

16. Nguyen TT, Vable AM, Glymour MM, et al. Trends for reported discrimination in health care in a national Sample of older adults with chronic conditions. J Gen Intern Med 2018;33(3):291–7. https://doi.org/10.1007/s11606-017-4209-5.

17. Erickson SE, Shlipak MG, Martin GS, et al. Racial and ethnic disparities in mortality from acute lung injury. Crit Care Med 2009;37(1):1–6. https://doi.org/10.1097/CCM.0b013e31819292ea.

18. Erickson SE, Vasilevskis EE, Kuzniewicz MW, et al. The effect of race and ethnicity on outcomes among patients in the intensive care unit: a comprehensive study involving socioeconomic status and resuscitation preferences. Crit Care Med 2011;39(3):429–35. https://doi.org/10.1097/CCM.0b013e318206b3af.

19. Williams JF, Zimmerman JE, Wagner DP, et al. African-American and white patients admitted to the intensive care unit: is there a difference in therapy and outcome? Crit Care Med 1995;23(4):626–36.

20. Mayr FB, Yende S, D'Angelo G, et al. Do hospitals provide lower quality of care to black patients for pneumonia? Crit Care Med 2010;38(3):759–65. https://doi.org/10.1097/CCM.0b013e3181c8fd58.

21. Jha AK, Orav EJ, Li Z, et al. Concentration and quality of hospitals that care for elderly black patients. Arch Intern Med 2007;167(11):1177–82. https://doi.org/10.1001/archinte.167.11.1177.

22. Asch DA, Islam MN, Sheils NE, et al. Patient and hospital factors associated with differences in mortality rates among black and white US Medicare beneficiaries hospitalized with COVID-19 infection. JAMA Netw Open 2021;4(6):e2112842. https://doi.org/10.1001/jamanetworkopen.2021.12842.

23. Hechenbleikner EM, Zheng C, Lawrence S, et al. Do hospital factors impact readmissions and mortality after colorectal resections at minority-serving hospitals? Surgery 2017;161(3):846–54. https://doi.org/10.1016/j.surg.2016.08.041.

24. Shen YC, Hsia RY. Do patients hospitalised in high-minority hospitals experience more diversion and poorer outcomes? A retrospective multivariate analysis of Medicare patients in California. BMJ Open 2016;6(3):e010263. https://doi.org/10.1136/bmjopen-2015-010263.

25. Rush B, Danziger J, Walley KR, et al. Treatment in disproportionately minority hospitals is associated with increased risk of mortality in sepsis: a national analysis. Crit Care Med 2020;48(7):962–7. https://doi.org/10.1097/CCM.0000000000004375.

26. Gaskin DJ, Spencer CS, Richard P, et al. Do minority patients use lower quality hospitals? *Inquiry.* Fall 2011;48(3):209–20. https://doi.org/10.5034/inquiryjrnl_48.03.06.

27. Ashana DC, Anesi GL, Liu VX, et al. Equitably allocating resources during crises: racial differences in mortality prediction models. Am J Respir Crit Care Med 2021. https://doi.org/10.1164/rccm.202012-4383OC.

28. Roy S, Showstark M, Tolchin B, et al. The potential impact of triage protocols on racial disparities in clinical outcomes among COVID-positive patients in a large academic healthcare system. PLoS One 2021;16(9):e0256763. https://doi.org/10.1371/journal.pone.0256763.

29. Riviello ED, Dechen T, O'Donoghue AL, et al. Assessment of a crisis standards of care scoring system for resource prioritization and estimated excess mortality by race, ethnicity, and socially vulnerable area during a regional surge in COVID-19. JAMA Netw Open 2022;5(3):e221744. https://doi.org/10.1001/jamanetworkopen.2022.1744.

30. Jones JM, Fingar KR, Miller MA, et al. Racial disparities in sepsis-related in-hospital mortality: using a broad case capture method and multivariate controls for clinical and hospital variables, 2004-2013. Crit Care Med 2017;45(12): e1209–17. https://doi.org/10.1097/CCM.0000000000002699.

31. Esper AM, Moss M, Lewis CA, et al. The role of infection and comorbidity: factors that influence disparities in sepsis. Crit Care Med 2006;34(10):2576–82. https://doi.org/10.1097/01.CCM.0000239114.50519.0E.

32. DiMeglio M, Dubensky J, Schadt S, et al. Factors underlying racial disparities in sepsis management. Healthcare (Basel) 2018;6(4). https://doi.org/10.3390/healthcare6040133.

33. Mayr FB, Yende S, Linde-Zwirble WT, et al. Infection rate and acute organ dysfunction risk as explanations for racial differences in severe sepsis. JAMA 2010;303(24):2495–503. https://doi.org/10.1001/jama.2010.851.

34. Soto GJ, Martin GS, Gong MN. Healthcare disparities in critical illness. Crit Care Med 2013;41(12):2784–93. https://doi.org/10.1097/CCM.0b013e3182a84a43.

35. Taylor SP, Karvetski CH, Templin MA, et al. Hospital differences drive antibiotic delays for black patients compared with white patients with suspected septic shock. Crit Care Med 2018;46(2):e126–31. https://doi.org/10.1097/CCM.0000000000002829.

36. Falvey JR, Murphy TE, Leo-Summers L, et al. Neighborhood socioeconomic disadvantage and disability after critical illness. Crit Care Med 2022;50(5): 733–41. https://doi.org/10.1097/CCM.0000000000005364.

37. Galiatsatos P, Follin A, Alghanim F, et al. The association between neighborhood socioeconomic disadvantage and readmissions for patients hospitalized with sepsis. Crit Care Med 2020;48(6):808–14. https://doi.org/10.1097/CCM.0000000000004307.

38. Chesley CF, Lane-Fall MB. What socioeconomic disadvantage means for critical illness recovery, clinical care, and research. Crit Care Med 2022;50(5):876–8. https://doi.org/10.1097/CCM.0000000000005414.

39. Donnelly JP, Lakkur S, Judd SE, et al. Association of neighborhood socioeconomic status with risk of infection and sepsis. Clin Infect Dis 2018;66(12): 1940–7. https://doi.org/10.1093/cid/cix1109.

40. Xie S, Hubbard RA, Himes BE. Neighborhood-level measures of socioeconomic status are more correlated with individual-level measures in urban areas compared with less urban areas. Ann Epidemiol 2020;43:37–43.e4. https://doi.org/10.1016/j.annepidem.2020.01.012.

41. Kind AJH, Buckingham WR. Making neighborhood-disadvantage metrics accessible - the neighborhood atlas. N Engl J Med 2018;378(26):2456–8. https://doi.org/10.1056/NEJMp1802313.

42. Hsia RY, Asch SM, Weiss RE, et al. California hospitals serving large minority populations were more likely than others to employ ambulance diversion. Health Aff 2012;31(8):1767–76. https://doi.org/10.1377/hlthaff.2011.1020.

43. Joynt KE, Sarma N, Epstein AM, et al. Challenges in reducing readmissions: lessons from leadership and frontline personnel at eight minority-serving hospitals. Jt Comm J Qual Patient Saf 2014;40(10):435–7. https://doi.org/10.1016/s1553-7250(14)40056-4.

44. Prieto-Centurion V, Gussin HA, Rolle AJ, et al. Chronic obstructive pulmonary disease readmissions at minority-serving institutions. Ann Am Thorac Soc 2013; 10(6):680–4. https://doi.org/10.1513/AnnalsATS.201307-223OT.

45. Zogg CK, Thumma JR, Ryan AM, et al. Medicare's hospital acquired condition reduction program disproportionately affects minority-serving hospitals: variation by race, socioeconomic status, and disproportionate share hospital payment receipt. Ann Surg 2020;271(6):985–93. https://doi.org/10.1097/SLA.0000000000003564.

46. Shih T, Ryan AM, Gonzalez AA, et al. Medicare's hospital readmissions reduction program in surgery may disproportionately affect minority-serving hospitals. Ann Surg 2015;261(6):1027–31. https://doi.org/10.1097/SLA.0000000000000778.

47. Shashikumar SA, Waken RJ, Luke AA, et al. Association of stratification by proportion of patients dually enrolled in Medicare and medicaid with financial penalties in the hospital-acquired condition reduction program. JAMA Intern Med 2021;181(3):330. https://doi.org/10.1001/jamainternmed.2020.7386.

48. Chaiyachati KH, Qi M, Werner RM. Changes to racial disparities in readmission rates after medicare's hospital readmissions reduction program within safety-net and non–safety-net hospitals. JAMA Netw Open 2018;1(7):e184154. https://doi.org/10.1001/jamanetworkopen.2018.4154.

Race, Ethnicity, and Gender Disparities in Acute Myocardial Infarction

Mridul Bansal, MD[a,1], Aryan Mehta, MD[b,1],
Akshay Machanahalli Balakrishna, MD[c], Marwan Saad, MD, PhD[d,e],
Corey E. Ventetuolo, MD, MS[f,g], Robert O. Roswell, MD[h],
Athena Poppas, MD[d,e], Jinnette Dawn Abbott, MD[e,i],
Saraschandra Vallabhajosyula, MD, MSc[d,e,*]

KEYWORDS

- Acute myocardial infarction • Cardiogenic shock • Cardiac arrest • Disparities • Sex
- Race

KEY POINTS

- Women and racial minorities continue to have worse outcomes highlighting the need to make health care more accessible and equitable.
- Despite national and societal efforts, clinical trials continue to have under representation of women and minorities, further limiting the full range of benefits from novel therapies for this population.
- An in-depth, comprehensive, and integrated understanding of the gender and racial disparities with particular attention to their social determinants of health to help in cardiovascular disease prevention and appropriate secondary prevention after incident acute myocardial infarction event are the need of the hour.

Sources of funding: None.
[a] Department of Medicine, East Carolina University Brody School of Medicine, Greenville, NC, USA; [b] Department of Medicine, University of Connecticut School of Medicine, Farmington, CT, USA; [c] Section of Cardiovascular Medicine, Department of Medicine, Creighton University School of Medicine, Omaha, NE, USA; [d] Division of Cardiology, Department of Medicine, Warren Alpert Medical School of Brown University, Providence, RI, USA; [e] Lifespan Cardiovascular Institute, Providence, RI, USA; [f] Division of Pulmonary, Critical Care and Sleep Medicine, Department of Medicine, Warren Alpert Medical School of Brown University, Providence, RI, USA; [g] Department of Health Services, Policy and Practice, Brown University, RI, USA; [h] Department of Cardiology, Zucker School of Medicine at Hofstra/Northwell, Hempstead, NY, USA; [i] Division of Cardiology, Department of Medicine, Warren Alpert Medical School of Brown University, Brown Medical School, Providence, RI, USA
[1] Drs M. Bansal and A. Mehta contributed equally as co-first authors.
* Corresponding author. 2 Dudley Street, Suite 360, Providence, Rhode Island 02905.
E-mail address: svallabhajosyula@lifespan.org

Crit Care Clin 40 (2024) 685–707
https://doi.org/10.1016/j.ccc.2024.05.005
0749-0704/24/© 2024 Elsevier Inc. All rights are reserved, including those for text and data mining, AI training, and similar technologies.

criticalcare.theclinics.com

INTRODUCTION

Cardiovascular disease (CVD) continues to be the leading cause of morbidity and mortality in the United States and worldwide, with over 17.9 million deaths from CVD in 2019.[1,2] There are persistent racial and gender disparities in the diagnosis, treatment, and prognosis of individuals with CVD, despite multiple advances in this field.[3–5] Women and people from racial and ethnic minority groups (black race, Hispanic ethnicity, Asian and Native Americans) are disproportionately affected by discrepancies in CVD diagnosis, treatment, and outcomes.[6] These racial and gender disparities are further exaggerated in the acute care setting, such as in patients with acute myocardial infarction (AMI), due to the additional time-sensitive nature.[7] Identifying and mitigating these vulnerabilities in conjunction with addressing structural racism and bias and encouraging suitable representation could result in better outcomes.[8] Unlike other reasons for admission to the intensive care unit (ICU) with a critical syndrome (such as sepsis or acute respiratory distress syndrome), AMI constitutes the end-result of failure of both primary and secondary prevention techniques. Further, the impact of lifestyle interventions and the social determinant of health is very pronounced in CVD. Therefore, when faced with these critically ill patients in the ICU, the critical care physician should seek to address both the acute health care disparities and the prevalent long-standing disparities to ensure durability of the ICU interventions.

In this narrative review, the differences in pathophysiology, clinical course, risk profile, and in management and outcomes of AMI patients across gender, racial, and ethnic groups will be discussed (**Table 1**). We also highlight demographic and psychosocial perspectives that might undergird disparities in cardiovascular care and provide recommendations for earlier identification of novel risk factors that increase the risk of adverse outcomes.

BACKGROUND

Extensive scientific literature describing differences in patterns of health care delivered to vulnerable populations dates back many decades. In the mid-19th century, German physician Rudolph Virchow suggested the presence of variations in health care-related outcomes and attributed these differences to several societal factors.[9] In the early to mid-20th century, CVD became one of the leading causes of death worldwide and was described to affect men, women, all races, and age groups equally.[10] In 1927, a study by Stone and Vanzant noted heart disease to be different in the Southern United States compared to the Eastern and Northern United States.[11] They attributed the larger population of black in the Southern United States to be one of the contributing factors and described the incidence of CVD in the black race to be 1.8 times more than the white race. A prospective cohort study done in Northern California that included patients who experienced acute AMI between 1995 and 2002, found the age-adjusted risk of AMI recurrence to be significantly higher in black men, black women, and Asian/Native American women when compared with white men.[12] Age-adjusted all-cause mortality was also significantly higher in black men and women compared with white men. These differences, attributed to gender, race, and ethnicity, were attenuated when certain variables including sociodemographic background were accounted for.[12] Differences in the incidence of AMI or recurrence of AMI were also being attributed to differences in risk factors for the development of CVD. Black and Hispanic Americans in the study population were more likely to be physically inactive, have poorer hypertensive and glycemic control, and were less likely to be informed by their health care professional that they were

Table 1
Summary of health care disparities in acute myocardial infarction and related states

Condition	Disparities Stratification[a]	Epidemiology and Risk Factors	Management	Outcomes
Acute myocardial infarction	Race and Ethnicity	Minority group have higher rates of dyslipidemia, obesity, chronic renal disease, insulin resistance, hypertension, and diabetes mellitus due to social factors	Minority groups are less likely to receive guideline-directed medications overall, and invasive procedures in non-ST-segment-elevation acute myocardial infarction	Minority group have higher readmission rates, increased adverse outcomes and long-term mortality
	Gender	Women are older and have higher prevalence of hypertension, and diabetes mellitus, have delayed time to first medical contact and increased rates of in-hospital and transfer times	Women have lower rates of reperfusion therapies, lower likelihood of receiving optimal medical therapy, longer delay to first medical contact and longer door-to-balloon time	Women have higher mortality
Cardiogenic shock	Race and Ethnicity	Minority groups have lower socio-economic status, higher rate of comorbidity in non-ST-segment-elevation acute myocardial infarction-cardiogenic shock	Minority group have lower rates of guideline-directed therapy and revascularization therapies	Minority group have higher mortality
	Gender	Women are older and with higher comorbidity	Older women have lower rates of invasive hemodynamic monitoring, revascularization therapies, and mechanical circulatory support utilization	Women have higher rates of morbidity, morbidity, and vascular complications
Cardiac arrest	Race and Ethnicity	Lower rates of receiving bystander cardiopulmonary resuscitation in minority group neighborhoods, variable emergency medical services arrival time	Minority groups have lower likelihood of receiving reperfusion therapies in post resuscitation treatment and lower utilization of targeted temperature management strategies	Minority group have higher mortality and poorer neurologic outcomes
	Gender	Women have lower rates of bystander cardiopulmonary resuscitation	Lower likelihood of receiving reperfusion therapies in post resuscitation treatment and lower utilization of targeted temperature management strategies	Variable results on mortality and neurologic outcomes

a Black race and Hispanic ethnicity are the most studied minority groups, with limited information on other sub-groups (Asian, Native American).

overweight.[13] In an analysis done in 1997, black patients were found to be less likely to undergo coronary revascularization procedures when compared to white patients, and this was not explained by the differences in clinical features of their CVD.[14] They were 13% less likely to receive angioplasty and 32% less likely to undergo coronary artery bypass grafting (CABG).[14] A similar but less significant trend was observed between coronary revascularization procedures between Hispanic and non-Hispanic white patients from 1975 to 1999 by Yarzebski and colleagues[15] This was also noted to be present in 2014, when Albert and colleagues explored the impact of Massachusetts enacted legislation that required all the residents to have health insurance.[16] Compared with white patients in the pre-legislature period, black and Hispanic patients were found to have lower rates of CABG or percutaneous coronary intervention (PCI) while Asians/Native Americans were found to have a higher rate of revascularization.[16] Similarly, during the post-legislature period lower rates of revascularization therapies were observed in black and Hispanic patients with higher rates in Asians/Native Americans when compared to white patients. In this analysis, men were also more likely to receive cardiovascular revascularization procedures when compared to women. Hence, a reduction in barriers to insurance did not eliminate pre-existing disparities in access to cardiovascular procedures.[16] Glance and colleagues in their analysis on effect of Medicaid expansion noted reduction of uninsured black patients as compared to uninsured white patients. However, this was not associated with reduction in disparities in AMI revascularization therapies.[17] The concerns of AMI care disparities on being less sensitive to insurance, was also noted in another similar study on Medicaid expansion.[18]

Apart from racial disparities, differences in outcomes due to gender have been studied extensively. In 1997, Herman and colleagues analyzed the population admitted from 1985 to 1990 and included in World Health Organization multinational monitoring of trends and determinants in CVD-Bremen AMI Registry for 28-day mortality difference among men and women.[19] They noted that even after adjusting for age, women had 20.9% mortality post-AMI versus 16.8% in men ($P=$ .04). After adjusting for cardiac impairment and therapies however no difference was observed. The Minnesota Heart Study also showed higher age-adjusted mortality in women less than 65 years (12.5% of women vs 6.5% of men, $P<.01$).[20] The increased risk was driven by young women, which has been shown in other studies as well.

Multivariate analysis also showed that among those less than 65 years, female gender was a strong and independent predictor of early death (odds ratio [OR] 2.0; 95% confidence interval [CI] 1.2–3.5; $P<.01$). Another large database study consisting greater than 15,000 patients noted that female gender was an independent predictor of operative mortality after CABG surgery.[21] Additionally, women and minorities have also historically been underrepresented in human subject research. In a mandate in 1993 through the National Institute of Health (NIH) Revitalization Act, the NIH established guidelines to include minorities and women in clinical research trials.[22] Furthermore, in 2016 NIH enacted a policy to list sex as a biological variable.[23]

Despite the pervasive disparities and the attempt to improve these efforts by NIH guidelines, studies continue to note the under-representation of women and minorities in cardiovascular clinical trials. In an analysis of clinical trials, Gong and colleagues noted that women comprised less than 40% of all subjects (37% non-coronary artery disease vascular, 30% coronary artery disease, 28% heart failure, 28% arrhythmia) during 1986 to 2015.[24] Although the enrollment increased in recent years, it still represented lower than expected disease population proportions. Another analysis of cardiovascular clinical trials in Canada between 1997 and 2009 found that the enrollment rates for women were lower than expected by 5% in coronary artery disease,

13% in heart failure, 9% in arrhythmia, and 3% in primary prevention.[25] A recent 10-year analysis on different cardiometabolic drugs noted that the majority of the trials only had 36% women and they were grossly under-represented compared to their disease burden.[26] Similar disparities have also existed among the minority and non-white population. When stratified by race, there were 81% white subjects enrolled compared to just 4% black subjects in this study. These findings were also observed by Purasana and colleagues who noted that between years 2000 and 2019 among the clinical trials registered in ClinicalTrials.gov only 21% of trials defined a recruitment target for underrepresented groups.[27]

CHARACTERISTICS OF DISPARITIES

In this section, we will seek to address the basis for clinical and health care disparities in the care of AMI patients. While AMI, and certainly cardiogenic shock (CS) and cardiac arrest (CA) complicating AMI, are frequently seen in the ICU, the health care disparities associated with these conditions are grounded in the baseline characteristics. In this section, we will highlight gender disparities in presentation, sex differences in biology, and the interaction of gender, race, and ethnicity.

Misclassification and Misdiagnosis Associated with Gender

The major misclassification and misdiagnosis biases stem from the prevalence of symptoms considered atypical of AMI in women. Women present less frequently with classical sub-sternal chest discomfort with radiation to the jaw and shoulder. A recent study by Milner and colleagues noted that only 54% of women had chest pain as their chief complaint when they had an AMI compared to 69% of men ($P<.001$).[28] These differences are more marked in the younger population, where women significantly were less likely to report chest pain. The same study reported that respiratory symptoms like shortness of breath seemed to be the chief complaint of AMI among younger women. Brush and colleagues elucidated how women have a broader and more heterogeneous phenotype of symptoms across the spectrum of AMI that further confounds the initial diagnosis.[29] They showed that women had 426 interview-symptom phenotypes as compared to 280 phenotypes in men. Women were also more broadly distributed in interview-symptoms phenotype.[29] Shin and colleagues investigated the interview styles when assessing for symptoms of AMI and found that if questions were open-ended then women and men had similar reporting of chest pain but if a narrowed line of questioning was adopted, then men reported more chest pain.[30] Recently the role of prodromal symptoms has been explored prior to an AMI. A study in Germany observed that more than 50% of women had prodromal symptoms of sleep disturbance versus 32% of men before an AMI.[31]

Often misclassification of the pathology leads to a domino effect. In an Australian STEMI registry, Stehli and colleagues noted that women had longer delays to primary reperfusion and higher 30-day mortality than their men counterparts (OR 1.38; 95% CI 1.06–1.79; $P=.02$).[32] In a similar analysis, Coventry and colleagues also reported that women who had less chest pain than their men counterparts were less likely to be allocated a priority one ambulance response (men 98.3% vs women 95.5%).[33] A study from New York City noted that 62% of women did not complain of chest pain while having an STEMI as compared to 36% of men ($P=.01$).[34] This eventually led to 72% of women having an estimated time gap of more than 90 minutes between symptom onset and hospital presentation versus 54% of men ($P=.03$).[34] All these studies further consolidate the fact that women present with more nonspecific and atypical symptoms that can often lead to overlooking the diagnosis of acute AMI in women. This ultimately can lead to delays in presentation to the hospital and receiving timely care.

Pathophysiologic Variations by Sex

In addition to differences in clinical care, certain nuances in pathophysiology differ in biological males and females that may account for variations in outcomes of acute cardiovascular conditions. Studies have reported that women's hearts have increased pro-inflammatory markers compared to men.[35] Fietcher and colleagues used vertebral bone marrow metabolism as a surrogate marker of inflammation and noted that females had increased 18-fluerodexoy glucose bone marrow uptake.[36] They found a significant association between increased bone marrow metabolism and impaired myocardial function (P=.04) and perfusion (P=.014) in females.[36] This association was non-existent in males (P=.28). The role of vascular dysfunction and its higher prevalence in biological females with obstructive coronary artery disease may contribute to the differences in outcomes.[37] Merz and colleagues proposed that myocardial ischemia might result when symptoms occur in an acute stress state in the setting of impaired blood flow reserve and endothelial dysfunction among small arterial lumen vessels.[37]

Multiple analyses have observed that females have less atherosclerotic burden than males when presenting with AMI. Berger and colleagues noted that biological females had more nonobstructive coronary artery disease (14% vs 8%) along with reduced 2-vessel (25% vs 28%) and 3-vessel coronary artery disease (23% vs 26%).[38] Another study done on young people with fatal ischemic heart disease noted that females who died of ischemic heart disease had only a 63% chance of having obstructive disease compared to 77% in biological males (P=.002).[39] Females also tend to have a higher incidence of plaque erosion compared to males, who have more plaque rupture that contributes to increased mortality.[40] Han and colleagues also noted that females have more disease of microcirculation, although males have a higher atherosclerotic burden.[41] In light of these findings and worse outcomes in females, the role of microvascular and endothelial dysfunction has been increasingly studied and recognized in females, especially in myocardial infarction with no obstructive coronary arteries (MINOCA). MINOCA prevalence has been noted to be about 5% to 6%.[42] Up to 50% of MINOCA patients are females. This is a considerable difference form the AMI with coronary artery disease population proportion where females make up only 25% of the population.[43] It is also more likely to be seen in black, Pacific Islander, or Hispanic populations.[43] Although, the pathophysiology remains poorly understood at present.

Intersection of Age, Race, and Gender

Health disparities are mostly caused by the distribution of CVD and associated risk factors, which differ among racial, ethnic, and gender groups. While men tend to have a higher prevalence of CVD risk factors at earlier ages, postmenopausal women have higher blood pressure, cholesterol, and weight compared to men of similar age.[44] Variable concentrations of endogenous estrogens, which have a protective but pleiotropic impact on the cardiovascular system, especially before menopause, are partly responsible for better cardiovascular health in biological females compared to males among white adults.[45] However, black adults do not follow similar trends which argues that the intersectionality framework–a social stratification which includes age, gender, and race and ethnicity–forms an interconnected system of oppression that restricts opportunities for people with underprivileged social status due to structural racism.[46] Therefore, more than just 1 inferior position, having several subordinate positions may be linked to worse health ramifications. An intersectionality framework stresses that being a black woman is more than simply the sum of being black and a woman in terms of CVD risk, challenging a belief that women are a homogenous group with similar life experiences and outcomes. Black women may encounter greater challenges than other intersectional groups in accomplishing ideal cardiovascular health because they may be more likely to encounter a series of life hardships and social or material challenges, and may have fewer available resources to deal with these obstacles.[47] The specific causes of varying racial and gender trends probably involve various environmental risks encountered during an individual's lifetime. There is increasing recognition that social determinants of general health which include health care access and quality, education access and quality, social and community context, economic stability, and neighborhood and built environment play an important role too.[48–50] Black adults are more likely to suffer the negative impacts of bias, such as restricted access to higher paying jobs, education, and health care, according to studies on the impact of communities.[51] In addition to offering fewer options for safe areas to exercise and less healthy food and drink options, low-income communities may also be responsible for obesity and a higher risk of CVD.[52] The intersectionality paradigm also illustrates how a person may be privileged in certain social systems of inequality while experiencing oppression in others. The multiplicative, additive, and amplified interaction between gender, race and ethnicity, and age described above has been demonstrated in a recent study by Kanchi and colleagues who found that the combined effects of gender and race and ethnicity on overweight/obesity and hypertension were greater than the sum of individual gender, race and ethnicity effects.[53] The group also found that white women had the lowest prevalence of CVD risk factors among the groups studied, while black women had the greatest prevalence.[53] These points highlight the significance of looking at gender and race concurrently, and they are consistent with a sizable but inconsistent body of research on social and environmental variations in CVD risk by race and gender as well as on hormonal variations by biological sex.[54] Recognizing the collective gender, racial, and ethnic differences across several CVD risk factors may lead to novel interesting etiologic questions, direct preventative initiatives, and emphasize the relative significance of racial, ethnic, and age differentiation within the same gender for CVD investigations.

ACUTE MYOCARDIAL INFARCTION AND RELATED STATES
ST and Non-ST-Segment Elevation Acute Myocardial Infarction

Disparities in management
Black patients continue to have a higher incidence of AMI including both ST-segment-elevation myocardial infarction (STEMI) and non-STEMI (NSTEMI).[55,56] Furthermore, black patients have higher rates of dyslipidemia, obesity, chronic renal disease, insulin resistance, hypertension, and diabetes mellitus, among other cardiovascular system-related comorbidities.[55] Hospital surveillance of NSTEMI in 4 United States areas over 15 years was evaluated by Arora and colleagues as part of the Atherosclerosis Risk in Communities surveillance investigation.[56] They noted that black patients had a 24% lower probability of receiving non aspirin anti-platelet therapies, 29% lower probability of coronary angiography and 45% lower probability of revascularization therapies. Previous studies found race associated with differential NSTEMI management, with black patients less likely than white patients to receive guideline-directed medications and invasive procedures.[55,57–60] According to studies like the Acute Coronary Treatment and Intervention Outcomes Network Registry-Get With The Guidelines database, even in risk-adjusted cases, black patients hospitalized with NSTEMI were

younger, less insured, and had a greater prevalence of comorbidities along with considerably lower likelihood of receiving invasive angiography (45% vs 61%) or revascularization (25% vs 45%) than white patients.[61]

Independent of race, compared to men, women are more likely to be placed in a lower risk category for CVD and to receive less intense medical care for the condition overall, including less invasive and pharmacologic treatments as well as lifestyle counseling.[62,63] Numerous studies have noted that women have lower treatment rates of traditional cardiovascular risk factors such as hypercholesterolemia and hypertension.[64,65] Women from racial and ethnic minority group backgrounds have reduced rates of statin utilization (primary and secondary prevention) and cholesterol goals compared to white women.[66,67] There has been a correlation found between being a women receiving invasive therapy for coronary obstruction and delay in care.[59,68] In the National Heart, Lung, and Blood Institute Dynamic Registry, compared to older women, young women less than 50 years, were more likely to experience adverse outcomes including target vessel and target lesion failure at 1 year, despite having less severe coronary artery disease by angiography.[69] The Variation in Recovery: Role of Gender on Outcomes of Young AMI patients study found that among young patients with STEMI, women experienced delay in reperfusion.[70]

Overall, disparities in treatment have been associated with lower education levels, single-marital status, and care interruptions.[65] Socioeconomic factors, such as lower income and lack of health insurance, physician prescribing tendencies, lower rates of specialist referrals, inadequate risk assessment, and poor patient-physician communication, are other potential explanations for the differences in cardiovascular treatment among women of racial and ethnic minorities.[71,72]

Disparities in outcomes

There have been conflicting data on significant differences in short term mortality rates among different racial and ethnic groups. In a recent observational study on patient with AMI post-PCI it was noted that black and women patients had increased risk of angina at 6 week and 1 year mark.[73] Similarly other analysis have noted that black individuals had increased rates of bleeding post-PCI/thrombolysis after an STEMI and also had increased risk of stent thrombosis.[74,75]

AMI has been associated with higher mortality in women, particularly in younger women with STEMI.[38,76] In 2016, women's overall CVD mortality (49%) was comparable to men's (51%).[6] However, there are still notable differences in subjective outcomes: women with ASCVD of all racial and ethnic origins report worse patient experiences, a worse self-reported perception of their health, and a lower quality of life.[77]

Analysis of cardiovascular outcomes over time has revealed long-lasting differences among women from racial and ethnic minority groups backgrounds. Compared to men or white women, the in-hospital mortality rate for acute AMI is considerably greater in black and Hispanic women, despite continuous efforts by various government organizations like the National Institute of Minority Health.[6,68] For instance, after controlling for age and comorbidities, a study discovered significantly higher odds of in-hospital mortality among younger Hispanic women compared to younger white men.[68] 1-year event rates for women in the Controlled Abciximab and Device Investigation to Lower Late Angioplasty Complications trial included higher rates of major adverse cardiac events (23.9% vs 15.3%), ischemic target-vessel revascularization (16.7% vs 12.1%), and mortality (7.6% vs 3.0%). Being a woman was an independent predictor of major adverse cardiovascular events and bleeding complications.[78] It has been repeatedly observed that after PCI, women and racial minorities experience greater rates of bleeding and vascular complications. Although rates of bleeding and vascular complications in this vulnerable population have decreased over time, data from the Northern New England PCI registry showed that being a woman was still a significant predictor of increased risk of bleeding and vascular complications even after baseline differences were considered.[79] A prospective study by Cai and colleagues, revealed that the incidence of major bleeding following PCI was higher in black patients compared to their white counterparts.[80] The disparate outcomes in women and racial and ethnic minority group backgrounds following AMI may be linked to biases in the provision of diagnosis, treatment (as discussed above), patient education, and an elevated burden of cardiovascular risk factors in certain groups.[81,82]

Cardiogenic Shock

Despite the significant therapeutic advances in management, AMI-CS accounts for significant morbidity and mortality.[4,83] CS accounts for one of the most common causes of death in patients with acute AMI with mortality approaching 50% within the first 48 hours after presentation[83] Despite significant research in the domain of acute cardiovascular care, there exist significant disparities in the management and outcomes of AMI-CS.[84] Studies have shown that patients of racial and ethnic minority group have higher mortality and lower rates of guideline-directed therapy and revascularization when compared to their white counterparts.[85–87] Also, women with acute AMI-CS have been found to have increased morbidity and mortality when compared to men.[88]

Koeth and colleagues evaluated 36,643 patients consisting of 66.8% men and 33.2% women with CS complicating STEMI. STEMI-CS was more frequently found in women when compared to men (adjusted OR 1.19; 95% CI 1.09–1.30).[89] Prior studies from our group have demonstrated gender-based health care disparities in the management and outcome of AMI-CS.[90–93] In one of the National Inpatient Sample analyses, being a woman was found to be a predictor of worse in-hospital outcomes including higher in-hospital mortality (adjusted OR, 1.05; 95% CI 1.02–1.08) and more frequent discharge to a skilled nursing facility.[90] Women with AMI-CS were noted to be older and of the Hispanic or non-white race. Older women had lower rates of PCI, CABG, invasive hemodynamic monitoring, and mechanical circulatory support utilization compared to men. Despite a higher risk of mortality and revascularization failure rate, Joseph and colleagues described a greater survival benefit to hospital discharge in women when compared to men with early initiation of hemodynamic support.[94] Similarly, early use of PCI was demonstrated to be an independent predictor of 1-year survival in women (hazards ratio 0.55; 95% CI 0.37–0.81), and no similar trend in men was noted.[95]

In a study by Ya'Qoub and colleagues in patients with AMI-CS, women of all races had higher in-hospital mortality when compared to men. Men who were of white, black, and Hispanic race and ethnicity had a mortality rate of 33.3%, 33.6%, and 34.7%, respectively.[96] In contrast, women who were of white, black, and Hispanic race and ethnicity had a higher mortality rate of 40.9%, 40%, and 45.4% even after adjusting for confounding factors (adjusted OR 1.11; 95% CI:1.06–1.16).[96] Similarly, men who were black and Hispanic had significantly higher in-hospital mortality compared to white men (black men: adjusted OR 1.18, 95% CI 1.04 to 1.34; Hispanic men: adjusted OR 1.19; 95% CI 1.06 to 1.33).[96] In a National Inpatient Sample analysis by Raheja and colleagues, mechanical circulatory support was utilized in 11.4% of the total 1,021,274 included patients.[97] White patients had significantly higher odds of getting mechanical circulatory support inserted (OR 1.18, 95% CI: 1.13–1.23) with significantly lower odds in black (OR: 0.65, 95% CI:0.61–0.69) and Hispanic (OR: 0.89; CI: 0.83–0.97) patients.[97,98] In a study demonstrating the utilization of extracorporeal life support for CS, Wang and colleagues noted women were more likely to be centrally cannulated.[99] They also noted women patients experienced more limb ischemia (7.5% vs 4.1%, $P<.001$) whereas men were more likely to receive renal replacement therapy (25.6% vs 31.3%, $P<.001$) and had longer hospital stays.[99] Women also had worse vascular compilations (8.8% vs 5.7%; $P<.001$), bleeding (7.1% vs 5.2%; $P=.01$), and limb ischemia (6.8% vs 4.5%; $P=.001$) per a recent Cardiogenic Shock Working Group report.[88]

Several studies have shown that being a woman and being from racial and ethnic minority groups to be independently associated with increased mortality. Trials adequately powered for pre-defined subgroup analysis based on gender and race should be promoted.[85] In addition, implementing STEMI and CS protocols will also aid in contributing to a reduction in health care disparities. Other potential solutions involve implicit bias training, social and familial support in patients with AMI-CS. The 6-point actionable framework by Sukhera and colleagues can help in better integration on implicit bias recognition and management to help improve racial and gender disparities.[100] In a recent analysis it was seen that black patients were less likely to be discharged home and more likely discharged to a skilled nursing facility.[101] Black patients in skilled nursing facility were more likely to be hospitalized than their white counterparts. Thus, addressing gaps in social support as part of post hospitalization care may be essential to addressing these disparities.[102]

Cardiac Arrest

It is estimated that every year, about 250,000 Americans suffer from out-of-hospital cardiac arrest (OHCA).[103] However, there are significant gender and racial differences in the incidence of witnessed arrests, resuscitation efforts, shockable rhythms, PCIs, and survival rates of cardiac arrest. Patients suffering from OHCA rely on lay rescuers to identify them, phone for assistance, start cardiopulmonary resuscitation (CPR), and perform early defibrillation.

Disparities in recipients of bystander cardiopulmonary resuscitation in out-of-hospital cardiac arrest

The most vital elements in the chain of survival for CA resuscitation are the identification of CA and provision of bystander CPR.[104] There is a difference in bystander CPR performance between genders.[105,106] Compared to women, men were more likely to get bystander CPR. This difference was not present in the home environment, but it was more notable in public settings.[107,108] Lower rates of women bystander CPR are caused by a variety of factors, including bias in instructional programs, modesty and social conventions surrounding touching or exposing a woman's chest, and a lack of awareness of cardiac disease in women.[105,106] Responders might be more motivated and less concerned about the legal ramifications of their acts while they are at home.[107] By using more realistic women patient simulators in CPR training, prejudice in training can be addressed, which could assist in overcoming social stigma related to the physical characteristics of patient gender or biological sex and lessen resistance to bystander CPR.[105] According to an Austrian study by Krammel and colleagues, women were less likely to administer an automated external defibrillator or do standby CPR on a person with CA.[109] This discrepancy may be lessened if women are encouraged, empowered, and trained to provide bystander CPR.[110]

Additionally, race and socio-economic status have an additive effect on the likelihood of receiving CPR. In a study by Sasson and colleagues, out of 14,225 adult CA patients, those from low-income, predominately black neighborhoods had a roughly 50% lower chance of receiving bystander CPR than those from high-income, predominately white communities. Higher income, on the other hand, attenuated the disparity in CPR provision for patients from integrated communities, but it only increased the likelihood of receiving CPR for a patient from a black community by 25%. Patients who were given bystander CPR had higher odds of being discovered in a shockable rhythm, requiring defibrillator treatment, and surviving to be admitted to and released from the hospital.[111] Similar findings were discovered for black patients in a different study that looked at 22,487 patients from the 2011 National Emergency Medical Services Information System. This study also found a curvilinear association between county socioeconomic status and bystander assistance.[112] A study by Naim and colleagues showed that black children were 50% less likely to receive bystander CPR if they lived in a neighborhood with the worst socioeconomic index than white children living in a community with the best index (based on a percentage of black race, employment rates, level of education until high school, and median income). Nonetheless, white children, irrespective of their residential neighborhood, were administered CPR at comparable rates.[113]

Being ethnically Hispanic may be associated with one's likelihood of receiving CPR in addition to race. Compared to non-Hispanic patients, a considerable number of studies have shown that Hispanic patients receive bystander CPR less frequently.[114,115] Moon and colleagues, found that in the state of Arizona, bystander CPR was given less frequently in Hispanic neighborhoods specifically and that an initial shockable rhythm during arrest was also less common within Hispanic neighborhoods when comparing CA by Hispanic versus. non-Hispanic neighborhoods. In Hispanic communities, there was also a significant decrease in survival to hospital discharge.[114]

Overall, the hypothesis that race, ethnicity, and socioeconomic factors like work and wages will collectively exacerbate gaps in OHCA bystander care and automated external defibrillator use is supported by both regional and national data. The least likely patients to obtain bystander help are black and Hispanic patients in the most socioeconomically challenged neighborhoods.

Baseline characteristics and prehospital care

In comparison to men, women patients with OHCA are often older, have a larger number of comorbidities, are more likely to be in private settings, have witnessed fewer arrests, and are more likely to have a non-shockable rhythm.[116] For both men and women, the time between collapsing and the ambulance arriving was comparable.[117] One possible explanation for women presenting with non-shockable rhythms more frequently than men could be the frequency of non-ASCVD as the cause of CA.[116] Compared to males, biological females have higher chest wall compliance, which facilitates and improves the effectiveness of chest compressions and resuscitation techniques.[108] Prior data suggest that females who are or will become pregnant have a higher chance of surviving a CA event even though they are more likely to have arrest features that are linked to worse outcomes.[118]

Regarding racial differences, black and Hispanic people with CA were younger, more frequently women, and were more likely to have an arrest in a low-income and black or Hispanic neighborhood. Different results on emergency medical services (EMS) arrival times for patients from low-income and minority group backgrounds have been reported in studies specifically examining variations in EMS response based on neighborhood socio-economic status and race. One study found that EMS arrival times for black neighborhoods were similar to or shorter than those for white neighborhoods, while another study found that EMS arrival times in the poorest neighborhoods were longer than national benchmarks.[119] Starks and colleagues, discovered that the duration of EMS treatments was longer in communities with a high concentration of black residents, but so did the duration to the first defibrillation. If cardiac arrests are happening in cities with high-rise buildings, it could take longer to defibrillate the patient because of the longer travel time.[120] A retrospective cohort study involving over 850,000 Medicare enrollees also revealed that, in comparison to black or Hispanic patients, a greater percentage of white patients were taken to the reference emergency department for the zip code following an acute event, such as CA. According to the American College of Emergency Medicine, EMS providers should provide transfer to the nearest suitable facility as a top priority. But compared to white patients, black and Hispanic patients in large United States cities were more likely to be sent to safety-net emergency rooms, that is, not to the closest referent emergency room for the zip code.[121] Such procedures could delay necessary post-resuscitation care, lowering overall odds of survival after OHCA, even if they might also be influenced by other variables, such as the facility where a patient has previously received care.

In-hospital management

In CA with STEMI, immediate coronary angiography and PCI lead to better results.[122] Therefore, emergent coronary angiography is advised for patients with OHCA who have STEMI, as well as for patients who have CS or recurrent ventricular arrhythmias.[123] In a recent multi-year national database analysis it was noted that women with CA post AMI, received less frequent coronary angiography (56.0% vs 66.2%), PCI (40.4% vs 49.7%), mechanical circulatory devices support (17.6% vs 22.0%), and CABG (8.3% vs 10.8%), with a longer median time to angiography.[124] Other studies in women with OHCA have also noted similar finding of less frequent coronary angiography (28% vs 50%), PCI (17% vs 30%), and CABG (0.4% vs 30%) in post-resuscitation treatment.[116,122,125] While limited, there appear to be gender differences in targeted temperature management (TTM) use.[126] TTM was employed less frequently in women in both non-shockable and non-shockable rhythms, according to a national database study conducted in the United States.[116] Compared to men, TTM was utilized less frequently in women (47% vs 61% $P<.01$), as shown by Winther-Jensen and colleagues.[125]

A retrospective analysis of hospitalizations following OHCA in California revealed that, while more life-sustaining treatments like percutaneous endoscopic gastrostomy tubes, tracheostomies, and, dialysis were administered to black and Hispanic patients, they received significantly fewer guideline-directed post resuscitation therapies (cardiac catheterization after ventricular fibrillation/tachycardia, therapeutic hypothermia). Also, black patients were more likely to be women with higher comorbidities and increased rates of neurologic and renal failure. Black patients underwent less coronary angiography and PCI.[127] Furthermore, it has been demonstrated that many hospitals treating the Hispanic/Latino community offer a lower level of guideline-directed TTM after OHCA.[128]

Outcomes

There are conflicting data on the impact of gender on survival after OHCA.[108,118,129] Women had lower unadjusted odds of survival, according to prior registry studies; however, on multivariate analysis, after controlling for therapy and baseline variables, women were linked to higher odds of survival.[118,129] The differences in baseline characteristics and interventions seen in the studies provide the most compelling explanation for the higher survival on multivariate analysis. In particular, women had lower rates of coronary angiography, PCI, and TTM; they were also older, less likely to have an

OHCA outside the home, and less frequently received bystander CPR, therefore, diminishing the sign of higher mortality in women.[130] It is possible that geographic difference in gender outcomes might exist in those experiencing AMI-CA. A Swedish study found that women had greater survival rates, and a Canadian study found no gender-specific variance in survival.[108,131] Disparities in prehospital care, risk factors, demography, and health care systems across different nations may account for the contradictory survival outcomes.

In the Cardiac Arrest Registry to Enhance Survival registry (2013–2017), of 250,000 patients, residents in census tracts with a preponderance of black people or those with low-to-middle-class incomes had a lower chance of surviving the OHCA after being released from the hospital or of surviving without suffering from a serious neurologic impairment. In these data they performed as well as their white, wealthier peers when it came to surviving until hospital admittance. The authors challenge the belief that poor survival rates in low-income and minority group areas are primarily caused by subpar CPR performance in the field.[113] According to Chan and colleagues hypothesis, survival differences based on race, ethnicity, and income might be connected to other, sporadically studied aspects of resuscitation care, like hospital post-resuscitation efforts and EMS procedures.[132]

To tackle the barriers in cardiac arrest disparities, it is important to implement public health initiatives to increase the number of women performing CPR as bystanders and to promptly send eligible women for internal defibrillator placement.[108] The lack of authentic women patient simulators could skew research and training in patient care.[105] The observed racial differences in CA outcomes may be reduced by optimizing baseline outpatient medical comorbidities and facilitating quick access to medical care during cardiac arrest. Regardless of gender and race, aggressive post-resuscitation care, which includes TTM and emergency coronary angiography, should be prioritized as it is likely to have positive effects.

FUTURE DIRECTIONS

There is a pressing need for future acute cardiovascular care research to develop strategies to modify social determinants of health. Social determinants of health are described as the conditions in an individual's environment that may affect health, quality of life, outcomes, and risks. This includes but is not limited to the individual's race, ethnicity, income, and health care access.[133] In recent literature, multiple studies have shown the effect of different components of social determinants of health on the outcomes of acute cardiovascular conditions.[48–50] Dupre and colleagues in their analysis noted AMI to be significantly higher among the unemployed (hazard ratio 1.35, 95% CI 1.10–1.66), and the risk increased incrementally with job losses highest being with 4 job losses when compared to no job loss.[134] This was further complemented by a large study in the Netherlands that observed a higher rate of mortality in the lowest income quartile as compared to the highest income quartile (hazard ratio 1.17, 95% CI 1.11–1.25).[135] They also were less likely to receive appropriate reperfusion strategies within the first 24 hours.[135] As described earlier, studies have noted racial disparities, especially among the non-white population who often have worse outcomes as compared to their counterparts. In summary, the current literature has repeatedly noted low economic status, less social support, reduced health care literacy, and limited health care access to be associated with increased CVDs and worse outcomes. Building upon this the American College of Cardiology/American Heart Association guidelines in 2019, published guidelines that recommended clinical evaluation of these determinants to help in the prevention of CVDs[136] (**Fig. 1**).

Individual Variations	Clinical Presentation	Management	Outcomes
• Physiological differences in sexes • Comorbidities • Social Determinants of health	• Physiological differences in sexes • Comorbidities • Social Determinants of health • Pre-hospital healthcare delivery • Healthcare access	• Comorbidities • Implicit biases • Social Determinants of health • Healthcare delivery	• Comorbidities • Implicit biases • Social Determinants of health • Healthcare delivery

Continuum of critically ill acute myocardial infarction conditions

• Atypical symptoms like shortness of breath, nausea, vomiting, atypical sites of pain apart from chest pain • Increased myocardial infarction with no obstructive coronary arteries and microcirculation changes • Racial disparities • Low income populations • Reduced healthcare literacy • Unemployment	• Individual variations *plus* • Poor healthcare access • Increased time to call EMS • Delays in FMC • Low priority of ambulance levels	• Lower likelihood of receiving guideline directed medical therapies • Lower rate of revascularization strategies like PCI and CABG • Longer door to balloon contact times • Lower rates of invasive hemodynamic monitoring and mechanical circulatory support utilization • Lower utilization of targeted temperature management strategies • Higher rates of misdiagnosis	• Increased morbidity and mortality rates • Higher readmission rates • Increase adverse outcomes

Fig. 1. Health care disparities in the continuum of care for patients with acute myocardial infarction. CABG, coronary artery bypass grafting; EMS, emergency medical services; FMC, first medical contact; PCI, percutaneous coronary intervention.

Recently there also has been focus on the utility and application of standardized AMI protocols to reduce gender gaps.[137] In one such analysis, researchers at the Cleveland Clinic developed a comprehensive 4-step STEMI protocol that used standardized approach to treat patients with STEMI. They observed reduction in variations of care delivered to men and women along with improved outcomes for women.[138] Additional multidisciplinary teams for cardiogenic shock and cardiac arrest may aid in standardization of health care delivery to women and minority populations.[139,140] In addition, there remains a significant under-representation of women and racial minorities in the cardiovascular clinical trials as described above. This lack of diversity presents a dominant clinical concern apart from being a social issue as it limits generalizability and evaluation of various therapies for these vulnerable subpopulations. There are multiple steps to alleviate these issues ranging from strengthening community engagement with pragmatic trial designs, having diverse clinical investigators and staff to stratification of efficacy and adverse events outcomes into different subgroups. Although the NIH and the United States Food and Drug Administration have established guidelines to increase diversity of participants significant work remains to be done.

SUMMARY

In the contemporary era, there remain disparities in management and outcomes of patients with AMI. Women and racial minorities continue to have worse outcomes highlighting the need to make health care more accessible and equitable. Despite national and societal efforts, clinical trials continue to have under representation of women and minorities, further limiting the full range of benefits from novel therapies for this population. An in-depth, comprehensive, and integrated understanding of the gender and racial disparities with particular attention to their social determinants of health to help in CVD prevention and appropriate secondary prevention after incident AMI event are the need of the hour.[141]

CLINICS CARE POINTS

- Clinicians need to carefully evaluate implicit and explicit biases in the care of women and racial minorities.
- Attention to recruitment of women and racial minorities into clinical trials and studies is urgently needed.

DISCLOSURE

C.E. Ventetuolo reports consulting fees from Regeneron, Janssen, and Merck, outside of the submitted work. J.D. Abbott reports consulting fees from Abbott, Medtronic, Penumbra. Research Boston Scientific, Shockwave, Med Alliance, Microport. All other authors do not have any financial disclosures to report.

REFERENCES

1. World Health Organization (WHO). Fact sheet: cardiovascular disease. 2021. Available at: https://www.who.int/en/news-room/fact-sheets/detail/cardiovascular-diseases-(cvds). [Accessed 17 October 2023].
2. Available at: https://www.cdc.gov/nchs/fastats/leading-causes-of-death.htm. [Accessed 2 November 2023].
3. Vallabhajosyula S, El Hajj SC, Bell MR, et al. Intravascular ultrasound, optical coherence tomography, and fractional flow reserve use in acute myocardial infarction. Catheter Cardiovasc Interv 2020;96(1):E59–66.
4. Vallabhajosyula S, Prasad A, Dunlay SM, et al. Utilization of palliative care for cardiogenic shock complicating acute myocardial infarction: a 15-year national perspective on trends, disparities, predictors, and outcomes. J Am Heart Assoc 2019;8(15):e011954.
5. Vallabhajosyula S, Ya'Qoub L, Dunlay SM, et al. Sex disparities in acute kidney injury complicating acute myocardial infarction with cardiogenic shock. ESC Heart Fail 2019;6(4):874–7.
6. Benjamin EJ, Muntner P, Alonso A, et al. Heart disease and stroke statistics-2019 update: a report from the American heart association. Circulation 2019; 139(10):e56–528.
7. Vallabhajosyula S, Verghese D, Desai VK, et al. Sex differences in acute cardiovascular care: a review and needs assessment. Cardiovasc Res 2022;118(3): 667–85.
8. Machanahalli BA, Ismayl M, Butt DN, et al. Trends, outcomes, and management of acute myocardial infarction in patients with chronic viral hepatitis. Hosp Pract (1995) 2022;50(3):236–43.
9. Amick BC. Society and health. USA: Oxford University Press; 1995.
10. Braunwald E. Evolution of the management of acute myocardial infarction: a 20th century saga. Lancet 1998;352(9142):1771–4.

11. Stone CT, Vanzant FR. Heart disease as seen in a southern clinic: a clinical and pathologic survey. J Am Med Assoc 1927;89(18):1473–80.

12. Iribarren C, Tolstykh I, Somkin CP, et al. Sex and racial/ethnic disparities in outcomes after acute myocardial infarction: a cohort study among members of a large integrated health care delivery system in northern California. Arch Intern Med 2005;165(18):2105–13.

13. Peek ME, Cargill A, Huang ES. Diabetes health disparities. Med Care Res Rev 2007;64(5_suppl):101S–56S.

14. Effect of race on the presentation and management of patients with acute chest pain. Ann Intern Med 1993;118(8):593–601.

15. Yarzebski J, Bujor CF, Lessard D, et al. Recent and temporal trends (1975 to 1999) in the treatment, hospital, and long-term outcomes of hispanic and non-hispanic white patients hospitalized with acute myocardial infarction: a population-based perspective. Am Heart J 2004/04/01/2004;147(4):690–7.

16. Albert MA, Ayanian JZ, Silbaugh TS, et al. Early results of Massachusetts healthcare reform on racial, ethnic, and socioeconomic disparities in cardiovascular care. Circulation 2014;129(24):2528–38.

17. Glance LG, Thirukumaran CP, Shippey E, et al. Impact of medicaid expansion on disparities in revascularization in patients hospitalized with acute myocardial infarction. PLoS One 2020;15(12):e0243385.

18. Wadhera RK, Bhatt DL, Wang TY, et al. Association of state medicaid expansion with quality of care and outcomes for low-income patients hospitalized with acute myocardial infarction. JAMA Cardiol 2019;4(2):120–7.

19. Herman B, Greiser E, Pohlabeln H. A sex difference in short-term survival after initial acute myocardial infarction. The MONICA-Bremen Acute Myocardial Infarction Register, 1985-1990. Eur Heart J 1997;18(6):963–70.

20. Demirovic J, Blackburn H, McGovern PG, et al. Sex differences in early mortality after acute myocardial infarction (the Minnesota Heart Survey). Am J Cardiol 1995;75(16):1096–101.

21. Blankstein R, Ward RP, Arnsdorf M, et al. Female gender is an independent predictor of operative mortality after coronary artery bypass graft surgery. Circulation 2005;112(9_supplement):I323–7.

22. Available at: https://grants.nih.gov/grants/funding/women_min/guidelines_update.htm. [Accessed 1 November, 2023].

23. Miller LR, Marks C, Becker JB, et al. Considering sex as a biological variable in preclinical research. Faseb J 2017;31(1):29–34.

24. Gong IY, Tan NS, Ali SH, et al. Temporal trends of women enrollment in major cardiovascular randomized clinical trials. Can J Cardiol 2019;35(5):653–60.

25. Tsang W, Alter DA, Wijeysundera HC, et al. The impact of cardiovascular disease prevalence on women's enrollment in landmark randomized cardiovascular trials: a systematic review. J Gen Intern Med 2012;27(1):93–8.

26. Khan MS, Shahid I, Siddiqi TJ, et al. Ten-year trends in enrollment of women and minorities in pivotal trials supporting recent US food and drug administration approval of novel cardiometabolic drugs. J Am Heart Assoc 2020;9(11):e015594.

27. Prasanna A, Miller HN, Wu Y, et al. Recruitment of black adults into cardiovascular disease trials. J Am Heart Assoc 2021;10(17):e021108.

28. Milner KA, Vaccarino V, Arnold AL, et al. Gender and age differences in chief complaints of acute myocardial infarction (Worcester Heart Attack Study). Am J Cardiol 2004;93(5):606–8.

29. Brush JE Jr, Krumholz HM, Greene EJ, et al. Sex differences in symptom phenotypes among patients with acute myocardial infarction. Circ Cardiovasc Qual Outcomes 2020;13(2):e005948.
30. Ju Young S, Martin R, Bryant Howren M. Influence of assessment methods on reports of gender differences in AMI symptoms. West J Nurs Res 2009;31(5): 553–68.
31. Nairz F, Meisinger C, Kirchberger I, et al. Association of sleep disturbances within 4 weeks prior to incident acute myocardial infarction and long-term survival in male and female patients: an observational study from the MONICA/KORA Myocardial Infarction Registry. BMC Cardiovasc Disord 2018;18(1):235.
32. Stehli J, Dinh D, Dagan M, et al. Sex differences in prehospital delays in patients with ST-segment-elevation myocardial infarction undergoing percutaneous coronary intervention. J Am Heart Assoc 2021;10(13):e019938.
33. Coventry LL, Bremner AP, Jacobs IG, et al. Myocardial infarction: sex differences in symptoms reported to emergency dispatch. Prehosp Emerg Care Apr--Jun 2013;17(2):193–202.
34. Weininger D, Cordova JP, Wilson E, et al. Delays to hospital presentation in women and men with ST-segment elevation myocardial infarction: a multi-center analysis of patients hospitalized in New York city. Therapeut Clin Risk Manag 2022;18:1–9.
35. Barcena de Arellano ML, Pozdniakova S, Kühl AA, et al. Sex differences in the aging human heart: decreased sirtuins, pro-inflammatory shift and reduced anti-oxidative defense. Aging (Albany NY) 2019;11(7):1918–33.
36. Fiechter M, Haider A, Bengs S, et al. Sex differences in the association between inflammation and ischemic heart disease. Thromb Haemostasis 2019;119(9): 1471–80.
37. Bairey Merz CN, Shaw LJ, Reis SE, et al. Insights from the NHLBI-Sponsored Women's Ischemia Syndrome Evaluation (WISE) Study: Part II: gender differences in presentation, diagnosis, and outcome with regard to gender-based pathophysiology of atherosclerosis and macrovascular and microvascular coronary disease. J Am Coll Cardiol 2006;47(3 Suppl):S21–9.
38. Berger JS, Elliott L, Gallup D, et al. Sex differences in mortality following acute coronary syndromes. JAMA 2009;302(8):874–82.
39. Smilowitz NR, Sampson BA, Abrecht CR, et al. Women have less severe and extensive coronary atherosclerosis in fatal cases of ischemic heart disease: an autopsy study. Am Heart J 2011;161(4):681–8.
40. Vaccarino V, Parsons L, Every NR, et al. Sex-based differences in early mortality after myocardial infarction. National Registry of Myocardial Infarction 2 Participants. N Engl J Med 1999;341(4):217–25.
41. Han SH, Bae JH, Holmes DR Jr, et al. Sex differences in atheroma burden and endothelial function in patients with early coronary atherosclerosis. Eur Heart J 2008;29(11):1359–69.
42. Pasupathy S, Air T, Dreyer RP, et al. Systematic review of patients presenting with suspected myocardial infarction and nonobstructive coronary arteries. Circulation 2015;131(10):861–70.
43. Tamis-Holland JE, Jneid H, Reynolds HR, et al. Contemporary diagnosis and management of patients with myocardial infarction in the absence of obstructive coronary artery disease: a scientific statement from the American heart association. Circulation 2019;139(18):e891–908.
44. Hu FB, Grodstein F, Hennekens CH, et al. Age at natural menopause and risk of cardiovascular disease. Arch Intern Med 1999;159(10):1061–6.

45. Groban L, Lindsey SH, Wang H, et al. Chapter 5 - sex and gender differences in cardiovascular disease. In: Neigh GN, Mitzelfelt MM, editors. Sex differences in physiology. Cambridge, MA: Academic Press; 2016. p. 61–87.

46. Choo HY, Ferree MM. Practicing intersectionality in sociological research: a critical analysis of inclusions, interactions, and institutions in the study of inequalities. Socio Theor 2010;28(2):129–49.

47. Bowleg L. The problem with the phrase women and minorities: intersectionality-an important theoretical framework for public health. Am J Publ Health 2012; 102(7):1267–73.

48. Stabellini N, Dmukauskas M, Bittencourt MS, et al. Social determinants of health and racial disparities in cardiac events in breast cancer. J Natl Compr Cancer Netw 2023;21(7):705–14.e17.

49. Matsushita M, Shirakabe A, Hata N, et al. Social determinants are crucial factors in the long-term prognosis of severely decompensated acute heart failure in patients over 75 years of age. J Cardiol 2018;72(2):140–8.

50. Javed Z, Haisum Maqsood M, Yahya T, et al. Race, racism, and cardiovascular health: applying a social determinants of health framework to racial/ethnic disparities in cardiovascular disease. Circ Cardiovasc Qual Outcomes 2022; 15(1):e007917.

51. Williams DR, Jackson PB. Social sources of racial disparities in health. Health Aff (Millwood) 2005;24(2):325–34.

52. Mobley LR, Root ED, Finkelstein EA, et al. Environment, obesity, and cardiovascular disease risk in low-income women. Am J Prev Med 2006;30(4):327–32.

53. Kanchi R, Perlman SE, Chernov C, et al. Gender and race disparities in cardiovascular disease risk factors among New York city adults: New York city health and nutrition examination survey (NYC HANES) 2013-2014. J Urban Health 2018;95(6):801–12.

54. Rosen SE, Henry S, Bond R, et al. Sex-specific disparities in risk factors for coronary heart disease. Curr Atherosclerosis Rep 2015;17(8):49.

55. Graham G. Racial and ethnic differences in acute coronary syndrome and myocardial infarction within the United States: from demographics to outcomes. Clin Cardiol 2016;39(5):299–306.

56. Arora S, Stouffer GA, Kucharska-Newton A, et al. Fifteen-year trends in management and outcomes of non-ST-segment-elevation myocardial infarction among black and white patients: the ARIC community surveillance study, 2000-2014. J Am Heart Assoc 2018;7(19):e010203.

57. Sonel AF, Good CB, Mulgund J, et al. Racial variations in treatment and outcomes of black and white patients with high-risk non-ST-elevation acute coronary syndromes: insights from CRUSADE (can rapid risk stratification of unstable angina patients suppress adverse outcomes with early implementation of the ACC/AHA guidelines?). Circulation 2005;111(10):1225–32.

58. Canto JG, Allison JJ, Kiefe CI, et al. Relation of race and sex to the use of reperfusion therapy in Medicare beneficiaries with acute myocardial infarction. N Engl J Med 2000;342(15):1094–100.

59. Vaccarino V, Rathore SS, Wenger NK, et al. Sex and racial differences in the management of acute myocardial infarction, 1994 through 2002. N Engl J Med 2005;353(7):671–82.

60. Peterson ED, Shah BR, Parsons L, et al. Trends in quality of care for patients with acute myocardial infarction in the National Registry of Myocardial Infarction from 1990 to 2006. Am Heart J 2008;156(6):1045–55.

61. Edmund Anstey D, Li S, Thomas L, et al. Race and sex differences in management and outcomes of patients after ST-elevation and non-ST-elevation myocardial infarct: results from the NCDR. Clin Cardiol 2016;39(10):585–95.

62. Mosca L, Linfante AH, Benjamin EJ, et al. National study of physician awareness and adherence to cardiovascular disease prevention guidelines. Circulation 2005;111(4):499–510.

63. Gulati M, Shaw LJ, Bairey Merz CN. Myocardial ischemia in women: lessons from the NHLBI WISE study. Clin Cardiol 2012;35(3):141–8.

64. Gu A, Kamat S, Argulian E. Trends and disparities in statin use and low-density lipoprotein cholesterol levels among US patients with diabetes, 1999-2014. Diabetes Res Clin Pract 2018;139:1–10.

65. Ngo-Metzger Q, Zuvekas S, Shafer P, et al. Statin use in the U.S. For secondary prevention of cardiovascular disease remains suboptimal. J Am Board Fam Med Nov-Dec 2019;32(6):807–17.

66. Peters SAE, Colantonio LD, Zhao H, et al. Sex differences in high-intensity statin use following myocardial infarction in the United States. J Am Coll Cardiol 2018;71(16):1729–37.

67. Nanna MG, Wang TY, Xiang Q, et al. Sex differences in the use of statins in community practice. Circ Cardiovasc Qual Outcomes 2019;12(8):e005562.

68. Rodriguez F, Foody JM, Wang Y, et al. Young hispanic women experience higher in-hospital mortality following an acute myocardial infarction. J Am Heart Assoc 2015;4(9):e002089.

69. Epps KC, Holper EM, Selzer F, et al. Sex differences in outcomes following percutaneous coronary intervention according to age. Circ Cardiovasc Qual Outcomes 2016;9(2 Suppl 1):S16–25.

70. Gupta A, Barrabes JA, Strait K, et al. Sex differences in timeliness of reperfusion in young patients with ST-segment-elevation myocardial infarction by initial electrocardiographic characteristics. J Am Heart Assoc 2018;7(6). https://doi.org/10.1161/jaha.117.007021.

71. Gamboa CM, Colantonio LD, Brown TM, et al. Race-sex differences in statin use and low-density lipoprotein cholesterol control among people with diabetes mellitus in the reasons for geographic and racial differences in stroke study. J Am Heart Assoc 2017;6(5). https://doi.org/10.1161/jaha.116.004264.

72. Safford MM, Gamboa CM, Durant RW, et al. Race-sex differences in the management of hyperlipidemia: the REasons for geographic and racial differences in stroke study. Am J Prev Med 2015;48(5):520–7.

73. Hess CN, Kaltenbach LA, Doll JA, et al. Race and sex differences in post-myocardial infarction angina frequency and risk of 1-year unplanned rehospitalization. Circulation 2017;135(6):532–43.

74. Collins SD, Torguson R, Gaglia MA Jr, et al. Does black ethnicity influence the development of stent thrombosis in the drug-eluting stent era? Circulation 2010;122(11):1085–90.

75. Mehta RH, Parsons L, Rao SV, et al. Association of bleeding and in-hospital mortality in black and white patients with st-segment-elevation myocardial infarction receiving reperfusion. Circulation 2012;125(14):1727–34.

76. De Luca G, Suryapranata H, Dambrink JH, et al. Sex-related differences in outcome after ST-segment elevation myocardial infarction treated by primary angioplasty: data from the Zwolle Myocardial Infarction study. Am Heart J 2004;148(5):852–6.

77. Okunrintemi V, Valero-Elizondo J, Patrick B, et al. Gender differences in patient-reported outcomes among adults with atherosclerotic cardiovascular disease. J Am Heart Assoc 2018;7(24):e010498.

78. Lansky AJ, Pietras C, Costa RA, et al. Gender differences in outcomes after primary angioplasty versus primary stenting with and without abciximab for acute myocardial infarction: results of the Controlled Abciximab and Device Investigation to Lower Late Angioplasty Complications (CADILLAC) trial. Circulation 2005;111(13):1611–8.

79. Ahmed B, Piper WD, Malenka D, et al. Significantly improved vascular complications among women undergoing percutaneous coronary intervention: a report from the Northern New England Percutaneous Coronary Intervention Registry. Circ Cardiovasc Interv 2009;2(5):423–9.

80. Cai A, Dillon C, Hillegass WB, et al. Risk of major adverse cardiovascular events and major hemorrhage among white and black patients undergoing percutaneous coronary intervention. J Am Heart Assoc 2019;8(22):e012874.

81. Ziaeian B, Kominski GF, Ong MK, et al. National differences in trends for heart failure hospitalizations by sex and race/ethnicity. Circ Cardiovasc Qual Outcomes 2017;10(7). https://doi.org/10.1161/circoutcomes.116.003552.

82. Sabatine MS, Blake GJ, Drazner MH, et al. Influence of race on death and ischemic complications in patients with non-ST-elevation acute coronary syndromes despite modern, protocol-guided treatment. Circulation 2005;111(10): 1217–24.

83. Vallabhajosyula S, Ya'Qoub L, Singh M, et al. Sex disparities in the management and outcomes of cardiogenic shock complicating acute myocardial infarction in the young. Circ Heart Fail 2020;13(10):e007154.

84. Kousa O, Addasi Y, Machanahalli Balakrishna A, et al. Elevated troponin in patients with acute gastrointestinal bleeding: prevalence, predictors and outcomes. Future Cardiol 2022;18(9):709–17.

85. Spaulding C. Racial, ethnic, and sex disparities in cardiogenic shock due to STEMI: act NOW. JACC Cardiovasc Interv 2021;14(6):661–3.

86. Vallabhajosyula S, Dunlay SM, Prasad A, et al. Acute noncardiac organ failure in acute myocardial infarction with cardiogenic shock. J Am Coll Cardiol 2019; 73(14):1781–91.

87. Vallabhajosyula S, Vallabhajosyula S, Dunlay SM, et al. Sex and gender disparities in the management and outcomes of acute myocardial infarction-cardiogenic shock in older adults. Mayo Clin Proc 2020;95(9):1916–27.

88. Ton VK, Kanwar MK, Li B, et al. Impact of female sex on cardiogenic shock outcomes: a cardiogenic shock working group report. JACC Heart Fail 2023. https://doi.org/10.1016/j.jchf.2023.09.025.

89. Koeth O, Zahn R, Heer T, et al. Gender differences in patients with acute ST-elevation myocardial infarction complicated by cardiogenic shock. Clin Res Cardiol 2009;98(12):781–6.

90. Vallabhajosyula S, Vallabhajosyula S, Dunlay SM, et al. Sex and gender disparities in the management and outcomes of acute myocardial infarction-cardiogenic shock in older adults. Mayo Clin Proc 2020;95(9):1916–27.

91. Vallabhajosyula S, Ya'Qoub L, Dunlay SM, et al. Sex disparities in acute kidney injury complicating acute myocardial infarction with cardiogenic shock. ESC Heart Failure 2019;6(4):874–7.

92. Vallabhajosyula S, Prasad A, Sandhu GS, et al. Ten-year trends, predictors and outcomes of mechanical circulatory support in percutaneous coronary

intervention for acute myocardial infarction with cardiogenic shock. EuroIntervention 2021;16(15):e1254–61.

93. Vallabhajosyula S, Arora S, Sakhuja A, et al. Trends, predictors, and outcomes of temporary mechanical circulatory support for postcardiac surgery cardiogenic shock. Am J Cardiol 2019;123(3):489–97.

94. Joseph SM, Brisco MA, Colvin M, et al. Women with cardiogenic shock derive greater benefit from early mechanical circulatory support: an update from the cVAD registry. J Intervent Cardiol 2016;29(3):248–56.

95. Isorni M-A, Aissaoui N, Angoulvant D, et al. Temporal trends in clinical characteristics and management according to sex in patients with cardiogenic shock after acute myocardial infarction: the FAST-MI programme. Archives of Cardiovascular Diseases 2018;111(10):555–63.

96. Ya'qoub L, Lemor A, Dabbagh M, et al. Racial, ethnic, and sex disparities in patients with STEMI and cardiogenic shock. JACC Cardiovasc Interv 2021;14(6): 653–60.

97. Raheja H, Waheed M, Harris C, et al. Racial disparities in the use of mechanical circulatory support devices in cardiogenic shock. Eur Heart J 2021; 42(Supplement_1). https://doi.org/10.1093/eurheartj/ehab724.1484.

98. Vallabhajosyula S, Dunlay SM, Barsness GW, et al. Sex disparities in the use and outcomes of temporary mechanical circulatory support for acute myocardial infarction-cardiogenic shock. CJC Open 2020;2(6):462–72.

99. Wang AS, Nemeth S, Vinogradsky A, et al. Disparities in the treatment of cardiogenic shock: does sex matter? Eur J Cardio Thorac Surg 2022;62(6). https://doi.org/10.1093/ejcts/ezac543.

100. Sukhera J, Watling C. A framework for integrating implicit bias recognition into health professions education. Acad Med 2018;93(1):35–40.

101. Patlolla SH, Shankar A, Sundaragiri PR, et al. Racial and ethnic disparities in the management and outcomes of cardiogenic shock complicating acute myocardial infarction. Am J Emerg Med 2022;51:202–9.

102. Li Y, Cai X, Glance LG. Disparities in 30-day rehospitalization rates among Medicare skilled nursing facility residents by race and site of care. Med Care 2015; 53(12):1058–65.

103. Roger VL, Go AS, Lloyd-Jones DM, et al. Executive summary: heart disease and stroke statistics–2012 update: a report from the American Heart Association. Circulation 2012;125(1):188–97.

104. Deakin CD. The chain of survival: not all links are equal. Resuscitation 2018; 126:80–2.

105. Kramer CE, Wilkins MS, Davies JM, et al. Does the sex of a simulated patient affect CPR? Resuscitation 2015;86:82–7.

106. Wallen R, Tunnage B, Wells S. The 12-lead ECG in the emergency medical service setting: how electrode placement and paramedic gender are experienced by women. Emerg Med J 2014;31(10):851–2.

107. Blewer AL, McGovern SK, Schmicker RH, et al. Gender disparities among adult recipients of bystander cardiopulmonary resuscitation in the public. Circ Cardiovasc Qual Outcomes 2018;11(8):e004710.

108. Safdar B, Stolz U, Stiell IG, et al. Differential survival for men and women from out-of-hospital cardiac arrest varies by age: results from the OPALS study. Acad Emerg Med 2014;21(12):1503–11.

109. Krammel M, Schnaubelt S, Weidenauer D, et al. Gender and age-specific aspects of awareness and knowledge in basic life support. PLoS One 2018; 13(6):e0198918.

110. Perman SM, Shelton SK, Knoepke C, et al. Public perceptions on why women receive less bystander cardiopulmonary resuscitation than men in out-of-hospital cardiac arrest. Circulation 2019;139(8):1060–8.
111. Sasson C, Magid DJ, Chan P, et al. Association of neighborhood characteristics with bystander-initiated CPR. N Engl J Med 2012;367(17):1607–15.
112. York Cornwell E, Currit A. Racial and social disparities in bystander support during medical emergencies on US streets. Am J Publ Health 2016;106(6): 1049–51.
113. Naim MY, Griffis HM, Burke RV, et al. Race/ethnicity and neighborhood characteristics are associated with bystander cardiopulmonary resuscitation in pediatric out-of-hospital cardiac arrest in the United States: a study from cares. J Am Heart Assoc 2019;8(14):e012637.
114. Moon S, Bobrow BJ, Vadeboncoeur TF, et al. Disparities in bystander CPR provision and survival from out-of-hospital cardiac arrest according to neighborhood ethnicity. Am J Emerg Med 2014;32(9):1041–5.
115. Blewer AL, Schmicker RH, Morrison LJ, et al. Variation in bystander cardiopulmonary resuscitation delivery and subsequent survival from out-of-hospital cardiac arrest based on neighborhood-level ethnic characteristics. Circulation 2020;141(1):34–41.
116. Kim LK, Looser P, Swaminathan RV, et al. Sex-based disparities in incidence, treatment, and outcomes of cardiac arrest in the United States, 2003-2012. J Am Heart Assoc 2016;5(6). https://doi.org/10.1161/jaha.116.003704.
117. Yiu KH, de Graaf FR, Schuijf JD, et al. Age- and gender-specific differences in the prognostic value of CT coronary angiography. Heart 2012;98(3):232–7.
118. Akahane M, Ogawa T, Koike S, et al. The effects of sex on out-of-hospital cardiac arrest outcomes. Am J Med 2011;124(4):325–33.
119. Hsia RY, Huang D, Mann NC, et al. A US national study of the association between income and ambulance response time in cardiac arrest. JAMA Netw Open 2018;1(7):e185202.
120. Starks MA, Schmicker RH, Peterson ED, et al. Association of neighborhood demographics with out-of-hospital cardiac arrest treatment and outcomes: where you live may matter. JAMA Cardiol 2017;2(10):1110–8.
121. Hanchate AD, Paasche-Orlow MK, Baker WE, et al. Association of race/ethnicity with emergency department destination of emergency medical services transport. JAMA Netw Open 2019;2(9):e1910816.
122. Geri G, Dumas F, Bougouin W, et al. Immediate percutaneous coronary intervention is associated with improved short- and long-term survival after out-of-hospital cardiac arrest. Circ Cardiovasc Interv 2015;8(10). https://doi.org/10.1161/circinterventions.114.002303.
123. Correction to: Part 8: post-cardiac arrest care: 2015 American heart association guidelines update for cardiopulmonary resuscitation and emergency cardiovascular care. Circulation 2017;136(10):e197.
124. Verghese D, Patlolla SH, Cheungpasitporn W, et al. Sex disparities in management and outcomes of cardiac arrest complicating acute myocardial infarction in the United States. Resuscitation 2022;172:92–100.
125. Winther-Jensen M, Hassager C, Kjaergaard J, et al. Women have a worse prognosis and undergo fewer coronary angiographies after out-of-hospital cardiac arrest than men. Eur Heart J Acute Cardiovasc Care 2018;7(5):414–22.
126. Wigginton JG, Pepe PE, Idris AH. Rationale for routine and immediate administration of intravenous estrogen for all critically ill and injured patients. Crit Care Med 2010;38(10 Suppl):S620–9.

127. Subramaniam AV, Patlolla SH, Cheungpasitporn W, et al. Racial and ethnic disparities in management and outcomes of cardiac arrest complicating acute myocardial infarction. J Am Heart Assoc 2021;10(11):e019907.
128. Morris NA, Mazzeffi M, McArdle P, et al. Hispanic/latino-serving hospitals provide less targeted temperature management following out-of-hospital cardiac arrest. J Am Heart Assoc 2021;10(24):e017773.
129. Wissenberg M, Hansen CM, Folke F, et al. Survival after out-of-hospital cardiac arrest in relation to sex: a nationwide registry-based study. Resuscitation 2014; 85(9):1212–8.
130. Adielsson A, Hollenberg J, Karlsson T, et al. Increase in survival and bystander CPR in out-of-hospital shockable arrhythmia: bystander CPR and female gender are predictors of improved outcome. Experiences from Sweden in an 18-year perspective. Heart 2011;97(17):1391–6.
131. Herlitz J, Engdahl J, Svensson L, et al. Is female sex associated with increased survival after out-of-hospital cardiac arrest? Resuscitation 2004;60(2):197–203.
132. Chan PS, McNally B, Vellano K, et al. Association of neighborhood race and income with survival after out-of-hospital cardiac arrest. J Am Heart Assoc 2020; 9(4):e014178.
133. Spruce L. Back to basics: social determinants of health. AORN J 2019; 110(1):60–9.
134. Dupre ME, George LK, Liu G, et al. The cumulative effect of unemployment on risks for acute myocardial infarction. Arch Intern Med 2012;172(22):1731–7.
135. Yong CM, Abnousi F, Asch SM, et al. Socioeconomic inequalities in quality of care and outcomes among patients with acute coronary syndrome in the modern era of drug eluting stents. J Am Heart Assoc 2014;3(6):e001029.
136. Arnett DK, Blumenthal RS, Albert MA, et al. 2019 ACC/AHA guideline on the primary prevention of cardiovascular disease: a report of the American College of Cardiology/American heart association task force on clinical practice guidelines. Circulation 2019;140(11):e596–646.
137. Solola Nussbaum S, Henry S, Yong Celina M, et al. Sex-specific considerations in the presentation, diagnosis, and management of ischemic heart disease. J Am Coll Cardiol 2022/04/12 2022;79(14):1398–406.
138. Huded Chetan P, Johnson M, Kravitz K, et al. 4-Step protocol for disparities in STEMI care and outcomes in women. J Am Coll Cardiol 2018/05/15 2018; 71(19):2122–32.
139. Vallabhajosyula S, Verghese D, Henry TD, et al. Contemporary management of concomitant cardiac arrest and cardiogenic shock complicating myocardial infarction. Mayo Clin Proc 2022;97(12):2333–54.
140. Tehrani BN, Sherwood MW, Rosner C, et al. A standardized and regionalized Network of care for cardiogenic shock. JACC Heart Fail 2022;10(10):768–81.
141. Gulati R, Behfar A, Narula J, et al. Acute myocardial infarction in young individuals. Mayo Clin Proc 2020;95(1):136–56.

Race, Ethnicity, and Gender Disparities in the Management and Outcomes of Critically Ill Adults with Acute Stroke

Fadar Oliver Otite, MD, SM[a],*, Nicholas Morris, MD[b]

KEYWORDS

- Acute ischemic stroke • Intensive care • Intravenous thrombolysis
- Mechanical thrombectomy • Disparity

KEY POINTS

- Racial, ethnicity and sex disparities are pervasive in the evaluation and acute care of ischemic stroke patients.
- Administration of intravenous thrombolysis and mechanical thrombectomy are the most critical steps in ischemic stroke treatment but compared to White patients, ischemic stroke patients from minority racial and ethnic groups are less likely to receive these potentially life-saving interventions.
- Sex and racial disparities in intracerebral hemorrhage or subarachnoid hemorrhage treatment have not been well studied.

INTRODUCTION

Stroke is the second leading cause of death and disability globally,[1,2] but marked disparity in incidence and outcome exists by race/ethnicity and by sex.[3] In the United States, stroke affects approximately 795,000 people annually but approximately equal to 55,000 excess strokes occur in women compared to men.[3] Stroke is the third leading cause of death in women in the United States compared to fifth in men.[4] In 2020, stroke was the underlying cause of 160,264 deaths in the United States,[3] and 56.5% of these deaths were in women.[3] Minority racial groups such as Black individuals have a disproportionately greater incidence and mortality from stroke when compared to non-Hispanic White individuals.[3] Variations in the acute and critical care of patients

[a] Cerebrovascular Division, Upstate Neurological Institute, Syracuse, NY, USA; [b] Neurocritical Care Division, Department of Neurology, University of Maryland, Baltimore, MD, USA
* Corresponding author. Department of Neurology, SUNY Upstate Medical University, 750 East Adams Street, Syracuse, NY 13210.
E-mail address: otitef@upstate.edu

Crit Care Clin 40 (2024) 709–740
https://doi.org/10.1016/j.ccc.2024.05.006   criticalcare.theclinics.com

with stroke by demographic factors may contribute to some of these differences in outcome. This review highlights key areas of disparities in the acute and critical care management of patients with stroke.

Race/ethnicity is not based on genotypic differences but implies a social construct based on phenotype, ethnicity, or other indicators of social differentiation that results in varying access to power and social and economic resources.[5] Therefore, our reference to race/ethnicity should be viewed within this framework. On the other hand, "sex" differences in the context of stroke encompasses biological/pathophysiological differences in stroke between male and female patients and gender differences imply sociocultural factors, such as education, power, and financial status that also influence stroke presentation and outcome.[6] Because it may be impossible to clearly delineate the contribution of biologic versus sociocultural factors to differences in stroke risk/presentation/management, our reference to "men" or "women" and "male" or "female" in this study assumes a combination of these biological and sociocultural factors.

In the United States, 87% of all strokes are ischemic stroke, 10% are intracerebral hemorrhage (ICH) while 3% are secondary to subarachnoid hemorrhage (SAH).[3] Because the paradigm for in-hospital management differs significantly between acute ischemic stroke (AIS) and hemorrhagic strokes (ICH and SAH), we describe demographic disparities separately for each subtype.

ACUTE ISCHEMIC STROKE
Disparities in Incidence

Stroke mortality is the product of incidence and case fatality rate,[7] so understanding demographic disparities in stroke incidence is critical to deciphering racial and/or sex disparities in stroke outcome. Globally, the lifetime risk of stroke is 25%, and this does not differ significantly between men and women.[8] However, within the United States, women may have a greater lifetime risk of stroke compared to men[9,10] likely because women live longer than men and stroke risk increases with age. The age-standardized incidence of AIS is approximately 30% higher in men compared to that of women.[11] But sex differences in the incidence of AIS vary across the age spectrum with higher incidence in women compared to men in young adults aged less than 35 years,[12] higher incidence in men in middle age, and overall similar/or higher incidence in women in older individuals aged 75 or older to 80 years.[11,13,14]

Black individuals in the United States have age and sex-standardized AIS incidence that is approximately equal to 1.5 times to 2.5 times that of White individuals.[15–17] Data from the Northern Manhattan Study (NOMAS) also report up to 2 times greater risk of stroke in Hispanic individuals compared to White US residents.[18] Whereas older studies from some cohorts suggest that the racial gaps may be more prominent in middle-aged individuals,[7,17] more recent data from NOMAS suggests that the AIS incidence gap may be driven mainly by higher incidence in older women aged older than 70 years.[19]

Differences in Stroke Subtypes and Stroke Severity

Partly because of older age of onset, cardioembolic strokes such as from atrial fibrillation (AF) tend to be more prevalent in women.[20] AIS due to cardioembolic etiologies are notoriously more severe and carry higher mortality risk compared to other AIS subtypes.[21] In contrast, AIS due to intracranial atherosclerosis disease (ICAD) may not show any sex predilection,[22] but extracranial large vessel atherosclerosis extracranial atherosclerotic disease (ECAD) may be more common in men.[22–24]

When looking at incidence data, most AIS subtypes occur at increased frequency in Black compared to White individuals,[19,25,26] but because of a disproportionately greater incidence of lacunar AIS in Black patients,[19] a greater percentage of AIS in Black patients may be lacunar when compared to White patients. In the Greater Cincinnati Northern Kentucky Stroke Study, lacunar strokes and AIS of undetermined source were twice as common, ECAD 40% more common and cardioembolic AIS just as common in Black compared to White individuals.[25] Older data from NOMAS also suggest that cardioembolic AIS were just as common in Hispanic and Black individuals compared to White individuals,[26] but more recent data from the same cohort suggest cardioembolic, lacunar, and ICAD AIS may actually be more common in Black and Hispanic compared to White individuals, while those from ECAD occurred less frequently in Black compared to White and Hispanic individuals.[19] In a cross-sectional analysis of 6,130,481 individuals evaluated with carotid Doppler ultrasound in 49 states of the United States over the period 2005 to 2019, the relative risk of high-grade carotid stenosis, defined as peak systolic velocity of 230 cm/s or greater was 60% lower in Black, 40% lower in Hispanic individuals, and 53% greater in Native American individuals when compared to White individuals.[27] This study provides indirect evidence of likely higher risk of ECAD-associated AIS in White individuals compared to other racial/ethnic groups.

Whether these subtype differences translate to differences in severity remains uncertain. Certain AIS types such as AF-associated AIS are more severe in women. As a consequence of advanced age, women with AIS are more likely to have greater comorbidity disease burden and higher prestroke disability, which may also contribute to differences in AIS outcome, but even after adjusting for these baseline differences, AF-associated AIS tend to be more severe in women.[28] Whether other AIS subtypes or AIS in general are more severe in women after accounting for confounding variables remains unknown. In the North East Melbourne Stroke Incidence Study of 1316 patients, women were older and had more severe AIS (median NIH Stroke Scale score 6 vs 5, $P < .01$), but these differences were completely attenuated after adjusting for age and comorbidity burden.[29] Among 4925 patients admitted in 2 academic medical centers in the United States from 2004 to 2011, no difference in AIS severity by race or sex was noted after adjusting for age and other covariates.[30] Another study done in a cohort of 984 US veterans reported marginally higher stroke severity in Black compared to White patients,[31] but this study did not differentiate AIS from ICH. A more contemporary study done among 45,459 Medicare beneficiaries aged 66 years or older from 2016 to 2017 found that Black and Hispanic patients with AIS had 21% and 54% greater multivariable-adjusted odds of presenting with severe stroke respectively, when compared to White patients with AIS.[32] Therefore, at least in this age group, minority subpopulations may likely have more severe strokes. Another study done in all age groups using the Get With the Guideline-Stroke (GWTG-S) registry showed Asian American patients may be more likely to present with severe strokes when compared to White patients after adjusting for baseline differences in age and covariates.[33]

Disparity in Prehospital Stroke Recognition, Clinical Presentation, and Mode of Transportation to the Hospital

Optimal acute care of patients with AIS begins well before patients arrive to the hospital, with prompt recognition of symptoms, first by lay persons and by emergency medical service (EMS) personnel.[34] Early recognition of AIS symptoms allows for early EMS prenotification of hospitals about potential patients with AIS, which in turn allows for more rapid triage, earlier evaluation, and faster door-to-imaging and door-to-treatment times for patients with AIS.[35,36] Prenotification is associated with reduced in-hospital death in AIS[37] but up to 1 in 3 strokes diagnosed in emergency department (ED) may be unrecognized in the prehospital setting.[34]

In the United States, disparity in prehospital stroke recognition by EMS personnel may exist by race and sex. In one analysis of greater than 3700 patients with stroke transported via EMS to hospitals in 2 Northern California counties, odds of accurate prehospital stroke recognition was 23% lower in Hispanic and Asian patients (odds ratio [OR] = 0.66, 95% confidence interval [CI] 0.55–0.80) when compared to White patients.[38] Correct stroke recognition was also lower in women compared to men (OR = 0.82, 95% CI = 0.71–0.94).[38]

Only 60% of patients with stroke in the United States arrive to the hospital by EMS,[37,39] but this proportion differs markedly by race/ethnicity and by sex with lower adjusted rates of utilization in men and individuals from minority population. Among approximately equal to 400,000 patients with stroke admitted to greater than 1600 GWTG-S participating hospitals from 2011 to 2014, Hispanic men had 23% lower and Asian men had 20% lower odds of EMS use compared to White men, but there was no difference in odds of EMS use between Black and White men after multivariable adjustment. Black women had 13% lower odds of EMS use and Hispanic and Asian women 29% lower odds of EMS use when compared to White women.[39] Similar lower odds of EMS use in Hispanic versus White patients and in men versus women was also noted in 500,829 stroke and transient ischemic attack (TIA) patients admitted to 682 hospitals participating in the Paul Coverdell National Acute Stroke Program from 2014 to 2019.[40]

Although women are more likely to present via EMS, men are still more likely to present within 3 hours of symptom onset. In the Brain Attack Surveillance in Corpus Christi project, women had 30% lower odds of presenting within 3 hours of symptom onset compared to men.[41] Women may be more likely to live alone, and this may lead to delayed recognition and hospital arrival.[42]

Some of the sex disparities in stroke recognition may be potentially explained by differences in stroke symptom presentation, as data have demonstrated that women with stroke have been more likely report nonfocal stroke symptoms compared to men.[43] In a recent meta-analysis of 60 studies, women were noted to have 24% greater odds of headache and 38% greater odds of mental status change at stroke presentation compared to men.[44] However, patients with AIS typically present with a constellation of symptoms with focal symptoms often being reported in addition to nonfocal symptoms.[43] In fact, pooled data from multiple meta-analyses suggest that women are just as likely as men to report focal symptoms,[44,45] including motor and speech deficits.[45] Even when women and men present with similar symptoms, another recent multicenter study of patients with minor ischemic cerebrovascular events or stroke mimics treated at multiple EDs in Canada, showed that women had 12% lower adjusted odds of being appropriately diagnosed with strokes.[46] This suggests that differences in stroke presentation may not account for all the disparity in EMS stroke recognition. Along the same lines, available evidence from the Atherosclerosis Risk in Communities Study suggests that some "classic" stroke symptoms such as facial droop and hemiparesis may be more prevalent in Black patients compared to White patients, which is discordant with the higher EMS misdiagnosis rate in this racial subgroup.[47] Differences in stroke presentation in other racial groups have not been studied extensively.

It remains unknown if differential reporting of stroke symptoms by sexes may contribute to sex differences in stroke recognition.[43] Similarly, cultural differences in the perception and reporting of stroke symptoms between minority versus White patients or unexplored biases in health care providers about women or ethnic minority patients may be potential contributing factors. Encouraging workforce diversification to include more women and ethnic minority workers may help foster cultural sensitivity and potentially contribute to eradication of noted disparities.

Data have demonstrated that women have better knowledge of stroke symptoms compared to men,[48] but compared to White patients, knowledge of stroke symptoms may be less in minority populations. Studies using multiple national surveys including the Behavioral Risk Factor Surveillance System Survey[49] and National Health Interview survey[50] show better awareness of stroke signs in women compared to men and in White compared to minority patients. These racial gaps in knowledge likely contribute to lower odds of EMS utilization by Black and other ethnic minority population but the root causes of knowledge gaps and of lower EMS utilization rates in ethnic minority patients extend beyond mere lack of knowledge to other systemic factors. Mistrust of the health care system based on past experiences and concerns for unaffordable EMS bills may make ethnic minority individuals more reluctant to call EMS.[34] Such financial vulnerability induced, in part, by socioeconomic inequity and structural racism may have downstream effect on EMS use and subsequent AIS care and outcome.

Disparity in Effectiveness of Intravenous Thrombolysis and Mechanical Thrombectomy

Restoration of cerebral blood flow to ischemic but noninfarcted brain regions either through intravenous thrombolysis (IVT) or mechanical thrombectomy (MT) is the most critical step in AIS management. IVT with recombinant tissue plasminogen activator (rtPA), alteplase, has been standard of care management for AIS for almost 3 decades.[51] The efficacy of this treatment of good AIS outcome has been established in multiple randomized trials for patients presenting within 4.5 hours of symptom onset.[52,53] However, the benefit of this medication is time-dependent, with more rapid treatment associated with bigger proportional benefit.[54,55] The enefits of stroke treatment delivered by a mobile stroke unit compared with standard management by Emergency Medical Services (BEST-MSU) trial showed that more rapid administration and better IVT outcome may be achieved by IVT administration in mobile stroke ambulances as opposed to waiting till hospital arrival.[56] More recently, another thrombolytic agent, tenecteplase, with greater fibrin specificity, faster onset of action, longer half-life,[57] and comparable efficacy to rtPA has emerged as an alternative to rtPA.

Following the publication of several overwhelmingly positive MT trials in 2015[58] and subsequent extended window trials,[59,60] MT is now the first-line treatment of the subset of AIS patients with anterior circulation strokes due to large vessel occlusion (LVO) presenting within 24 hours of symptom onset.[61] There is emerging evidence that AIS patients with posterior circulation LVO[62,63] and with large ischemic cores may also benefit from MT.[64–66] LVO-AIS make up the most severe AIS subgroup, carrying up to a 4.5 fold increased odds of death compared to non-LVO[67] and accounting for a disproportionately greater proportion of AIS-associated disability.[68] Depending on the population studied, LVO-AIS account for 13% to 52% of all AIS[69] but account for up to 90% of all AIS-related deaths.[68] However, MT is extremely efficacious in mitigating LVO-AIS-associated risk with number-needed-to-treat to reduce disability by at least one level on the modified Rankin Scale for one patient being just 2.6.[58]

Men and women benefit equally from IVT and MT. Pooled data from multiple meta-analyses of IVT randomized controlled clinical trials (RCCTs) show no heterogeneity of IVT effectiveness by sex.[70] Similarly, multiple pooled analyses of MT trials show no sex difference in MT outcome either in the early (<6 hours)[58,71,72] or late (6–24 hours) MT treatment windows.[73] However, clinical trials often have strict age and baseline inclusion/exclusion criteria that may limit their generalizability to all real-world patients. Observational studies of sex differences in MT have reported contrasting findings. Whereas one meta-analysis consisting mainly of observational studies reported poorer outcomes in women versus men following MT,[74] another more recent meta-analysis consisting of clinical trials and observational studies found no difference in MT outcome by sex.[75] However, these meta-analyses are fundamentally flawed by the lack of adjustment for potential confounding factors including age.[76] The limited available evidence, does not suggest any difference in MT effectiveness between White and Black patients.[77]

Racial and Sex Disparity in Intravenous Thrombolysis and Mechanical Thrombectomy Usage

Multiple studies over the last 2 decades have established lower IVT utilization in women.[78–80] In one recent meta-analysis of administrative database and hospital-based studies from multiple countries, women had 13% lower odds of receiving IVT compared to men[78] but subgroup analysis suggests some of these disparities may differ by geography with studies from the United States and Europe documenting 15% to 18% lower odds of utilization in women, while those from Asia report no sex gap in incidence.[78] Whereas multiple studies from Germany over the last decade[81,82] and from Spain over the period 2016 to 2019[83] show no sex difference in IVT utilization, National Inpatient Sample (NIS) studies in the United States over the 10 year period from 2008 to 2017 report lower adjusted utilization in women in the period 2008 to 2009, but the sex gap in utilization closed over time.[84] Interestingly, 2012 to 2019 statewide data from Ontario, Canada, showed a marginally significant 5% greater adjusted odds (OR 1.05, 95%CI 1.00–1.15) of IVT in women compared to men over this period suggesting that the sex disparity in the United States may not be generalizable to other countries.[85]

In the United States, several administrative database and registry-based studies have established lower rates of IVT usage in racial/ethnic minority populations compared to White individuals.[33,86] This disparity is irrespective of stroke center certification status[87,88] and is present in hospitals participating in quality improvement programs such as the GWTG-S program.[89] For example, AIS admissions in individuals of Black, Hispanic, and Asian/Pacific Islander descent in the NIS had 30%, 26%, and 23% lower odds of IVT in the period 2008 to 2009, respectively, when compared to White individuals.[84] This racial IVT gap declined significantly over time but Black and Asian/Pacific Islander individuals continue to have lower odds of use.[84] More contemporary NIS data restricted to the period 2017 to 2020 suggest this lower rate of utilization in Black individuals persists (**Fig. 1**). Whereas IVT utilization rate was well above 10% in all age/sex groups in other racial/ethnic groups, utilization rate in all age groups of Black men and women aged 60 years or older remain consistently less than 10% (see **Fig. 1**).

Multiple registry-based or administrative database studies have also documented lower odds of MT utilization in Black and ethnic minority patients.[84,90,91] However, these findings should be viewed with caution because these studies were unable to differentiate actual LVO from non-LVO AIS. Among patients with National Institutes of Health Stroke Scale (NIHSS) of 6 or greater presenting within 6 hours of symptom onset to GWTG-S hospitals from 2012 to 2019, MT utilization increased in all race/ethnic groups over time and disparity gaps narrowed over time, but Black patients continued to have lower odds of MT use even after 2015 when compared to White patients.[91] Odds of MT utilization did not differ between Hispanic or Asian patients with

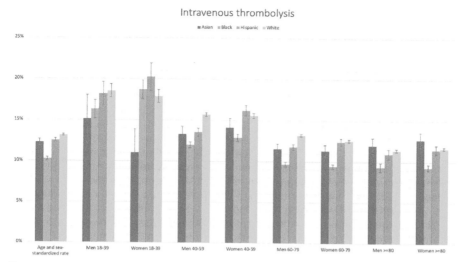

Fig. 1. Intravenous thrombolysis utilization in primary AIS admissions in the United States from 2017 to 2020 according to race and sex.

AIS when compared to White patients after 2015.[91] Current NIS data restricted to the period 2017 to 2020 demonstrate that these racial disparities persist with Black patients having lower MT utilization in all age and sex groups when compared to their White counterparts (**Fig. 2**). Still, studies evaluating whether minority racial subgroups are more/less susceptible to LVO-AIS or whether patients with LVO-AIS in these minority subgroups receive MT at similar frequency to White patients are lacking.

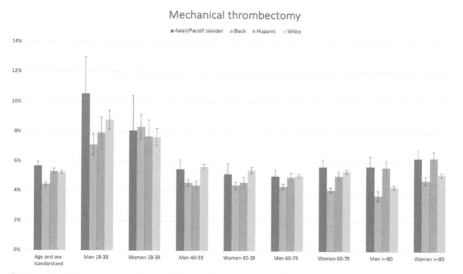

Fig. 2. MT utilization in primary AIS admissions in the United States from 2017 to 2020 according to race and sex.

In contrast to IVT, available data from contemporary studies suggest MT is used at greater frequency in women compared to men.[81,82,84,85] One administrative database study in the United States reported 20% greater odds of MT utilization in women in the period 2016 to 2017,[84] while another from Canada reported 35% greater odds of MT utilization in women compared to men over the period 2012 to 2017.[85] Multiple Germany-based stroke registries report 12% to 26% greater adjusted odds of MT utilization in women compared to men over the period 2000 to 2018.[81,82] These disparities are persistent after adjusting for differences in age and other covariates, so the exact underlying reasons for this disparity remain unknown. The one study to report on actual rates of LVO[83] found a higher proportion of women with AIS in Catalonia, Spain, had LVO (35.8%) compared to men (31.1%), but these estimates were unadjusted for age and other covariates. Additional studies may be needed in multiple populations to ascertain whether female patients with AIS are more predisposed to LVO.

Reasons underlying the lower utilization of IVT in women and ethnic minority patients are multifactorial, including such factors as time to diagnosis and treatment, contraindications to treatment, and patient preferences. First, late arrival to hospitals is the most common underlying reasons why patients with AIS do not receive IVT.[92,93] Due, in part, to previously mentioned and additional factors, Black patients and women are more likely to present late.[94] Even when women and Black patients present within treatment windows, they are still less likely to be treated due to contraindications but, in part, to additional factors. ED wait times are longer in Black compared to White but not in Hispanic compared to White patients after adjustment for differences in mode of transportation[95] particularly for those presenting with atypical symptoms.[96] Door to imaging times are longer in Black versus White and in female vs male patients.[97] Second, regarding contraindications, systolic/diastolic blood pressure greater than 185/110 mm Hg is a contraindication for IVT. Women[98] and Black patients[99] are more likely to have uncontrolled BP as a reason for not receiving IVT. Prior history of ICH may also be more prevalent in Black compared to White patients.[99] Regarding patient preferences, approximately 4% to 7% of IVT-eligible patients decline IVT but GWTG-S data suggest that female sex and Black race were associated with increased odds of IVT refusal.[100] Hispanic and Asian patients had similar odds of refusal but had lower odds of refusal compared to White patients.[100] Finally, up to 9% of AIS are initially misdiagnosed in the ED,[101] but odds of ED misdiagnosis is greater in women and in all minority patient subgroups,[102] leading to lost opportunities for treatment or delayed treatment.

Among IVT-treated patients, studies utilizing data from multiple hospitals in the United States demonstrate longer time-to-treatment in women and minority racial subgroups compared to men and White patients.[103,104]

Indications for Intensive Care Unit Admission in Acute Ischemic Stroke

About 15% to 20% of hospitalized patients with AIS are managed in an intensive care unit (ICU) at some point during hospitalization.[105] In 952,400 AIS admissions among Medicare beneficiaries aged 65 years or older in the United States from 2016 to 2019, 19.9% required ICU level care but marked variability exists by geographic regions.[106] Indications for ICU admissions in AIS include

- Symptomatic ICH (sICH)
- Large hemispheric infarction (LHI) with imminent or manifest malignant cerebral edema (MCE).
- Seizures/status epilepticus.

- Large cerebellar stroke (greater than one-third of the cerebellum) with risk of brainstem dysfunction from mass effect or fourth ventricular compression with accompanying obstructive hydrocephalus.
- Coma (indicates intubation/mechanical ventilation [MV] for airway protection). This will typically be in posterior circulation AIS causing dysfunction of the ascending arousal system in the upper pons or midbrain or involving bilateral regions of thalamus as may occur in basilar artery occlusion. A significant proportion of patients with anterior circulation AIS may present with some degree of impairment of consciousness,[107] but coma at presentation is atypical for anterior circulation AIS because the development of coma requires dysfunction of diffuse areas of bilateral cerebral hemispheres. When present, coma is usually in association with one of the earlier listed neurologic complications or other toxic/metabolic insults.
- Bulbar dysfunction with inability to clear secretions (indicates intubation/MV for airway protection).
- Because patients with severe strokes, typically NIHSS greater than 15 for right hemispheres or NIHSS greater than 20 for left hemisphere, are particularly at risk for these complications, patients with severe AIS are also closely monitored in the ICU in the acute period.
- Post-MT care, especially for patients whose MT were done under general anesthesia.
- Blood pressure management including hypotension or severe hypertension (>220/110 mm Hg in patients receiving no acute recanalization treatment or >180/105 mm Hg after IVT and/or MT)
- Other medical indications for ICU admission in non-AIS patients.

Sex and Race Disparities in Symptomatic Intracerebral Hemorrhage

SICH is one of the most feared complications of IVT but may also occur following MT and in patients receiving no recanalization treatment. Classification of post-IVT ICH as symptomatic requires radiological evidence (CT or MRI) of hemorrhage, either petechial hemorrhagic transformation into areas of known infarction or well-defined parenchymal hematomas, in conjunction with signs of neurologic deterioration.[108] Reported sICH rate following IVT from RCCTs and observational studies varies between 2% and 9% likely reflective of varying sICH definition among studies, differences in treatment time windows, and differences in underlying population studied.[109,110] Established predictors of sICH include increasing age, increasing NIHSS, increasing blood sugar, and increased time from AIS onset to treatment.[111] Comorbid AF, congestive heart failure, renal impairment, and previous antiplatelet use may each double the sICH risk.[111]

Male sex and Asian race are also associated with an increased sICH risk. In the Safe Implementation of Treatments in Stroke-International Stroke Thrombolysis Register of 45,079 receiving IVT, men had almost 20% greater adjusted odds of sICH compared to women. GWTG-S registry data demonstrate 36% greater odds of sICH in Asian American AIS compared to White patients.[33] In another GWTG-S study of 54,334 IVT-treated patients with AIS, Asian American patients also had 36% greater odds of any hemorrhagic complication and Black patients had 14% greater odds of hemorrhagic complications compared to White patients, but while the increased hemorrhagic risk in Asian patients was driven by excess sICH risk, that in Black patients was due to other forms of bleeding.[112] The GRASPS (glucose at presentation, race [Asian], age, sex [male], systolic blood pressure at presentation, and severity of stroke at presentation [NIHSS]) score for sICH prediction incorporates race and sex as score prediction variables,[113] but these factors should not be used as reasons to withhold IVT.

Over 85% of IVT-associated sICH occur within 24 hours of treatment,[108] so current American Heart Association (AHA) AIS treatment guidelines recommend close monitoring of IVT-treated patients in an ICU or stroke unit for 24 hours[114] with frequent examinations for neurologic symptoms/signs that may herald sICH.

Large Hemispheric Infarction and Malignant Cerebral Edema

LHI represents AIS typically following occlusion of the internal carotid artery or the trunk of the middle cerebral artery (MCA) that involves the total or subtotal territory of the MCA, affecting the basal ganglia at least partially, with or without involvement of the adjacent anterior cerebral or posterior cerebral artery territories.[115] MCE describes excessive space-occupying brain edema accompanied by brain herniation that results from the interplay of cytotoxic, ionic, and vasogenic edema that follows LHI.[116] Up to half of patients with LHI will develop MCE.[116]

Early clinical predictors of MCE include young age and higher admission NIHSS (median 17–20), while early radiological predictors include hypoattenuation of greater than 50% of the MCA territory on initial CT or MRI diffusion-weighted imaging at 6 hours with infarct volume of greater than 82 cc.[116,117] Vascular imaging with distal ICA, proximal MCA, or carotid T occlusion is also predictive of MCE but successful revascularization with IVT or MT is protective.[116,117]

Patients at risk of MCE require close ICU monitoring for signs of MCE including pupillary changes and altered mental status especially in the first few days following LHI, but MCE may sometimes develop later. Specific medical treatment of established MCE in LHI include those to treat mass effect and elevated intracranial pressure such as head of the bed elevation, aggressive fever management, cautious use of sedation, and hyperosmolar therapy utilizing mannitol or hypertonic sodium, but these medical measures are often inadequate. About 40% to 80% of patients with MCE still develop catastrophic cerebral herniation and die with these medical measures alone,[118] so early neurosurgical consultation for the evaluation of at-risk patients for possible surgical decompression is indicated.

Surgical decompression may be life-saving for patients with LHI and involves a frontal-temporal-parietal decompressive hemicraniectomy (DHC), with recommended anterior to posterior diameter of at least 12 cm and superior to inferior length of at least 9 cm, in addition to a durotomy,[119] allowing the brain to swell outward through the skull defect. Following DHC, patients continue to be monitored/managed in the ICU for post-DHC complications such as brain hemorrhage, brain herniation, cerebrospinal fluid disturbances, and seizures.[119] The benefits of DHC in patients with LHI was highlighted in one recent meta-analysis of 7 DHC RCCT trials showing 84% lower odds of in-hospital mortality and almost 3 fold greater odds of favorable outcome (mRS score ≤3) in the DHC group when compared to medical treatment group with no heterogeneity by age, sex, presence of aphasia, stroke severity, and involved vascular territories.[120] Patients with large cerebellar strokes with brainstem compression and hydrocephalus may also have excellent outcome with suboccipital craniectomy (SOC) and external ventricular drain placement in addition to medical measures.[114]

Current AHA AIS guidelines recommend shared decision between providers and patient families incorporating patient preferences when discussing treatment options in patients with LHI including DHC consideration,[114] but patient preferences for DHC may vary by sex and race. In one national study of anterior circulation AIS, women had 16% lower adjusted odds of DHC compared to men.[121] Whereas Hispanic patients had 28% greater odds of DHC compared to White patients, there was no difference in odds of DHC between Black and White patients.[121] Whether SOC utilization in patients with large cerebellar AIS differs by sex and race has not been studied extensively.

Some of the reported differences in DHC use may likely be due to racial or sex differences in aggressiveness of care. Ethnic minority patients are more likely to elect for life-sustaining treatment such as DHC, MV, tracheostomy, and percutaneous gastrostomy after AIS.[122] Women and White patients are more likely to have care limitations orders such as do-not-resuscitate orders during stroke hospitalization. Reasons for the racial disparities in care limitation orders may include factors such as mistrust of the health system by Black or ethnic minority patients leading to reduced willingness to forego life-sustaining treatment, poor patient–provider communication, or lack of access to quality end-of-life care.[123] Ethnic minority patients may also be less likely to forego life-sustaining treatment measures as a result of cultural and/or religious factors.[123]

Demographic Disparities in General Intensive Care Unit Care and Postacute Care

Studies evaluating demographic disparities in ICU care in the United States are sparse. In the derivation of the intensive care after thrombolysis score for predicting ICU need after thrombolysis, one single-center study identified male sex and Black race as important predictors.[124] However, this study is outdated as it predates the widespread use of MT that has occurred over the last decade. One large contemporary study of 67,442 patients in Ontario, Canada, found no difference in odds of ICU care between men and women, but female patients had 10% lower odds of MV when compared to men.[85] NIS data from 2017 to 2020 show 29% lower odds of MV utilization in women compared to men, while all minority racial/ethnic subgroups had greater odds of MV use compared to White admissions (**Table 1**). Pooled data from 19,652 participants enrolled in 5 multinational acute stroke randomized trials also demonstrated that women with AIS had 17% lower odds of ICU admission and 42% lower odds of intubation when compared to men.[125] These demographic disparities may likely, partly, due to differences in aggressiveness of care including racial difference in the use of care limitation orders such as do-not-resuscitate orders (see **Table 1**), but whether this is partly due to true disparity in care, that is, male and female patients being treated differently when in identical clinical scenarios remains unknown.

Female patients with AIS in the United States are less likely to receive defect-free stroke care when compared to male patients.[104,126] In a nationally representative sample of Medicare beneficiaries aged 65 years or older with AIS in the United States, women had lower odds of intracranial or extracranial vessel imaging, heart-rhythm monitoring, echocardiography, and evaluation by a neurologist or vascular neurologist, after adjustment for age, race, and comorbidities.[127] However, stroke care metrics do not differ between men and women hospitalized with AIS in Catalonia, Spain.[83]

Disparities in Acute Ischemic Stroke Outcome

Studies evaluating sex differences in AIS mortality have reported conflicting results.[42,43] Contemporary NIS data from 2017 to 2020, which is representative of inpatient mortality in the United States (**Table 2**), show that odds of unadjusted mortality is 11% greater in women versus men (**Table 3** model 1). This difference is attenuated in models adjusted for differences in age (see **Table 3**, model 2). Interestingly, in fully adjusted models that include differences in AIS severity and other covariates, mortality odds were 17% lower in women compared to men (see **Table 3** model 3), suggesting that when differences in stroke severity and other covariates are accounted for, in-

Table 1
Multivariable adjusted odds of utilization of acute recanalization therapies in acute ischemic stroke admissions in the United States from 2017 to 2020

	Odds Ratio	95% Confidence Interval	P-Value
Intravenous thrombolysis (weighted n = 2,057,310)			
Female vs male	1.01	0.99–1.03	.562
Race/ethnicity	—	—	—
Black vs White	0.73	0.71–0.76	<.001
Hispanic vs White	0.88	0.85–0.92	<.001
Asian/Pacific vs White	0.82	0.77–0.88	<.001
Other/unknown vs White	1.03	0.99–1.08	.150
MT (weighted n = 2,057,310)			
Female vs male	1.10	1.07–1.14	<.001
Race/ethnicity	—	—	—
Black vs White	0.76	0.71–0.79	<.001
Hispanic vs White	0.89	0.82–0.97	.007
Asian/Pacific vs White	0.96	0.87–1.06	.416
Other/unknown vs White	1.28	1.19–1.37	<.001

Patients with primary AIS and most covariates identified using International Classification of Diseases 10th revision (ICD-10) code using similar methods to that described previously in Otite et al.[84] Odds ratios obtained from logistic regression models (that take into account the survey design of the NIS through the use of relevant strata and discharge weights) with each outcome as dependent variables and with age, insurance status, income, coma, age, Elixhauser comorbidity score, prior stroke, coronary artery disease, AF, dementia, mechanical ventilation, hospital region, hospital location/teaching status, year of discharge, and dyslipidemia.

hospital mortality may be less in women. However, in-hospital mortality does not paint the full picture, as up to two-thirds of in-hospital deaths in the United States occur outside the hospital setting.[3]

Studies evaluating patient functional status at the time of discharge also yield conflicting results. Whereas 2017 to 2020 NIS data from the United States show that odds of good outcome at discharge, defined as routine home discharge, are worse in women compared to men (see **Table 3** model 3), data from Northern Germany from 2010 to 2018 suggest women may have more favorable outcome at the time of discharge. However, most studies evaluating AIS outcome beyond the acute hospitalization period report poorer short-term outcome in women compared to men. Women are more disabled and suffer more physical impairments in activities of daily living after AIS.[43,125,128,129] They have poorer quality of life,[125,130] experience more post-AIS depression,[43,131,132] and are more likely to be institutionalized after AIS compared to men.[129]

Most studies report lesser odds of in-hospital mortality[89] but greater odds of disability in Black and other ethnic minority population when compared to White patients.[133] NIS data over 2017 to 2020 are consistent with these findings (see **Table 3** model 3). It is likely that differential aggressiveness and utilization of limitations of care orders contribute to a significant proportion of these variations as up to 40% of short-term mortality in AIS may be reflective of patient/family wishes rather than disparities in provision of evidence-based care.[134] The lower utilization of withdrawal of care orders in patients of minority race/ethnicity groups allows for more patients

Table 2
Multivariable adjusted odds of utilization of mechanical ventilation and do-not-resuscitate orders in the United States from 2017 to 2020

Variable	Odds Ratio	95% Confidence Interval	P-Value
Mechanical ventilation (weighted n = 955,355[a])			
Female vs male	0.70	0.67–0.74	<0.001
Race/ethnicity	—	—	—
Black vs White	1.16	1.07–1.25	<.001
Hispanic vs White	1.39	1.27–1.52	<.001
Asian/Pacific vs White	1.25	1.00–1.35	.055
Other/unknown vs White	—	—	—
Do-not-resuscitate status (weighted n = 955,355[a])			
Female vs male	1.23	1.20–1.27	<.001
Race/ethnicity	—	—	—
Black vs White	0.44	0.42–0.47	<.001
Hispanic vs White	0.56	0.52–0.60	<.001
Asian/Pacific vs White	0.61	0.55–0.67	<.001
Other/unknown vs White	0.88	0.82–0.95	<.001

Patients with primary AIS and most covariates identified using ICD-10 code using similar methods to that described previously in Ahmed et al.[201] Do-not-resuscitate status determined using ICD-10-CM code Z66. Mechanical ventilation status determined using ICD-10 procedural codes09HN7BZ, 09HN8BZ, 0BH13EZ, 0BH17EZ, 0BH18EZ, 0CHY7BZ, 0CHY8BZ, 5A1935Z, 5A1945Z, and 5A1955Z. Odds ratios obtained from logistic regression models (that take into account the survey design of the NIS through use of relevant strata and discharge weights) with each outcome as dependent variables and with age, National Institute of Health Stroke Scale, stupor/coma, age, Elixhauser co-morbidity score, prior stroke, coronary artery disease, AF, dementia, hospital region, hospital location/teaching status, year of discharge, dyslipidemia, thrombolysis, and thrombectomy status. Model for mechanical ventilation and thrombolysis also included further adjustment for do-not-resuscitate status while that for do-not-resuscitate status included adjustment for mechanical ventilation status.

[a] Analysis restricted to admission with nonmissing NIHSS (48.4% of observations).

from these groups to live longer albeit with more disability. Therefore, unraveling how much of the racial/ethnic disparity in outcome may be due to differences in acute/critical care services as opposed to patient preferences still requires prospective evaluation but optimizing areas for potential improvement in prehospital and hospital care highlighted in **Table 4**, may possibly help improve outcomes for all demographic subgroups of patients.

HEMORRHAGIC STROKE

Compared to AIS, less is known about racial, ethnic, and sex disparities in the management and outcomes of patients with hemorrhagic stroke. Understanding and addressing disparities therein are important because the incidence of ICH[135] and SAH[136] are on the rise. In addition, disparities in incidence exist. Male patients have higher rates of ICH than female patients, while female patients have higher rates of SAH than male patients.[135,136] Non-Hispanic Black Americans have higher rates of ICH and SAH than non-Hispanic White Americans, and this disparity is rising over time.[135,136] These trends are particularly concerning because while mortality due to

Table 3
Multivariable adjusted odds of in-hospital mortality and home discharge in acute ischemic stroke admissions in the United States from 2017 to 2020

Variable	Odds Ratio	95% Confidence Interval	P-value	Odds Ratio	95% Confidence Interval	P-Value
		In-hospital Mortality			Routine Home Discharge	
Model 1 (weighted n = 2,057,310)						
Female vs male	1.11	1.07–1.15	<.001	0.65	0.65–0.66	<.001
Race/ethnicity	—	—	—	—	—	—
Black vs White	0.71	0.68–0.75	<.001	0.99	0.97–1.02	.631
Hispanic vs White	0.82	0.76–0.88	<.001	1.24	1.21–1.27	<.001
Asian/Pacific vs White	1.08	0.98–1.19	.087	1.00	0.95–1.04	.885
Other/ unknown vs White	1.31	1.22–1.40	<.001	1.02	0.99–1.05	.179
Model 2 (weighted n = 2,057,310)						
Female vs male	0.97	0.94–1.00	.063	0.77	0.76–0.78	<.001
Race/ethnicity	—	—	—	—	—	—
Black vs White	0.89	0.84–0.93	<.001	0.69	0.67–0.70	<.001
Hispanic vs White	0.94	0.88–1.01	.076	0.97	0.94–1.00	.076
Asian/Pacific vs White	1.14	1.04–1.25	.005	0.90	0.86–0.95	<.001
Other/ unknown vs White	1.44	1.34–1.54	<.001	0.86	0.83–0.89	<.001
Model 3 (weighted n = 955,355[a])						
Female vs male	0.80	0.75–0.85	<.001	0.84	0.82–0.86	<.001
Race/ethnicity	—	—	—	—	—	—
Black vs White	0.78	0.70–0.87	<.001	0.78	0.75–0.81	<.001
Hispanic vs White	0.84	0.74–0.95	.006	0.98	0.94–1.03	.461
Asian/Pacific vs White	0.83	0.70–1.00	.047	0.85	0.79–0.92	<.001
Other/ unknown vs White	1.08	0.95–1.23	.242	0.93	0.88–0.97	.003

Patients with primary AIS and most covariates identified using ICD-10 code using similar methods to that described previously in Ahmed et al.[201] Model 1: unadjusted model. Model 2: Model 1 + age. Model 3: Model 2 + National Institute of Health Stroke Scale, stupor/coma, age, Elixhauser comorbidity score, prior stroke, coronary artery disease, AF, dementia, hospital region, hospital location/teaching status, year of discharge, dyslipidemia, thrombolysis, and thrombectomy status. Model for mechanical ventilation also included further adjustment for do-not-resuscitate status while that for do-not-resuscitate status included adjustment for mechanical ventilation status.

[a] Analysis restricted to admission with nonmissing NIHSS (48.4% of observations).

Table 4
Key areas of sex and racial/ethnic disparities in the epidemiology, prehospital, in-hospital care and outcome of acute ischemic stroke

Potential Areas of Disparities	Sex Disparity	Racial/Ethnic Disparity
IVT usage	Variable between countries. Older US studies report lower utilization in women, but more current NIS data from 2017–2020 show that this gap has closed. Contemporary studies from Germany, Spain, and Asia also show no difference in utilization while those from Canada suggest greater utilization in women	2017–2020 NIS data suggest lower odds of utilization in Black, Asian/Pacific Islander, and Hispanic patients compared to White patients
MT usage	2017–2020 NIS data and registry data from Germany, Canada, and Spain show greater MT utilization in women compared to men	2017–2020 NIS data suggest lower odds of utilization in Black, Asian/Pacific Islander, and Hispanic patients compared to White patients
Symptomatic ICH after thrombolysis	sICH risk greater in men compared to women	sICH risk greater in Asian compared to White patients. No difference in sICH risk between Black and Hispanic compared to White patients
DHC for MCE	NIS data suggest DHC used less frequently in women in the United States compared to men	NIS data suggest DHC used more frequently in Hispanic patients in the United States compared to White patients. No difference in utilization between Black and White patients
Overall ICU utilization	Pooled data from multinational acute stroke randomized trials suggest lower odds of ICU admission in women compared to men. Another large study from Canada shows no sex difference in utilization	Studies evaluating racial/ethnic differences in overall ICU utilization are sparse. One small study suggests higher ICU utilization rate in Black compared to White patients, but this study predated the MT era
Mechanical ventilation	Data from the NIS, Canada, and pooled data from multinational stroke trials show greater odds of mechanical ventilation in men compared to women	NIS data also show greater odds of mechanical ventilation in Black and Hispanic patients compared to White patients. Asian patients showed a trend toward higher but not significant

(*continued on next page*)

Table 4 (continued)		
Potential Areas of Disparities	**Sex Disparity**	**Racial/Ethnic Disparity**
Presence of do-not-resuscitate orders	NIS data suggest DNR orders more prevalent in women compared to men	NIS data suggest DNR orders are less prevalent in all ethnic minority patients compared to White patients
Unadjusted in-hospital mortality	NIS data suggest higher odds of mortality in women in the United States compared to men	NIS data suggest lower odds of unadjusted mortality in Black, Hispanic, and Asian patients compared to White patients
Adjusted in-hospital mortality	NIS data suggest lower odds of mortality in women in the United States compared to men	NIS data suggest lower odds of mortality in Black, Hispanic, and Asian patients compared to White patients
Long-term mortality	Variable	Variable
Functional outcome	Variable, but most studies report worse functional outcome in women compared to men	Worse in Black and Hispanic patients compared to White patients Outcome at discharge may be worse in Asian patients but long-term outcome not well studied

AIS is falling, mortality is not changing after hemorrhagic stroke, and morbidity is substantial.[137,138] In the following section, we will review disparities in the management and outcomes of ICH and SAH separately.

Intracerebral Hemorrhage

Investigations into prehospital, triage, and emergency evaluation disparities of ICH are inherently enmeshed with those of AIS as the 2 diagnoses cannot be differentiated on clinical grounds alone. Retrospective analyses of emergency medicine and stroke registries including both ischemic and hemorrhagic patients with stroke suggest that Black patients wait longer in the ED and are less likely to undergo CT imaging within guideline-recommended time limits compared to White patients.[95,139] A retrospective study from a single-institution found that female sex, but not race, was associated with decreased likelihood of activation of a stroke code.[140] Of note, Black patients with ICH are more likely than White patients to present directly to urban, academic centers; White patients are more likely to require interfacility transfer.[139]

Following diagnosis of ICH, critical and time-sensitive measures include blood pressure lowering and reversal of coagulopathy. Only blood pressure lowering has been assessed for disparity. Much of what we know about disparities in ICH care is derived from the Ethnic/Racial Variation of Intracerebral Hemorrhage (ERICH) study, multicenter prospective case-control study of ICH among Black patients, Hispanic patients, and White. An analysis from ERICH found that Black patients and Hispanic patients had higher prehospital and ED blood pressure than White patients and that Black patients continued to have higher blood pressure than Hispanic and White patients after 1 day of admission.[141] A post hoc analysis of the Antihypertensive Treatment of Acute Cerebral Hemorrhage II trial found that White but not Black patients with intensive blood pressure reduction had worse outcomes than those with conservative treatment.[142] A similar post hoc analysis of the same study did not find an interaction of blood pressure management strategy and sex on outcomes following ICH.[143] A post hoc study of pooled data from the Intensive Blood Pressure Reduction in Acute Cerebral Haemorrhage trials (INTERACT 1 and 2) found that although male and female patients had comparable baseline blood pressure, male patients had slightly increased blood pressure compared to women at 1 and 7 days with no significant interaction with outcome.[144]

Surgical management of ICH is not generally recommended but can be considered on a case-by-case basis. Treatment of symptomatic hydrocephalus, however, requires insertion of an external ventricular drain. Studies of disparity in surgical management reveal conflicting results. An analysis from ERICH did not find evidence of racial or ethnic disparity in utilization of surgical procedures.[145] In contrast, a retrospective study from a large administrative database found that craniectomy utilization for some racial and ethnic minorities (Hispanic patients, Asian patients) but not Black patients was increased compared to craniectomy utilization for White patients after adjustment for other variables.[146] The same study determined that external ventricular drain utilization was higher in Black than in White patients and that minority patients in general received higher rates of life-saving (ie, craniectomy) or life-sustaining (ie, tracheostomy or gastrostomy) procedures. A study of sex differences from ERICH found that male patients with ICH are more likely to receive external ventricular drains, but not other surgical procedures, compared to female patients.[147] The propensity for male patients to receive more external ventricular drains has been corroborated in a separate cohort.[148]

Other care processes were explored in the GWTG-S registry from 2003 to 2012.[139] In that period, after adjustment for patient and hospital characteristics, Black patients were more likely to receive venous thromboembolism prophylaxis, dysphagia screening, stroke education, and rehabilitation assessment than White patients. White patients were more likely to receive smoking cessation counseling than Black patients. Like Black patients, Asian and Hispanic patients were more likely to receive dysphagia screening and less likely to receive smoking cessation counseling compared to White patients.

Several other studies have evaluated for disparities in gastrostomy tube placement in patients with ICH. Most suggest that Black and Hispanic patients are more likely to receive gastrostomy tubes than White patients.[149–151] Studies of sex disparities in gastrostomy placement after ICH offer conflicting findings.[147,151]

Life-sustaining procedures reflect goals of care decisions in severe disease. Disparities in care limitations and palliative care services occur following ICH. Asian patients seem to opt for life-sustaining interventions more than White patients and receive less palliative care.[152–154] So too do Hispanic patients and Black patients when compared to White patients.[139,152–155] While palliative care use after ICH is increasing in all races and ethnicities, the disparity compared to White patients is closing over time in Hispanic patients, but not Black patients.[156] The presence of sex disparities in goals of care decisions after ICH is uncertain. While some studies report that females patients are more likely to receive early care limitations compared to males patients after ICH,[157,158] others do not.[147,154,159]

Disparities in intracerebral hemorrhage outcome

As for AIS, ICH outcomes disparities are difficult to disentangle from disparities in goals of care. Registry studies suggest Black, Hispanic, and Asian patients with ICH all have lower in-hospital risk-adjusted mortality than White patients despite more severe presentations.[160] Post hoc analysis of a randomized controlled trial (RCT) similarly determined that White patients had lower survival than Asian patients, as well as lower quality of life, but not functional outcomes at 3 months.[161] An adjusted analysis of only young patients with supratentorial ICH from ERICH found that Black and Hispanic patients had better 3 month functional outcomes compared to White patients. The effect of race and ethnicity did not persist in an adjusted analysis of the entire ERICH cohort.[162] A recent single-center retrospective study did not find any differences in ED care delivery, discharge outcomes, or 3 month mortality by race or ethnicity.[163]

Some studies suggest no sex differences in outcomes after ICH after adjustment for premorbid status, ICH severity, and age.[164] Other studies suggest that either male or female patients with ICH fare better.[138,143,144,148,158,164] Post hoc analysis of 2 large RCTs found that among patients with poor outcome at 1 month, male sex was associated with a good outcome at 1 year, suggesting a sex disparity in recovery trajectory.[165] No such disparity was found for race or ethnicity in that study. A retrospective study from 11 inpatient rehab facilities found that among patients with hemorrhagic stroke, functional independence disparities not present at hospital discharge emerged at 3 months and persisted to 1 year, with White patients showing better recovery than Black and especially Hispanic patients in fully adjusted models.[166]

Racial and ethnic disparity exists in the risk of ICH recurrence, with Asian, Black, and Hispanic patients all at higher risk than White patients.[167,168,35,36] Inadequately controlled hypertension, mostly due to undertreatment, partially drives the disparity.[168–170,36–38] So too does increased blood pressure variability, which contributes to an increased risk of all major adverse cardiovascular and cerebrovascular events following ICH, particularly among Black patients.[168,171] In a retrospective study from a high-resource setting with near universal medical insurance coverage, Asian, Black, and Hispanic patients were more likely to have minimal blood pressure improvement after ICH as compared to White patients, and this disparity was exacerbated by neighborhood poverty.[172] In a separate study, patients from the same cohort from areas with more socioeconomic disadvantage, as measured by the area deprivation index, were less likely to have their blood pressure, cholesterol, and hemoglobin A1c measured before ICH, but not after.[173] These results suggest that acute inpatient hospitalizations can help mitigate disparities among ICH survivors. There does not appear to be a disparity in ICH recurrence risk by sex.[174,175]

Subarachnoid Hemorrhage

Over 85% of SAH are aneurysmal and even less is known about disparities in the evaluation, management, and outcomes of aneurysmal and nonaneurysmal SAH. Black and Hispanic patients are more likely than White patients to present directly to centers where they are managed, while White patients are more likely to be transferred.[176,177] A retrospective study of an administrative database found that among patients who presented to an ED with a headache, non-Hispanic White race and male sex were associated with a missed diagnosis of life-threatening illness, including SAH.[178] Other studies have not found an association between sex and misdiagnosis of SAH.[179,180]

Disparities in blood pressure
Although the optimal blood pressure target after aneurysmal SAH remains unknown, excessively high blood pressure is associated with increased risk of rebleeding before

aneurysms are secured. Current SAH treatment guidelines recommend blood pressure control as part of medical measures to prevent rebleeding.

Retrospective review from an academic tertiary care center found that Black patients had higher admission blood pressure than White patients with SAH and that the time to blood pressure control was longer in Black patients even after adjusting for initial blood pressure disparities.[181] The study did not find any sex disparities in hyperacute blood pressure control after SAH.

Disparities in aneurysm treatment

To minimize risk of aneurysmal rebleeding, current guidelines recommend early definitive treatment of aneurysms via open microsurgical clipping or endovascular coiling as soon as possible but preferably within 24 hours of symptom onset.[182]

Time to aneurysm securement may be an important area of disparities in SAH management. Studies from a large, national administrative database have found that Hispanic patients may have longer delays in aneurysm treatment than White patients.[183,184] Asian or Pacific Islander patients have longer time to aneurysm securement than White patient as well, while Black patients may not.[184] A smaller institutional analysis and a post hoc analysis from 2 RCTs did not find any evidence of racial or ethnic disparity in time to aneurysm treatment.[185,186] Female sex has been associated with earlier time to aneurysm securement than male sex.[184,187]

There may also be disparities in the modality of aneurysm securement. White patients are more likely than patients of other races and ethnicities to undergo endovascular coiling versus open clipping,[188] but this study may not be reflective of changes in SAH practices that occurred over the last decade. Overall, the rates of endovascular coiling have increased across all races and ethnicities; however, the trend of relative increase of coiling to clipping is much more pronounced for White patients than for Asian, Black, and Hispanic patients.[189] The trend is completely absent for Native American patients.[189] A previous trend toward increased coiling to clipping in male patients compared to female patients has dissipated over time.[188,189] Not much is known about disparities in other care processes.

Disparities in vasospasm and delayed cerebral ischemia

Cerebral vasospasm associated with delayed cerebral ischemia may occur in up to 30% of patients with SAH. Clinical deterioration due to delayed cerebral ischemia (DCI) defined as the occurrence of focal neurologic impairment or a decrease of at least 2 points on the Glasgow Coma Scale (GCS) occurs typically at days 4 to 14 following SAH with peak at day 10 and may be associated with poor SAH outcome.[182] Established predictors of DCI include SAH clinical and radiological grade, young age, and aneurysm size, but female sex may be associated with an increased risk. Although older studies suggest no sex difference in risk of vasospasm and DCI after SAH, more recent studies suggest that female patients may possibly carry higher risk. One of the largest studies to evaluate this question utilized data from 6713 patients contained in 10 studies included in the SAHIT (SAH International Trialists) consortium to show 29% higher risk of DCI in women compared to men but no difference in risk of cerebral infarction was noted between women and men.[131] A recent single-center observational study of 328 patients noted higher rates of clinical deterioration, radiological vasospasm, DCI, and cerebral infarction in women versus men, but no difference in modified Rankin Scale (mRS) was noted at 6 to 12 months.[190]

Disparities in clinical goals of care and outcome

Regarding goals of care, data from a national administrative dataset and from a prospectively enrolled single-center cohort suggest that White patients or their surrogates accept more care limitations than Black and Hispanic patients or their surrogates.[191,192] Single-center studies have not demonstrated sex-based disparities in care limitations after SAH.[192,193]

Two recent, large retrospective analyses from a national administrative database found that both Black and Hispanic patients had lower mortality than White patients after SAH.[189,194] One of those analyses found that Black patients had the highest odds of poor outcome (defined by discharge destination), and Hispanic patients had higher odds of an excellent outcome than White patients. The same analysis determined that female patients had lower odds of good clinical outcome compared to male patients. These results persisted after adjustment for age, medical comorbidities, and SAH severity. A similar analysis of the nationwide inpatient sample found that Black patients had lower in-hospital mortality than White patients but not improved discharge rates of discharge to home.[195] It also reported that women were not more likely than men to have a home discharge after adjustment for covariables. Data from a New York State administrative dataset that defined poor outcome as in-hospital death or discharge other than to home found that White patients had fewer poor outcomes than patients from other races and ethnicities.[196] These analyses from administrative datasets lack important information regarding goals of care.

An older analysis combining patients from 2 RCTs did not find an association of race with 3 month functional outcomes.[186] Retrospective, smaller studies of racial and ethnic disparities neither have generally uncovered any[185,197] nor have they revealed significant sex disparities in outcome after SAH.[198–200] The reason for discordance between smaller clinical cohort studies and large administrative studies is uncertain but may relate to statistical power or covariate adjustment.

CLINICS CARE POINTS

- Intravenous thrombolysis and mechanical thrombectomy treatment gaps by race and ethnicity may involve the interplay of personal and systemic factors at several steps in the acute stroke chain of survival.

- Demographic disparities in the need for subsequent ICU care for ischemic stroke patients may be predicated on some of these disparities in acute care.

- However, the landscape of sex and racial or ethnic disparities in the critical care and outcome of ischemic and hemorrhagic stroke patients appears to be a complex tangled web of variations in incidence, clinical presentation, acute care and patient preferences.

DISCLOSURE

F. Otite has no relevant disclosures or conflict of interest. N. Morris has no relevant disclosures or conflict of interest.

REFERENCES

1. Feigin VL, Owolabi MO, Abd-Allah F, et al. Pragmatic solutions to reduce the global burden of stroke: a world stroke organization–lancet neurology commission. Lancet Neurol 2023;22(12):1160–206.
2. Krishnamurthi RV, Ikeda T, Feigin VL. Global, regional and country-specific burden of ischaemic stroke, intracerebral haemorrhage and subarachnoid haemorrhage: a systematic analysis of the global burden of disease study 2017. Neuroepidemiology 2020;54(2):171–9. https://doi.org/10.1159/000506396.

3. Tsao CW, Aday AW, Almarzooq ZI, et al. Heart disease and stroke statistics—2023 update: a report from the American Heart Association. Circulation 2023; 147(8):e93–621.

4. Heron M. Deaths: leading causes for 2018. Natl Vital Stat Rep 2021;70(4):1–115.

5. Churchwell K, Elkind MS, Benjamin RM, et al. Call to action: structural racism as a fundamental driver of health disparities: a presidential advisory from the American Heart Association. Circulation 2020;142(24):e454–68.

6. Ospel J, Singh N, Ganesh A, et al. Sex and gender differences in stroke and their practical implications in acute care. Journal of Stroke 2023;25(1):16–25.

7. Howard G, Moy CS, Howard VJ, et al. Where to focus efforts to reduce the black-white disparity in stroke mortality: incidence versus case fatality? Stroke 2016;47(7):1893–8. https://doi.org/10.1161/strokeaha.115.012631.

8. GLRoS Collaborators. Global, regional, and country-specific lifetime risks of stroke, 1990 and 2016. N Engl J Med 2018;379(25):2429–37.

9. Petrea RE, Beiser AS, Seshadri S, et al. Gender differences in stroke incidence and poststroke disability in the Framingham heart study. Stroke 2009;40(4): 1032–7.

10. Seshadri S, Beiser A, Kelly-Hayes M, et al. The lifetime risk of stroke: estimates from the Framingham Study. Stroke 2006;37(2):345–50. https://doi.org/10.1161/01.STR.0000199613.38911.b2.

11. Appelros P, Stegmayr B, Terént A. Sex differences in stroke epidemiology: a systematic review. Stroke 2009;40(4):1082–90.

12. Leppert MH, Burke JF, Lisabeth LD, et al. Systematic review of sex differences in ischemic strokes among young adults: are young women disproportionately at risk? Stroke 2022;53(2):319–27.

13. Howard VJ, Madsen TE, Kleindorfer DO, et al. Sex and race differences in the association of incident ischemic stroke with risk factors. JAMA Neurol 2019; 76(2):179–86.

14. Yoon CW, Bushnell CD. Stroke in women: a review focused on epidemiology, risk factors, and outcomes. J Stroke 2023;25(1):2–15. https://doi.org/10.5853/jos.2022.03468.

15. Howard VJ, Kleindorfer DO, Judd SE, et al. Disparities in stroke incidence contributing to disparities in stroke mortality. Ann Neurol 2011;69(4):619–27.

16. Rosamond WD, Folsom AR, Chambless LE, et al. Stroke incidence and survival among middle-aged adults: 9-year follow-up of the Atherosclerosis Risk in Communities (ARIC) cohort. Stroke 1999;30(4):736–43. https://doi.org/10.1161/01.str.30.4.736.

17. Kissela B, Schneider A, Kleindorfer D, et al. Stroke in a biracial population: the excess burden of stroke among blacks. Stroke 2004;35(2):426–31. https://doi.org/10.1161/01.Str.0000110982.74967.39.

18. Collaborators NMSS, Sacco RL, Boden-Albala B, et al. Stroke incidence among white, black, and Hispanic residents of an urban community: the Northern Manhattan Stroke Study. Am J Epidemiol 1998;147(3):259–68.

19. Gardener H, Sacco RL, Rundek T, et al. Race and ethnic disparities in stroke incidence in the Northern Manhattan Study. Stroke 2020;51(4):1064–9.

20. Niewada M, Kobayashi A, Sandercock PA, et al. Influence of gender on baseline features and clinical outcomes among 17,370 patients with confirmed ischaemic stroke in the international stroke trial. Neuroepidemiology 2005;24(3):123–8.

21. Kamel H, Healey JS. Cardioembolic stroke. Circ Res 2017;120(3):514–26.

22. Voigt S, van Os H, van Walderveen M, et al. Sex differences in intracranial and extracranial atherosclerosis in patients with acute ischemic stroke. Int J Stroke 2021;16(4):385–91. https://doi.org/10.1177/1747493020932806.
23. Mitta N, Sreedharan SE, Sarma SP, et al. Women and stroke: different, yet similar. Cerebrovasc Dis Extra 2021;11(3):106–11.
24. van Dam-Nolen DH, van Egmond NC, Koudstaal PJ, et al. Sex differences in carotid atherosclerosis: a systematic review and meta-analysis. Stroke 2023;54(2): 315–26.
25. Schneider AT, Kissela B, Woo D, et al. Ischemic stroke subtypes: a population-based study of incidence rates among blacks and whites. Stroke 2004;35(7): 1552–6. https://doi.org/10.1161/01.STR.0000129335.28301.f5.
26. White H, Boden-Albala B, Wang C, et al. Ischemic stroke subtype incidence among whites, blacks, and Hispanics: the Northern Manhattan Study. Circulation 2005;111(10):1327–31.
27. Lal BK, Meschia JF, Brott TG, et al. Race differences in high-grade carotid artery stenosis. Stroke 2021;52(6):2053–9.
28. Lang C, Seyfang L, Ferrari J, et al. Do women with atrial fibrillation experience more severe strokes? Results from the Austrian stroke unit registry. Stroke 2017;48(3):778–80.
29. Gall S, Donnan G, Dewey H, et al. Sex differences in presentation, severity, and management of stroke in a population-based study. Neurology 2010;74(12): 975–81.
30. Boehme AK, Siegler JE, Mullen MT, et al. Racial and gender differences in stroke severity, outcomes, and treatment in patients with acute ischemic stroke. J Stroke Cerebrovasc Dis 2014;23(4):e255–61. https://doi.org/10.1016/j.jstrokecerebrovasdis.2013.11.003.
31. Jones MR, Horner RD, Edwards LJ, et al. Racial variation in initial stroke severity. Stroke 2000;31(3):563–7.
32. Bosch PR, Karmarkar AM, Roy I, et al. Association of Medicare-Medicaid dual eligibility and race and ethnicity with ischemic stroke severity. JAMA Netw Open 2022;5(3):e224596.
33. Song S, Liang L, Fonarow GC, et al. Comparison of clinical care and in-hospital outcomes of Asian American and white patients with acute ischemic stroke. JAMA Neurol 2019;76(4):430–9.
34. Zachrison KS, Nielsen VM, De La Ossa NP, et al. Prehospital stroke care part 1: emergency medical services and the stroke systems of care. Stroke 2023;54(4): 1138–47.
35. Lin CB, Peterson ED, Smith EE, et al. Emergency medical service hospital prenotification is associated with improved evaluation and treatment of acute ischemic stroke. Circulation: Cardiovascular quality and outcomes 2012;5(4): 514–22.
36. Abdullah AR, Smith EE, Biddinger PD, et al. Advance hospital notification by EMS in acute stroke is associated with shorter door-to-computed tomography time andincreased likelihood of administration of tissue-plasminogen activator. Prehosp Emerg Care 2008;12(4):426–31.
37. Nielsen VM, Song G, DeJoie-Stanton C, et al. Emergency medical services Prenotification is associated with reduced odds of in-hospital mortality in stroke patients. Prehosp Emerg Care 2023;27(5):639–45.
38. Govindarajan P, Friedman BT, Delgadillo JQ, et al. Race and sex disparities in prehospital recognition of acute stroke. Acad Emerg Med 2015;22(3):264–72.

39. Mochari-Greenberger H, Xian Y, Hellkamp AS, et al. Racial/ethnic and sex differences in emergency medical services transport among hospitalized US stroke patients: analysis of the National Get with the Guidelines–Stroke Registry. J Am Heart Assoc 2015;4(8):e002099.
40. Asaithambi G, Tong X, Lakshminarayan K, et al. Emergency medical services utilization for acute stroke care: analysis of the Paul coverdell national acute stroke program, 2014-2019. Prehosp Emerg Care 2022;26(3):326–32.
41. Smith MA, Lisabeth LD, Bonikowski F, et al. The role of ethnicity, sex, and language on delay to hospital arrival for acute ischemic stroke. Stroke 2010; 41(5):905–9.
42. Bushnell CD, Chaturvedi S, Gage KR, et al. Sex differences in stroke: challenges and opportunities. J Cerebr Blood Flow Metabol 2018;38(12):2179–91.
43. Rexrode KM, Madsen TE, Yu AY, et al. The impact of sex and gender on stroke. Circ Res 2022;130(4):512–28.
44. Ali M, van Os HJ, van der Weerd N, et al. Sex differences in presentation of stroke: a systematic review and meta-analysis. Stroke 2022;53(2):345–54.
45. Shajahan S, Sun L, Harris K, et al. Sex differences in the symptom presentation of stroke: a systematic review and meta-analysis. Int J Stroke 2023;18(2): 144–53.
46. Amy Y, Penn AM, Lesperance ML, et al. Sex differences in presentation and outcome after an acute transient or minor neurologic event. JAMA Neurol 2019;76(8):962–8.
47. Rathore SS, Hinn AR, Cooper LS, et al. Characterization of incident stroke signs and symptoms: findings from the atherosclerosis risk in communities study. Stroke 2002;33(11):2718–21.
48. Stroebele N, Mueller-Riemenschneider F, Nolte CH, et al. Knowledge of risk factors, and warning signs of stroke: a systematic review from a gender perspective. Int J Stroke 2011;6(1):60–6.
49. Madsen TE, Baird KA, Silver B, et al. Analysis of gender differences in knowledge of stroke warning signs. J Stroke Cerebrovasc Dis 2015;24(7):1540–7.
50. Jackson SL, Legvold B, Vahratian A, et al. Sociodemographic and geographic variation in awareness of stroke signs and symptoms among adults—United States, 2017. MMWR (Morb Mortal Wkly Rep) 2020;69(44):1617.
51. Adams HP, Brott TG, Furlan AJ, et al. Guidelines for thrombolytic therapy for acute stroke: a supplement to the guidelines for the management of patients with acute ischemic stroke: a statement for healthcare professionals from a Special Writing Group of the Stroke Council, American Heart Association. Circulation 1996;94(5):1167–74.
52. Hacke W, Kaste M, Bluhmki E, et al. Thrombolysis with alteplase 3 to 4.5 hours after acute ischemic stroke. N Engl J Med 2008;359(13):1317–29.
53. Disorders NIoN, Group Sr-PSS. Tissue plasminogen activator for acute ischemic stroke. N Engl J Med 1995;333(24):1581–8.
54. Emberson J, Lees KR, Lyden P, et al. Effect of treatment delay, age, and stroke severity on the effects of intravenous thrombolysis with alteplase for acute ischaemic stroke: a meta-analysis of individual patient data from randomised trials. Lancet 2014;384(9958):1929–35.
55. Atlantis T. Association of outcome with early stroke treatment: pooled analysis of ATLANTIS, ECASS, and NINDS rt-PA stroke trials. Lancet 2004;363(9411): 768–74.
56. Grotta JC, Yamal J-M, Parker SA, et al. Prospective, multicenter, controlled trial of mobile stroke units. N Engl J Med 2021;385(11):971–81.

57. Mahawish K, Gommans J, Kleinig T, et al. Switching to tenecteplase for stroke thrombolysis: real-world experience and outcomes in a regional stroke network. Am Heart Assoc 2021;52(10):e590–3.

58. Goyal M, Menon BK, Van Zwam WH, et al. Endovascular thrombectomy after large-vessel ischaemic stroke: a meta-analysis of individual patient data from five randomised trials. Lancet 2016;387(10029):1723–31.

59. Nogueira RG, Jadhav AP, Haussen DC, et al. Thrombectomy 6 to 24 hours after stroke with a mismatch between deficit and infarct. N Engl J Med 2018;378(1): 11–21.

60. Albers GW, Lansberg MG, Kemp S, et al. A multicenter randomized controlled trial of endovascular therapy following imaging evaluation for ischemic stroke (DEFUSE 3). London, England: SAGE Publications Sage UK; 2017.

61. Nguyen TN, Castonguay AC, Siegler JE, et al. Mechanical thrombectomy in the late presentation of anterior circulation large vessel occlusion stroke: a guideline from the Society of Vascular and Interventional Neurology guidelines and Practice Standards Committee. Stroke: Vascular and Interventional Neurology 2023; 3(1):e000512.

62. Tao C, Nogueira RG, Zhu Y, et al. Trial of endovascular treatment of acute basilar-artery occlusion. N Engl J Med 2022;387(15):1361–72.

63. Jovin TG, Li C, Wu L, et al. Trial of thrombectomy 6 to 24 hours after stroke due to basilar-artery occlusion. N Engl J Med 2022;387(15):1373–84.

64. Sarraj A, Hassan AE, Abraham MG, et al. Trial of endovascular thrombectomy for large ischemic strokes. N Engl J Med 2023;388(14):1259–71.

65. Huo X, Ma G, Tong X, et al. Trial of endovascular therapy for acute ischemic stroke with large infarct. N Engl J Med 2023;388(14):1272–83.

66. Bendszus M, Fiehler J, Subtil F, et al. Endovascular thrombectomy for acute ischaemic stroke with established large infarct: multicentre, open-label, randomised trial. Lancet 2023;402(10414):1753–63.

67. Smith WS, Lev MH, English JD, et al. Significance of large vessel intracranial occlusion causing acute ischemic stroke and TIA. Stroke 2009;40(12):3834–40.

68. Malhotra K, Gornbein J, Saver JL. Ischemic strokes due to large-vessel occlusions contribute disproportionately to stroke-related dependence and death: a review. Front Neurol 2017;8:651.

69. Asif KS, Otite FO, Desai SM, et al. Mechanical thrombectomy global access for stroke (MT-GLASS): a mission thrombectomy (MT-2020 Plus) study. Circulation 2023;147(16):1208–20.

70. Bushnell C, Howard VJ, Lisabeth L, et al. Sex differences in the evaluation and treatment of acute ischaemic stroke. Lancet Neurol 2018;17(7):641–50.

71. Sheth SA, Lee S, Warach SJ, et al. Sex differences in outcome after endovascular stroke therapy for acute ischemic stroke. Stroke 2019;50(9):2420–7.

72. Chalos V, de Ridder IR, Lingsma HF, et al. Does sex modify the effect of endovascular treatment for ischemic stroke? A subgroup analysis of 7 randomized trials. Stroke 2019;50(9):2413–9.

73. Bala F, Casetta I, Nannoni S, et al. Sex-related differences in outcomes after endovascular treatment of patients with late-window stroke. Stroke 2022;53(2): 311–8.

74. Dmytriw A, Ku J, Yang V, et al. Do outcomes between women and men differ after endovascular thrombectomy? A meta-analysis. Am J Neuroradiol 2021; 42(5):910–5.

75. Ouyang M, Shajahan S, Liu X, et al. Sex differences in the utilization and outcomes of endovascular treatment after acute ischemic stroke: a systematic review and meta-analysis. Frontiers in Global Women's Health 2023;3:1032592.

76. Deb-Chatterji M, Schlemm E, Flottmann F, et al. Sex differences in outcome after thrombectomy for acute ischemic stroke are explained by confounding factors. Clin Neuroradiol 2021;31:1101–9.

77. Bouslama M, Rebello LC, Haussen DC, et al. Endovascular therapy and ethnic disparities in stroke outcomes. Interv Neurol 2018;7(6):389–98. https://doi.org/10.1159/000487607.

78. Strong B, Lisabeth LD, Reeves M. Sex differences in IV thrombolysis treatment for acute ischemic stroke: a systematic review and meta-analysis. Neurology 2020;95(1):e11–22.

79. Asdaghi N, Romano JG, Wang K, et al. Sex disparities in ischemic stroke care: FL-PR CReSD study (Florida–Puerto Rico Collaboration to Reduce Stroke Disparities). Stroke 2016;47(10):2618–26.

80. Reeves M, Bhatt A, Jajou P, et al. Sex differences in the use of intravenous rt-PA thrombolysis treatment for acute ischemic stroke: a meta-analysis. Stroke 2009; 40(5):1743–9.

81. Bonkhoff AK, Karch A, Weber R, et al. Female stroke: sex differences in acute treatment and early outcomes of acute ischemic stroke. Stroke 2021;52(2): 406–15.

82. Weber R, Krogias C, Eyding J, et al. Age and sex differences in ischemic stroke treatment in a nationwide analysis of 1.11 million hospitalized cases. Stroke 2019;50(12):3494–502.

83. Silva Y, Sánchez-Cirera L, Terceño M, et al. Sex and gender differences in acute stroke care: metrics, access to treatment and outcome. A territorial analysis of the Stroke Code System of Catalonia. European Stroke Journal 2023;8(2): 557–65.

84. Otite FO, Saini V, Sur NB, et al. Ten-year trend in age, sex, and racial disparity in tPA (Alteplase) and thrombectomy use following stroke in the United States. Stroke 2021;52(8):2562–70.

85. Yu AYX, Austin PC, Rashid M, et al. Sex differences in intensity of care and outcomes after acute ischemic stroke across the age continuum. Neurology 2023; 100(2):e163–71.

86. Ikeme S, Kottenmeier E, Uzochukwu G, et al. Evidence-based disparities in stroke care metrics and outcomes in the United States: a systematic review. Stroke 2022;53(3):670–9.

87. Aparicio HJ, Carr BG, Kasner SE, et al. Racial disparities in intravenous recombinant tissue plasminogen activator use persist at primary stroke centers. J Am Heart Assoc 2015;4(10):e001877.

88. Bhattacharya P, Mada F, Salowich-Palm L, et al. Are racial disparities in stroke care still prevalent in certified stroke centers? J Stroke Cerebrovasc Dis 2013; 22(4):383–8. https://doi.org/10.1016/j.jstrokecerebrovasdis.2011.09.018.

89. Schwamm LH, Reeves MJ, Pan W, et al. Race/ethnicity, quality of care, and outcomes in ischemic stroke. Circulation 2010;121(13):1492–501.

90. Rinaldo L, Rabinstein AA, Cloft H, et al. Racial and ethnic disparities in the utilization of thrombectomy for acute stroke: analysis of data from 2016 to 2018. Stroke 2019;50(9):2428–32.

91. Sheriff F, Xu H, Maud A, et al. Temporal trends in racial and ethnic disparities in endovascular therapy in acute ischemic stroke. J Am Heart Assoc 2022;11(6): e023212.

92. Barber PA, Zhang J, Demchuk AM, et al. Why are stroke patients excluded from TPA therapy? An analysis of patient eligibility. Neurology 2001;56(8):1015–20. https://doi.org/10.1212/wnl.56.8.1015.

93. Reiff T, Michel P. Reasons and evolution of non-thrombolysis in acute ischaemic stroke. Emerg Med J 2017;34(4):219–26. https://doi.org/10.1136/emermed-2015-205140.

94. Springer MV, Labovitz DL, Hochheiser EC. Race-ethnic disparities in hospital arrival time after ischemic stroke. Ethn Dis 2017;27(2):125.

95. Karve SJ, Balkrishnan R, Mohammad YM, et al. Racial/ethnic disparities in emergency department waiting time for stroke patients in the United States. J Stroke Cerebrovasc Dis Jan-Feb 2011;20(1):30–40. https://doi.org/10.1016/j.jstrokecerebrovasdis.2009. 10.006.

96. Neves G, DeToledo J, Morris J, et al. An analysis of racial inequities in emergency department triage among patients with stroke-like symptoms in the United States. BMC Emerg Med 2023;23(1):90. https://doi.org/10.1186/s12873-023-00865-z.

97. Polineni SP, Perez EJ, Wang K, et al. Sex and race-ethnic disparities in door-to-CT time in acute ischemic stroke: the Florida stroke registry. J Am Heart Assoc 2021;10(7):e017543.

98. Madsen TE, Khoury JC, Alwell KA, et al. Analysis of tissue plasminogen activator eligibility by sex in the Greater Cincinnati/Northern Kentucky Stroke Study. Stroke 2015;46(3):717–21. https://doi.org/10.1161/strokeaha.114.006737.

99. Hsia AW, Edwards DF, Morgenstern LB, et al. Racial disparities in tissue plasminogen activator treatment rate for stroke: a population-based study. Stroke 2011;42(8):2217–21.

100. Mendelson SJ, Zhang S, Matsouaka R, et al. Race-ethnic disparities in rates of declination of thrombolysis for stroke. Neurology 2022;98(16):e1596–604.

101. Tarnutzer AA, Lee SH, Robinson KA, et al. ED misdiagnosis of cerebrovascular events in the era of modern neuroimaging: a meta-analysis. Neurology 2017; 88(15):1468–77. https://doi.org/10.1212/wnl.0000000000003814.

102. Newman-Toker DE, Moy E, Valente E, et al. Missed diagnosis of stroke in the emergency department: a cross-sectional analysis of a large population-based sample. Diagnosis (Berl) 2014;1(2):155–66. https://doi.org/10.1515/dx-2013-0038.

103. Fonarow GC, Smith EE, Saver JL, et al. Timeliness of tissue-type plasminogen activator therapy in acute ischemic stroke: patient characteristics, hospital factors, and outcomes associated with door-to-needle times within 60 minutes. Circulation 2011;123(7):750–8.

104. Asdaghi N, Romano JG, Wang K, et al. Sex disparities in ischemic stroke care: FL-PR CReSD study (Florida-Puerto Rico collaboration to reduce stroke disparities). Stroke 2016;47(10):2618–26. https://doi.org/10.1161/strokeaha.116.013059.

105. Coplin WM. Critical care management of acute ischemic stroke. Continuum: Lifelong Learning in Neurology 2012;18(3):547–59.

106. Santos D, Maillie L, Dhamoon MS. Patterns and outcomes of intensive care on acute ischemic stroke patients in the US. Circulation: Cardiovascular Quality and Outcomes 2023;16(3):e008961.

107. Cucchiara B, Kasner S, Wolk D, et al. Lack of hemispheric dominance for consciousness in acute ischaemic stroke. J Neurol Neurosurg Psychiatr 2003;74(7): 889–92.

108. Yaghi S, Willey JZ, Cucchiara B, et al. Treatment and outcome of hemorrhagic transformation after intravenous alteplase in acute ischemic stroke: a scientific

statement for healthcare professionals from the American Heart Association/ American Stroke Association. Stroke 2017;48(12):e343–61.

109. Score IHR. Predicting the Risk of Symptomatic Intracerebral Hemorrhage in Ischemic Stroke Treated With Intravenous Alteplase. 2012.

110. Sussman ES, Connolly Jr ES. Hemorrhagic transformation: a review of the rate of hemorrhage in the major clinical trials of acute ischemic stroke. Front Neurol 2013;4:69.

111. Whiteley WN, Slot KB, Fernandes P, et al. Risk factors for intracranial hemorrhage in acute ischemic stroke patients treated with recombinant tissue plasminogen activator: a systematic review and meta-analysis of 55 studies. Stroke 2012;43(11):2904–9.

112. Mehta RH, Cox M, Smith EE, et al. Race/ethnic differences in the risk of hemorrhagic complications among patients with ischemic stroke receiving thrombolytic therapy. Stroke 2014;45(8):2263–9.

113. Menon BK, Saver JL, Prabhakaran S, et al. Risk score for intracranial hemorrhage in patients with acute ischemic stroke treated with intravenous tissue-type plasminogen activator. Stroke 2012;43(9):2293–9.

114. Powers WJ, Rabinstein AA, Ackerson T, et al. Guidelines for the early management of patients with acute ischemic stroke: 2019 update to the 2018 guidelines for the early management of acute ischemic stroke: a guideline for healthcare professionals from the American Heart Association/American Stroke Association. Stroke 2019;50(12):e344–418.

115. Torbey MT, Bösel J, Rhoney DH, et al. Evidence-based guidelines for the management of large hemispheric infarction: a statement for health care professionals from the Neurocritical Care Society and the German Society for Neuro-intensive Care and Emergency Medicine. Neurocritical Care 2015;22: 146–64.

116. Liebeskind DS, Jüttler E, Shapovalov Y, et al. Cerebral edema associated with large hemispheric infarction: implications for diagnosis and treatment. Stroke 2019;50(9):2619–25.

117. Wu S, Yuan R, Wang Y, et al. Early prediction of malignant brain edema after ischemic stroke: a systematic review and meta-analysis (P3. 9-010). AAN Enterprises 2019.

118. Wijdicks EF, Sheth KN, Carter BS, et al. Recommendations for the management of cerebral and cerebellar infarction with swelling: a statement for healthcare professionals from the American Heart Association/American Stroke Association. Stroke 2014;45(4):1222–38.

119. Lin J, Frontera JA. Decompressive hemicraniectomy for large hemispheric strokes. Stroke 2021;52(4):1500–10.

120. Reinink H, Jüttler E, Hacke W, et al. Surgical decompression for space-occupying hemispheric infarction: a systematic review and individual patient meta-analysis of randomized clinical trials. JAMA Neurol 2021;78(2):208–16.

121. Lekoubou A, Tankam C, Bishu KG, et al. Decompressive hemicraniectomy for stroke by race/ethnicity in the United States. Eneurologicalsci 2022;29:100421.

122. Faigle R, Urrutia VC, Cooper LA, et al. Racial differences in utilization of life-sustaining vs curative inpatient procedures after stroke. JAMA Neurol 2016; 73(9):1151–3.

123. Ornstein KA, Roth DL, Huang J, et al. Evaluation of racial disparities in hospice use and end-of-life treatment intensity in the REGARDS cohort. JAMA Netw Open 2020;3(8):e2014639.

124. Faigle R, Marsh EB, Llinas RH, et al. ICAT: a simple score predicting critical care needs after thrombolysis in stroke patients. Crit Care 2015;20:1–8.

125. Carcel C, Wang X, Sandset EC, et al. Sex differences in treatment and outcome after stroke: pooled analysis including 19,000 participants. Neurology 2019; 93(24):e2170–80.

126. Overwyk KJ, Yin X, Tong X, et al. Defect-free care trends in the Paul Coverdell National acute stroke program, 2008-2018. Am Heart J 2021;232:177–84.

127. Bruce SS, Merkler AE, Bassi M, et al. Differences in diagnostic evaluation in women and men after acute ischemic stroke. J Am Heart Assoc 2020;9(5): e015625. https://doi.org/10.1161/jaha.119.015625.

128. Reeves MJ, Bushnell CD, Howard G, et al. Sex differences in stroke: epidemiology, clinical presentation, medical care, and outcomes. Lancet Neurol 2008; 7(10):915–26.

129. McCullough LD, Lichtman JH. Comparable care, worse outcomes for women with stroke. Nat Rev Neurol 2014;10(7):367–8.

130. Bushnell CD, Reeves MJ, Zhao X, et al. Sex differences in quality of life after ischemic stroke. Neurology 2014;82(11):922–31. https://doi.org/10.1212/wnl. 0000000000000208.

131. Germans MR, Jaja BN, de Oliviera Manoel AL, et al. Sex differences in delayed cerebral ischemia after subarachnoid hemorrhage. J Neurosurg 2017;129(2): 458–64.

132. Dong L, Sánchez BN, Skolarus LE, et al. Sex difference in prevalence of depression after stroke. Neurology 2020;94(19):e1973–83. https://doi.org/10.1212/wnl. 0000000000009394.

133. Buie JN, Zhao Y, Burns S, et al. Racial disparities in stroke recovery persistence in the post-acute stroke recovery phase: evidence from the health and retirement study. Ethn Dis 2020;30(2):339.

134. Kelly AG, Hoskins KD, Holloway RG. Early stroke mortality, patient preferences, and the withdrawal of care bias. Neurology 2012;79(9):941–4. https://doi.org/10. 1212/WNL.0b013e318266fc40.

135. Bako AT, Pan A, Potter T, et al. Contemporary trends in the nationwide incidence of primary intracerebral hemorrhage. Stroke 2022;53(3):e70–4.

136. Xia C, Hoffman H, Anikpezie N, et al. Trends in the incidence of spontaneous subarachnoid hemorrhages in the United States, 2007–2017. Neurology 2023; 100(2):e123–32.

137. Waziry R, Heshmatollah A, Bos D, et al. Time trends in survival following first hemorrhagic or ischemic stroke between 1991 and 2015 in the Rotterdam study. Stroke 2020;51(3):824–9.

138. Toyoda K, Yoshimura S, Nakai M, et al. Twenty-year change in severity and outcome of ischemic and hemorrhagic strokes. JAMA Neurol 2022;79(1):61–9.

139. Xian Y, Holloway RG, Smith EE, et al. Racial/ethnic differences in process of care and outcomes among patients hospitalized with intracerebral hemorrhage. Stroke 2014;45(11):3243–50.

140. Doelfel SR, Kalagara R, Han EJ, et al. Gender disparities in stroke code activation in patients with intracerebral hemorrhage. J Stroke Cerebrovasc Dis 2021; 30(12):106119.

141. Koch S, Elkind MS, Testai FD, et al. Racial-ethnic disparities in acute blood pressure after intracerebral hemorrhage. Neurology 2016;87(8):786–91.

142. Anadani M, Qureshi AI, Menacho S, et al. Race/ethnicity and response to blood pressure lowering treatment after intracerebral hemorrhage. European Stroke Journal 2021;6(4):343–8.

143. Fukuda-Doi M, Yamamoto H, Koga M, et al. Sex differences in blood pressure–lowering therapy and outcomes following intracerebral hemorrhage: results from ATACH-2. Stroke 2020;51(8):2282–6.

144. Sandset EC, Wang X, Carcel C, et al. Sex differences in treatment, radiological features and outcome after intracerebral haemorrhage: pooled analysis of intensive blood pressure reduction in acute cerebral haemorrhage trials 1 and 2. European stroke journal 2020;5(4):345–50.

145. Chen C-J, Ding D, Ironside N, et al. Predictors of surgical intervention in patients with spontaneous intracerebral hemorrhage. World neurosurgery 2019;123: e700–8.

146. Cruz-Flores S, Rodriguez GJ, Chaudhry MRA, et al. Racial/ethnic disparities in hospital utilization in intracerebral hemorrhage. Int J Stroke 2019;14(7):686–95.

147. Guha R, Boehme A, Demel SL, et al. Aggressiveness of care following intracerebral hemorrhage in women and men. Neurology 2017;89(4):349–54.

148. Wang SS-Y, Bögli SY, Nierobisch N, et al. Sex-related differences in patients' characteristics, provided care, and outcomes following spontaneous intracerebral hemorrhage. Neurocritical Care 2022;37(1):111–20.

149. Faigle R, Bahouth MN, Urrutia VC, et al. Racial and socioeconomic disparities in gastrostomy tube placement after intracerebral hemorrhage in the United States. Stroke 2016;47(4):964–70.

150. Hwang DY, George BP, Kelly AG, et al. Variability in gastrostomy tube placement for intracerebral hemorrhage patients at US hospitals. J Stroke Cerebrovasc Dis 2018;27(4):978–87.

151. Faigle R, Carrese JA, Cooper LA, et al. Minority race and male sex as risk factors for non-beneficial gastrostomy tube placements after stroke. PLoS One 2018;13(1):e0191293.

152. Faigle R, Ziai WC, Urrutia VC, et al. Racial differences in palliative care use after stroke in majority-white, minority-serving, and racially integrated US hospitals. Crit Care Med 2017;45(12):2046.

153. Murthy SB, Moradiya Y, Hanley DF, et al. Palliative care utilization in nontraumatic intracerebral hemorrhage in the United States. Crit Care Med 2016; 44(3):575–82.

154. McFarlin J, Hailey CE, Qi W, et al. Associations between patient characteristics and a new, early do-not-attempt resuscitation order after intracerebral hemorrhage. J Palliat Med 2018;21(8):1161–5.

155. Fraser SM, Torres GL, Cai C, et al. Race is a predictor of withdrawal of life support in patients with intracerebral hemorrhage. J Stroke Cerebrovasc Dis 2018; 27(11):3108–14.

156. Suolang D, Chen BJ, Faigle R. Temporal trends in racial and ethnic disparities in palliative care use after intracerebral hemorrhage in the United States. Stroke 2022;53(3):e85–7.

157. Nakagawa K, Vento MA, Seto TB, et al. Sex differences in the use of early do-not-resuscitate orders after intracerebral hemorrhage. Stroke 2013;44(11): 3229–31.

158. Craen A, Mangal R, Stead TG, et al. Gender differences in outcomes after nontraumatic intracerebral hemorrhage. Cureus 2019;11(10).

159. Lillemoe K, Lord A, Torres J, et al. Factors associated with DNR status after nontraumatic intracranial hemorrhage. Neurohospitalist 2020;10(3):168–75.

160. Kalasapudi L, Williamson S, Shipper AG, et al. Scoping review of racial, ethnic, and sex disparities in the diagnosis and management of hemorrhagic stroke. Neurology 2023;101(3):e267–76.

161. Krishnan K, Beishon L, Berge E, et al. Relationship between race and outcome in asian, black, and caucasian patients with spontaneous intracerebral hemorrhage: data from the virtual international stroke trials archive and efficacy of nitric oxide in stroke trial. Int J Stroke 2018;13(4):362–73.

162. Woo D, Comeau ME, Venema SU, et al. Risk factors associated with mortality and neurologic disability after intracerebral hemorrhage in a racially and ethnically diverse cohort. JAMA Netw Open 2022;5(3):e221103.

163. Su CM, Warren A, Kraus C, et al. Lack of racial and ethnic-based differences in acute care delivery in intracerebral hemorrhage. Int J Emerg Med 2021; 14(1):1–7.

164. Roquer J, Rodríguez-Campello A, Jiménez-Conde J, et al. Sex-related differences in primary intracerebral hemorrhage. Neurology 2016;87(3):257–62.

165. Shah VA, Thompson RE, Yenokyan G, et al. One-year outcome trajectories and factors associated with functional recovery among survivors of intracerebral and intraventricular hemorrhage with initial severe disability. JAMA Neurol 2022; 79(9):856–68.

166. Simmonds KP, Luo Z, Reeves M. Race/ethnic and stroke subtype differences in poststroke functional recovery after acute rehabilitation. Arch Phys Med Rehabil 2021;102(8):1473–81.

167. Leasure AC, King ZA, Torres-Lopez V, et al. Racial/ethnic disparities in the risk of intracerebral hemorrhage recurrence. Neurology 2020;94(3):e314–22.

168. Rodriguez-Torres A, Murphy M, Kourkoulis C, et al. Hypertension and intracerebral hemorrhage recurrence among white, black, and Hispanic individuals. Neurology 2018;91(1):e37–44.

169. Biffi A, Teo KC, Castello JP, et al. Impact of uncontrolled hypertension at 3 months after intracerebral hemorrhage. J Am Heart Assoc 2021;10(11):e020392.

170. Walsh KB, Woo D, Sekar P, et al. Untreated hypertension: a powerful risk factor for lobar and nonlobar intracerebral hemorrhage in whites, blacks, and Hispanics. Circulation 2016;134(19):1444–52.

171. Castello JP, Teo KC, Abramson JR, et al. Long-term blood pressure variability and major adverse cardiovascular and cerebrovascular events after intracerebral hemorrhage. J Am Heart Assoc 2022;11(6):e024158.

172. Abramson JR, Castello JP, Keins S, et al. Biological and social determinants of hypertension severity before vs after intracerebral hemorrhage. Neurology 2022;98(13):e1349–60.

173. Mayerhofer E, Zaba NO, Parodi L, et al. Disparities in brain health comorbidity management in intracerebral hemorrhage. Front Neurol 2023;14:1194810.

174. Schmidt LB, Goertz S, Wohlfahrt J, et al. Recurrent intracerebral hemorrhage: associations with comorbidities and medicine with antithrombotic effects. PLoS One 2016;11(11):e0166223.

175. Casolla B, Moulin S, Kyheng M, et al. Five-year risk of major ischemic and hemorrhagic events after intracerebral hemorrhage. Stroke 2019;50(5):1100–7.

176. Roark C, Case D, Gritz M, et al. Nationwide analysis of hospital-to-hospital transfer in patients with aneurysmal subarachnoid hemorrhage requiring aneurysm repair. J Neurosurg 2018;131(4):1254–61.

177. Shah D, Patel U, Kellner C, et al. National trends of interhospital transfers for aneurysmal subarachnoid hemorrhage in the United States. Stroke: Vascular and Interventional Neurology 2023;3(1):e000462.

178. Dubosh NM, Edlow JA, Goto T, et al. Missed serious neurologic conditions in emergency department patients discharged with nonspecific diagnoses of headache or back pain. Ann Emerg Med 2019;74(4):549–61.

179. Ois A, Vivas E, Figueras-Aguirre G, et al. Misdiagnosis worsens prognosis in subarachnoid hemorrhage with good Hunt and Hess score. Stroke 2019; 50(11):3072–6.
180. Vermeulen MJ, Schull MJ. Missed diagnosis of subarachnoid hemorrhage in the emergency department. Stroke 2007;38(4):1216–21.
181. Zhou X, Bates AH, Mahajan UV, et al. Racial differences in time to blood pressure control of aneurysmal subarachnoid hemorrhage patients: a single-institution study. PLoS One 2023;18(2):e0279769.
182. Hoh BL, Ko NU, Amin-Hanjani S, et al. 2023 guideline for the management of patients with aneurysmal subarachnoid hemorrhage: a guideline from the American Heart Association/American Stroke Association. Stroke 2023;54(7):e314–70.
183. Attenello FJ, Wang K, Wen T, et al. Health disparities in time to aneurysm clipping/coiling among aneurysmal subarachnoid hemorrhage patients: a national study. World neurosurgery 2014;82(6):1071–6.
184. Donoho DA, Patel A, Buchanan IA, et al. Treatment at safety-net hospitals is associated with delays in coil embolization in patients with subarachnoid hemorrhage. World neurosurgery 2018;120:e434–9.
185. Eden SV, Morgenstern LB, Sekar P, et al. The role of race in time to treatment after subarachnoid hemorrhage. Neurosurgery 2007;60(5):837–43.
186. Rosen D, Novakovic R, Goldenberg FD, et al. Racial differences in demographics, acute complications, and outcomes in patients with subarachnoid hemorrhage: a large patient series. J Neurosurg 2005;103(1):18–24.
187. Siddiq F, Chaudhry SA, Tummala RP, et al. Factors and outcomes associated with early and delayed aneurysm treatment in subarachnoid hemorrhage patients in the United States. Neurosurgery 2012;71(3):670–8.
188. Lin N, Cahill KS, Frerichs KU, et al. Treatment of ruptured and unruptured cerebral aneurysms in the USA: a paradigm shift. J Neurointerventional Surg 2018; 10(Suppl 1):i69–76.
189. Schupper AJ, Hardigan TA, Mehta A, et al. Sex and racial disparity in outcome of aneurysmal subarachnoid hemorrhage in the United States: a 20-year analysis. Stroke 2023;54(5):1347–56. https://doi.org/10.1161/strokeaha.122.041488.
190. Lai PMR, Gormley WB, Patel N, et al. Age-dependent radiographic vasospasm and delayed cerebral ischemia in women after aneurysmal subarachnoid hemorrhage. World neurosurgery 2019;130:e230–5.
191. Qureshi AI, Adil MM, Suri MFK. Rate of use and determinants of withdrawal of care among patients with subarachnoid hemorrhage in the United States. World neurosurgery 2014;82(5):e579–84.
192. Choi HA, Fernandez A, Jeon S-B, et al. Ethnic disparities in end-of-life care after subarachnoid hemorrhage. Neurocritical Care 2015;22:423–8.
193. Kowalski RG, Chang TR, Carhuapoma JR, et al. Withdrawal of technological life support following subarachnoid hemorrhage. Neurocritical Care 2013;19: 269–75.
194. Wahood W, Rizvi AA, Alexander AY, et al. Trends in admissions and outcomes for treatment of aneurysmal subarachnoid hemorrhage in the United States. Neurocritical Care 2022;37(1):209–18. https://doi.org/10.1007/s12028-022-01476-5.
195. Mahajan UV, Khan HA, Zhou X, et al. Predictors of in-hospital mortality and home discharge in patients with aneurysmal subarachnoid hemorrhage: a 4-year retrospective analysis. Neurocritical Care 2023;38(1):85–95. https://doi.org/10.1007/s12028-022-01596-y.

196. Zacharia BE, Grobelny BT, Komotar RJ, et al. The influence of race on outcome following subarachnoid hemorrhage. J Clin Neurosci 2010;17(1):34–7. https://doi.org/10.1016/j.jocn.2009.05.015.
197. Larrew T, Pryor W, Weinberg J, et al. Aneurysmal subarachnoid hemorrhage: a statewide assessment of outcome based on risk factors, aneurysm characteristics, and geo-demography. J Neurointerventional Surg 2015;7(11):855–60.
198. Hamdan A, Barnes J, Mitchell P. Subarachnoid hemorrhage and the female sex: analysis of risk factors, aneurysm characteristics, and outcomes. J Neurosurg 2014;121(6):1367–73.
199. Pegoli M, Mandrekar J, Rabinstein AA, et al. Predictors of excellent functional outcome in aneurysmal subarachnoid hemorrhage. J Neurosurg 2015;122(2):414–8.
200. Galea JP, Dulhanty L, Patel HC. Predictors of outcome in aneurysmal subarachnoid hemorrhage patients: observations from a multicenter data set. Stroke 2017;48(11):2958–63.
201. Ahmed R, Mhina C, Philip K, et al. Age-and sex-specific trends in medical complications after acute ischemic stroke in the United States. Neurology 2023;100(12):e1282–95./

Race, Ethnicity, and Gender Disparities in Management and Outcomes of Critically Ill Adults with Sepsis

Panagis Galiatsatos, MD, MHS[a,b],*, Henry Brems, MD[a],
Carlie N. Myers, MD[c], Kristina Montemayor, MD[a]

KEYWORDS

- Sepsis • Health equity • Health disparities • Race • Ethnicity • Gender

KEY POINTS

- Sepsis is a disease of biological disarray and one of health disparities, warranting further understanding of the social risk factors and impact of sepsis.
- Disparities regarding sepsis occur across race, ethnicity, and gender, with complex factors that impact these outcomes, from incidence to outcomes.
- Mitigating sepsis-related disparities will take both community-health and population-health approaches for health systems, in an attempt to modify certain risk factors for sepsis along with sepsis-related interventions.

INTRODUCTION

To establish the concepts regarding health equity and health disparities, an assessment of what is meant by both should be reviewed, especially as they apply to the acute, pathologic syndrome that is sepsis. In regard to *health equity*, this notion is rooted in complex sociologic understandings that center on how an individual and/or social network views health and certain priorities of health. Meaning, health equity is more than a goal but also reflects the fair treatment of each person aiming to achieve health equity and aims to result in the best health an individual and a society can achieve, achieved without barriers or discrimination. In regard to health disparities, this reflects the

[a] Division of Pulmonary and Critical Care Medicine, Department of Medicine, Johns Hopkins School of Medicine, Baltimore, MD, USA; [b] Office of Diversity, Inclusion, and Health Equity, Johns Hopkins Health System, Baltimore, MD, USA; [c] Division of Critical Care Medicine, Cincinnati Children's Hospital Medical Center, University of Cincinnati School of Medicine, Cincinnati, OH, USA
* Corresponding author. 4940 Eastern Avenue, 4th Floor, Asthma & Allergy Building, Baltimore, MD 21224.
E-mail address: pgaliat1@jhmi.edu

Crit Care Clin 40 (2024) 741–752
https://doi.org/10.1016/j.ccc.2024.06.001   **criticalcare.theclinics.com**

differences recognized between groups that are seen as socially advantaged against groups that are socially disadvantaged.[1] Specifically the definition, *health disparities* represent differences across socially privileged groups versus socially marginalized groups that, as a society, these differences are modifiable, avoidable, and unjust.[2] When attempting to mitigate the disparity between two populations, the interventions affect influential factors that are modifiable and overrepresented in the marginalized groups.[2,3] Therefore, the challenge around the objective recognition of differences between two groups before being designated as a disparity is that such differences must also go through a social review, reflecting on judgment on an inequitable outcome that is preventable, regardless if the factor was intentional or unintentional.

With such views, critical care pathologies such as sepsis have the ability to offer unique perspectives in regard to a person's and a society's goal of health equity and health disparities. By evaluating sepsis-related incidence and outcomes, an understanding of the mechanisms that drive this life-threatening pathology will provide insight into various aspects of the disease, with a focus on risk factors for its incidence and outcomes. In this review, we explore health disparities regarding sepsis as it aligns with certain social factors—race, ethnicity, and gender—when taking into account incidence, management, and outcomes. Further, we offer discussions on how a region's incidence of sepsis can be used as a population health target, whereby reduction in sepsis in order to close its own health disparity gaps may also assist in health equity goals beyond sepsis. Finally, this review on sepsis and health disparities will provide an understanding for clinicians involved in critical care to understand their role promoting health equity.

ETHNICITY AND RACE
Ethnicity

Both race and ethnicity are social constructs that assist in organizing populations by specific features, cultures, and/or other sociodemographic defining variables. They are created without scientific or biological meaning, though their influence in medical and health outcomes is substantial.[4] However, before exploring these topics with regard to sepsis and sepsis-related outcomes, several factors must be established. First such sociodemographic characterizations of populations are social terms that often change overtime, warranting any research in medicine and science on diverse populations to assure that the language and terminology around race and ethnicity is accurate, fair, and precise and reflects equity and consistency.[4] For instance, race in the past had been considered to be a biological construct, a notion now that has been debunked.[4,5] Next, recognize that race and ethnicity, depending on how they are used, may be factors that serve more than their sociodemographic descriptor, whereby, they may be used to be proxies toward more complicated social understandings that are often not captured in medical research, such socioeconomic position, and wealth.[6] Such a recognition is often cited for the reason there are inconsistent outcomes when exploring sepsis and the influence of race and ethnicity.[7] Finally, these terms vary globally, warranting that any evaluation of race and ethnicity must be met with the recognition that it will be evaluated through the lens of a specific region to minimize heterogeneity of the terms. Therefore, we have selected to assess race and ethnicity in the United States, where race and ethnicity are consistently found to be associated with variable health outcomes across these social groups.[8]

Ethnicity is a social construct that encompasses characteristics that reinforce a sense of homophily in a population, characteristics that include nationality, language, religion, geographic, or ancestry origin.[9] In the United States, using the 2020 US

Census definitions, ethnicity was focused on standards that require to collect and report data on minimum of 2 ethnicities: "Hispanic or Latino" and "Not Hispanic or Latino."[10] In addition to the dichotomized categories, the US Census recognizes that ethnicity is not a biological or genetic reference, but one of social, cultural, and ancestry, as set forth by the Office of Management and Budget in 1997. Therefore, as we explore ethnicity and its influence on sepsis, we will use the same categories, comparing the majority ethnicity in the United States (not Hispanic or Latino) against Hispanic or Latino populations.[11]

In one of the first epidemiologic studies on sepsis in the United States, conducted from 1979 to 2000 using ICD-9 codes (1979 was the first year using such coding), differences in race and gender were found.[12] While the study discussed racial findings (adult Black males fared worse in regard to sepsis-related outcomes as compared to other genders and White persons), and the method section notes ethnicity was collected, there is no report on ethnic groups in the final report.[12] Barnato and colleagues years later conducted another large, retrospective population-based cohort study using hospital discharge and 2000 US Census data, spanning 68 hospitals and 71,102,655 persons.[13] In this epidemiologic study, Black persons had higher rate of severe sepsis as compared to White persons; however, Hispanic ethnicity was found to be associated with lower incidence rates of severe sepsis, conditional on similar regional urbanicity and poverty.[13] Of note, in this study, Hispanic ethnicity was compared to Black and White racial populations, and sepsis definitions were using the now outdated definitions of sepsis (Sepsis-1 and Sepsis-2).[14]

A decade later, Jones and colleagues found that minority groups, including Hispanic/Latino persons, had higher rates of sepsis mortality compared to White persons.[15] The study used Healthcare Cost and Utilization Project (HCUP) State Inpatient Databases from the United States, reviewing data from 2004 to 2013. The study found that in 2004, sepsis-related mortality was similar between White persons hospitalized with sepsis and Hispanic persons hospitalized with sepsis: 178.2 deaths per 1000 sepsis-related hospitalizations for White patients versus 168.6 deaths per 1000 sepsis-related hospitalizations for Hispanic patients. And while sepsis-related mortality decreased for these subgroups over the next decade, it was not an equitable decrease. By 2013, a disparity emerged, with 91.2 deaths per 1000 sepsis-related hospitalizations for White patients being statistically significantly lower than Hispanic patients (97.9 deaths per 1000 sepsis-related hospitalizations) ($P<.001$). However, Jones and colleagues found that when controlling for hospital-level characteristics, Black, White, and Hispanic patients had similar sepsis-related mortality, with only estimates of Asian/Pacific Islanders remaining comparatively elevated.[15] Therefore, this study reaffirmed a trend found in the 2000s of Hispanic populations fairing as well as White populations in regard to sepsis outcomes, then deviating into health care-related disparities a decade later.

More recently, during the surge of the COVID-19 pandemic in its early years, Hispanic/Latino populations were disproportionately impacted.[16–18] Given severe COVID-19 has similarities in its pathophysiology with sepsis and septic shock,[19] recognizing the complexities around social patterns and behaviors that influenced the disparities in Hispanic/Latino persons around COVID-19-induced sepsis may have a significant amount of public health insight. Specifically, how sepsis impacts minority populations disproportionately may have more to do with non-biological factors (eg, access to nutritious foods, primary care and health care services, and transportation) that drive certain comorbidities of diabetes and hypertension,[20] which are influential to sepsis and sepsis-related mortality. Such insight was evident during the surge of severe COVID-19 in Hispanic/Latino populations.[21]

As the categorization of ethnicity becomes its own distinction, owing in part to a growing population presently in the United States, this will lead to new epidemiologic insights of sepsis similar to what was evident with severe COVID-19 research, where ethnicities were compared against each other (eg, non-Hispanic/Latino vs Hispanic/Latino). This will break from research of the past where ethnic groups were often compared with racial groups,[12,13,22] reaffirming how such social categories are viewed evolves overtime.[23] Therefore, future research is warranted to fully understand how changing social phenotypes (and changing perspectives on how best to evaluate such social categories) will contribute to identifying sepsis-related disparities among diverse ethnicities in the United States.

Race

In the United States, Black and other non-White individuals experience the highest incidence of sepsis.[12,13,24] Given the disproportionate burden of disease faced by racial minority groups, significant efforts have been made to understand (1) where disparities exist in sepsis-related management and outcomes and (2) what factors underlie those disparities.

Similar to incidence, mortality from sepsis appears higher for Black compared to White patients. While some studies have found either no difference or a higher mortality among White patients with sepsis, these may have been influenced geographic distribution and various adjustments in methodology.[25–31] Higher sepsis-related mortality among Black and other racial minority groups has been demonstrated several times, including among several large, nationally representative cohorts.[12,15,24,32–41] Parallel to mortality, other data demonstrate that non-White patients also face a longer length of stay and a higher 30 day readmission rate after sepsis-related hospitalization.[25,42–45] Nonetheless, most prior studies investigating disparities in sepsis-related outcomes have focused on mortality.

Despite the observed racial variation in unadjusted mortality, the difference by race frequently disappears in adjusted models. Most notably, a prior meta-analysis found no association between race and sepsis-related mortality when pooling results from adjusted analyses of 6 trials.[7] Importantly, this finding reinforces that the observed disparity is not due to something genetic or inherent to race, which is a social rather than a biologic construct.[4,46] Often, adjusted variables in the models include behaviors or socioeconomic factors, such as educational status, income, preferred language spoken, tobacco and substance abuse, and obesity[7] This reaffirms that a variety of other factors may explain the observed disparity in sepsis-related mortality, which necessitate further exploration.

Comorbidities and a higher severity of illness at presentation may partially explain differences in mortality. In multiple large retrospective cohort studies, Black patients with sepsis were more likely to have a higher severity of illness and degree of comorbidities, which accounted for observed differences in mortality.[33,47]

Social, economic, and geographic factors (centered on neighborhood composition that provides insight into the proximity of health and lifestyle that influence sepsis-related outcomes) also appear to contribute to differences in mortality by race. Geographic analyses have documented regional variation in sepsis-related mortality and suggest that socioeconomic indicators and access to care may strongly influence the higher mortality among Black communities.[39,48–51] Lack of insurance and residence in a medically underserved area also appear to contribute to increased mortality among Black patients with sepsis.[34,52] Further, community-level poverty and socioeconomic status are strongly associated with sepsis-attributable mortality.[35] Lastly, cultural factors may contribute to care preferences that may in turn influence outcomes, as 2 prior studies have suggested Black patients in the intensive care unit (ICU) with sepsis may be less likely to seek palliative or comfort-oriented care.[53,54]

In addition, differences in quality of care and management strategies may also explain disparities in outcomes. In a large study across 18 states over 10 years, higher sepsis mortality rates persisted for racial minorities when accounting for patient-level characteristics, but there were no differences when accounting for hospital characteristics.[15] Other studies have investigated specific management strategies, and racial disparities have been documented in antibiotic administration,[55,56] ICU admission,[33,57] interhospital transfer,[58,59] and implementation of protocol-based care.[60]

Notably, these disparities in management are likely attributable to between-hospital differences.[56,58,60] Specifically, hospitals that treat a greater proportion of Black patients have been found to have lower adherence to sepsis protocols or timely antibiotic administration.[56,60] Within centers, capacity strain has not been found to modify ICU admission,[57] and differences in time to antibiotics may be accounted for by infectious source and severity of illness.[55] Further, there do not appear to be differences in use of vasopressors, mechanical ventilation, and renal replacement therapy in sepsis, although data are limited.[29] Together, these data suggest that racial disparities in sepsis care are driven by structural and societal factors related to where patients seek care—and the quality of care delivered at those hospitals—rather than differences in treatment by race at a given hospital.

Race may also impact individual-level care among patients with sepsis. One study of end-of-life care found that physicians may be less likely to discuss prognosis and more likely to recommend withdrawal of life support among non-White patients.[61] Given prior evidence that suggests racial biases influence physician decision-making in other areas of medicine,[62,63] further research to understand the impact of race on physician decision-making in sepsis is warranted and may identify opportunities to improve care and address racial disparities.

Overall, Black and other non-White individuals with sepsis in the United States face worse outcomes and may receive less optimal care. Like many other illnesses, disparities in sepsis appear most likely a result of multiple interwoven structural factors, including socioeconomic disadvantages, chronic disease burden, and access to care. While a broader solution to sepsis-related disparities would therefore be complex, some steps can be taken now. For example, community-based or hospital-based interventions aimed at quality improvement can be developed to explicitly account for racial equity as an outcome.[64,65] Regardless, continued efforts both to understand the causes and to develop interventions for racial disparities in sepsis are warranted.

SEX AND GENDER

Sex and gender have been found to impact health outcomes in both acute and chronic medical conditions, and while they are often used interchangeably, it is important to understand how sex and gender differ. Sex commonly refers to biological attributes and characteristics while gender refers to social and cultural constructs.[66] Although women have historically been excluded or underrepresented in clinical trials, emerging evidence has shown the impact of sex and gender on critical care outcomes.[66,67]

Globally, men have a higher incidence of sepsis and are more likely to be admitted to an ICU for sepsis management.[68] In a study of 750 million hospitalizations in the United States, Martin and colleagues demonstrated men consistently were more likely to have sepsis compared to women.[12] Further studies have also shown comparable results as men are more likely than women to be admitted to the ICU for sepsis and develop severe sepsis and septic shock compared to women and these disparities remained consistent overtime.[66]

Several mechanisms have been investigated to understand the noted sex disparities in sepsis, including potential biological factors, immune-mediated effects, and endogenous sex hormones.[68–70] Animal models demonstrate that female sex appears to offer protective advantages regarding sepsis susceptibility. Female individuals have been shown to exhibit a less reactive inflammatory response compared to male individuals, and researchers have shown that female individuals exhibit higher bacterial clearance rates compared to male individuals.[71] In human studies, the pro-inflammatory cytokine, interleukin-6, is significantly elevated in men compared to women. Furthermore, researchers have demonstrated that androgens, male sex hormones, can attenuate the immune response, in contrast to estradiol, female sex hormones, which have been associated with immunoprotective effects.[71] Trauma as well as sepsis-related outcomes in premenopausal women are better when compared to men of the same age group supporting the protective effects of estrogen.[66] Understanding the association of endogenous sex hormones on critical care outcomes as well as how variations of hormone levels may impact outcomes is of paramount concern as future targeted therapies may reduce disparities. Finally, as more people identify with a gender different from their assigned sex at birth and explore gender transition, understanding the impact of exogenous gender-affirming hormone therapies on critical care outcomes is needed.

While it is important to recognize the innate biological differences that could explain the observed sex disparity in sepsis, it is imperative to understand whether gender differences in treatment and management of sepsis exist. Two interventions that have been shown to improve mortality in sepsis and septic shock are the implementation of sepsis bundles and the rapid initiation of empiric antibiotics. Sepsis bundles are less likely to be implemented and completed in the emergency room if the patient identifies as female.[66,68] Furthermore, women are more likely to have a delay in antibiotic initiation and authors have shown that women were treated more conservatively and less likely to receive hemodialysis catheters, mechanical ventilation, deep venous thrombosis (DVT) prophylaxis, and use of vasopressors.[66,68]

Gender may also impact individual-level care with regard to code status discussions and identification of treatment preferences as decisions to withhold or withdraw life-sustaining treatment are more commonly observed in women which may introduce bias and impact the allocation of ICU resources.[66] Furthermore, gender differences in symptom perception may further contribute to underrepresentation of women in the ICU. Women may be presenting with atypical symptoms that may lead to underdiagnosis. Moreover, women are often in caregiver roles and have household responsibilities that may delay evaluation and care.[66] Lastly, it remains unclear if sepsis-related outcomes differ based on the gender of the treating provider and further research is needed to address these inconsistencies and inequity of standard of care implementation. Overall, while men are more likely to have sepsis and require ICU admission, women receive less timely initiation of antibiotics as well as more conservative management. Gaining further insight into the sex and gender differences in sepsis and critical care outcomes is needed to eliminate disparities and promote the use of personalized care in medicine.

PEDIATRICS AND SEPSIS

The global incidence of pediatric severe sepsis represents a substantial proportion of pediatric critical care admissions, of which the burden of international mortality accounts for millions of pediatric deaths annually.[72,73] While advances in surveillance, early recognition tools and technology, and care delivery for pediatric sepsis have improved worldwide,[72,74] pediatric-related racial, ethnic, and socioeconomic disparities persist in sepsis.[75,76] These racial, ethnic, and socioeconomic disparities in sepsis-related health outcomes, including mortality, have become evident in fetal, neonatal, and pediatric health.[76] Access to health care, economic stability, quality education, social cohesion and community connectedness, and the built environment are critical drivers in pediatric sepsis-related disparities. In the context of structural racism and extreme poverty, mirroring disparities in the adult population, Black pediatric patients in the United States have higher odds of sepsis-related death than their White counterparts.[77] Within the emergency department setting, clinicians' decreased recognition of sepsis in Black pediatric patients leads to delays in treatment and escalation of care.[75] Racial disparities persist despite improvements in surveillance, early recognition tools, timely resuscitation, and antibiotic administration.[76] Additionally, Hispanic patients suffer higher sepsis-related mortality, representing persistent and pervasive racial and ethnic disparities in pediatric sepsis.[78]

Socioeconomic disparities in neonatal and pediatric sepsis have been associated with increased morbidity and mortality.[79] Patients with limited health care access and poverty have increased odds of death and health care utilization.[80] Children with limited or poor access to health care, using insurance status as a surrogate for both socioeconomic surrogate and health access, suffered higher odds of mortality than those with health insurance. After adjusting for variable patient demographics and illness severity, evidence suggests that insurance status and median household income are associated with neonatal and pediatric sepsis-related mortality.[79,80]

Pediatric health care should address sociomedical needs and eliminate unjust and preventable pediatric morbidity and mortality. Recognition of disparities in pediatric health, specifically sepsis, poses a unique opportunity for health professionals to affect the lifelong health and life course trajectory for marginalized and minoritized pediatric patients. Further, it reaffirms that initiating these interventions for sepsis-related disparities in children should occur in parallel to such interventions in adults.

SUMMARY

From both a health equity and health disparities points of view, sepsis impacts the promise of health for many sociodemographic populations, effecting many disproportionately by ethnicity, race, and gender. The high rates of sepsis occurrence in such specific populations identified by the aforementioned social standards are not random, and understanding how and why this occurs should be at the forefront of sepsis-related research. While management of sepsis has improved over the last few decades,[74] it does not negate the higher incidences of sepsis among such vulnerable populations based on social factors. Therefore, the need to have a comprehensive review at all stages of this pathologic syndrome, from onset to management to outcomes, is warranted in an effort to find the modifiable factors that plague vulnerable groups at the greatest rates.

An approach to impact sepsis from a health equity and population health standpoint would be to explore community-based and hospital-based interventions in parallel. Hospital-based interventions can explore aspects such as complying with the Surviving Sepsis Guidelines[74] as well as assuring tools meant to be objective evaluators of vital signs take into account any bias toward certain populations (eg, renal function using race-based calculations[81] or pulse oximeters that poorly perform for dark-skinned patients[82]); thereby, increasing the quality of the strategies meant to improve organ dysfunction in critically ill individuals. Further, recognizing diseases that contribute to sepsis incidence and poor outcomes (eg, diabetes, hypertension[20]) are well addressed as patients leave the critical care settings. Community-based interventions can focus on identifying risk factors to sepsis onset and prevention (eg, vaccine campaigns, identifying risk factors that create chronic diseases associated with sepsis), as well as discussions on advocacy to assist in neighborhoods and geographic regions to improve their respective health (access to nutritious foods, and green open spaces). For instance, a reduction in chronic diseases (obesity and cardiovascular diseases that are associated with sepsis) is associated with the presence and access to green spaces.[83]

If we begin to use sepsis as a disease not only of biological disarray, but also one of social justice, then health care professionals, especially critical care doctors, can begin to understand their roles in health equity and ending health disparities. Even before their patients ever step into their respective critical care units. Reaffirming medicine as a public trust in the present may come from impacting in positive ways an ancient pathologic condition, whereby its influence on vulnerable populations extends beyond the ICUs.

CLINICS CARE POINTS

- In the management of sepsis, recognizing that disparity gaps may exist in certain populations in both incidence and outcomes of sepsis is vital to achieving health equity for critical care patients.
- With such insight, proper sepsis clinical care must be matched with population health strategies to mitigate such disparity gaps between such populations respective hospitals serve and care for.

DISCLOSURE

The Authors have nothing to disclose.

REFERENCES

1. LaVeist TA. Disentangling race and socioeconomic status: a key to understanding health inequalities. J Urban Health 2005;82(2 Suppl 3):iii26–34.
2. Jackson JW. Meaningful causal decompositions in health equity research: definition, identification, and estimation through a weighting framework. Epidemiology 2021;32(2):282–90.
3. VanderWeele TJ. Mediation analysis: a practitioner's guide. Annu Rev Publ Health 2016;37:17–32.
4. Flanagin A, Frey T, Christiansen SL, Committee AMAMoS. Updated guidance on the reporting of race and ethnicity in medical and science journals. JAMA 2021; 326(7):621–7.
5. Ford ME, Kelly PA. Conceptualizing and categorizing race and ethnicity in health services research. Health Serv Res 2005;40(5 Pt 2):1658–75.
6. Egede LE. Race, ethnicity, culture, and disparities in health care. J Gen Intern Med 2006;21(6):667–9.
7. Galiatsatos P, Sun J, Welsh J, et al. Health disparities and sepsis: a systematic review and meta-analysis on the influence of race on sepsis-related mortality. J Racial Ethn Health Disparities 2019;6(5):900–8.

8. National Academies of Sciences, Engineering, and Medicine; Health and Medicine Division; Board on Population Health and Public Health Practice; Committee on Community-Based Solutions to Promote Health Equity in the United States. Communities in Action: Pathways to Health Equity. In: Baciu A, Negussie Y, Geller A, Weinstein JN, editors. National Academies Press (US); Washington, DC. 2017.

9. Lu C, Ahmed R, Lamri A, et al. Use of race, ethnicity, and ancestry data in health research. PLOS Glob Public Health 2022;2(9):e0001060.

10. United States Census Bureau. Additional instructions for respondents. Available at: https://www.census.gov/programs-surveys/decennial-census/technical-documentation/questionnaires/2020/response-guidance.html. [Accessed 3 October 2023].

11. Office of Management and Budget. Revisions to the standards for the classification of federal data on race and ethnicity. Fed Regist 1997;62(210):58782–90.

12. Martin GS, Mannino DM, Eaton S, et al. The epidemiology of sepsis in the United States from 1979 through 2000. N Engl J Med 2003;348(16):1546–54.

13. Barnato AE, Alexander SL, Linde-Zwirble WT, et al. Racial variation in the incidence, care, and outcomes of severe sepsis: analysis of population, patient, and hospital characteristics. Am J Respir Crit Care Med 2008;177(3):279–84.

14. Engoren M, Seelhammer T, Freundlich RE, et al. A comparison of sepsis-2 (systemic inflammatory response syndrome based) to sepsis-3 (sequential organ failure assessment based) definitions-a multicenter retrospective study. Crit Care Med 2020;48(9):1258–64.

15. Jones JM, Fingar KR, Miller MA, et al. Racial disparities in sepsis-related in-hospital mortality: using a broad case capture method and multivariate controls for clinical and hospital variables, 2004-2013. Crit Care Med 2017;45(12):e1209–17.

16. Gold JAW, Rossen LM, Ahmad FB, et al. Race, ethnicity, and age trends in persons who died from COVID-19 - United States, May-August 2020. MMWR Morb Mortal Wkly Rep 2020;69(42):1517–21.

17. Podewils LJ, Burket TL, Mettenbrink C, et al. Disproportionate incidence of COVID-19 infection, hospitalizations, and deaths among persons identifying as Hispanic or Latino - Denver, Colorado March-October 2020. MMWR Morb Mortal Wkly Rep 2020;69(48):1812–6.

18. Stokes EK, Zambrano LD, Anderson KN, et al. Coronavirus disease 2019 case surveillance - United States, January 22-May 30, 2020. MMWR Morb Mortal Wkly Rep 2020;69(24):759–65.

19. Zafer MM, El-Mahallawy HA, Ashour HM. Severe COVID-19 and sepsis: immune pathogenesis and laboratory markers. Microorganisms 2021;9(1).

20. Ahlberg CD, Wallam S, Tirba LA, et al. Linking sepsis with chronic arterial hypertension, diabetes mellitus, and socioeconomic factors in the United States: a scoping review. J Crit Care 2023;77:154324.

21. Chidambaram V, Tun NL, Haque WZ, et al. Factors associated with disease severity and mortality among patients with COVID-19: a systematic review and meta-analysis. PLoS One 2020;15(11):e0241541.

22. Soto GJ, Martin GS, Gong MN. Healthcare disparities in critical illness. Crit Care Med 2013;41(12):2784–93.

23. Tabb KM. Changes in racial categorization over time and health status: an examination of multiracial young adults in the USA. Ethn Health 2016;21(2):146–57.

24. Mayr FB, Yende S, Linde-Zwirble WT, et al. Infection rate and acute organ dysfunction risk as explanations for racial differences in severe sepsis. JAMA 2010;303(24):2495–503.

25. Esper AM, Moss M, Lewis CA, et al. The role of infection and comorbidity: factors that influence disparities in sepsis. Crit Care Med 2006;34(10):2576–82.

26. Guillamet MCV, Dodda S, Liu L, et al. Race does not impact sepsis outcomes when considering socioeconomic factors in multilevel modeling. Crit Care Med 2022;50(3):410–7.

27. Sammon JD, Klett DE, Sood A, et al. Sepsis after major cancer surgery. J Surg Res 2015;193(2):788–94.

28. Plurad DS, Lustenberger T, Kilday P, et al. The association of race and survival from sepsis after injury. Am Surg 2010;76(1):43–7.

29. Koköfer A, Mamandipoor B, Flamm M, et al. The impact of ethnic background on ICU care and outcome in sepsis and septic shock – a retrospective multicenter analysis on 17,949 patients. BMC Infect Dis 2023;23:194.

30. Moore JX, Donnelly JP, Griffin R, et al. Black-white racial disparities in sepsis: a prospective analysis of the REasons for Geographic and Racial Differences in Stroke (REGARDS) cohort. Crit Care 2015;19(1):279.

31. Sandoval E, Chang DW. Association between race and case fatality rate in hospitalizations for sepsis. J Racial Ethn Health Disparities 2016;3(4):625–34.

32. Firempong AO, Shaheen MA, Pan D, et al. Racial and ethnic disparities in the incidence and mortality from septic shock and respiratory failure among elective neurosurgery patients. Neurol Res 2014;36(10):857–65.

33. Barnato AE, Alexander SL, Linde-Zwirble WT, et al. Racial variation in the incidence, care, and outcomes of severe sepsis. Am J Respir Crit Care Med 2008; 177(3):279–84.

34. Goodwin AJ, Nadig NR, McElligott JT, et al. Where you live matters. Chest 2016; 150(4):829–36.

35. Galiatsatos P, Brigham EP, Pietri J, et al. The effect of community socioeconomic status on sepsis-attributable mortality. J Crit Care 2018;46:129–33.

36. Vogel TR, Dombrovskiy VY, Lowry SF. Trends in postoperative sepsis: are we improving outcomes? Surg Infect 2009;10(1):71–8.

37. Bime C, Poongkunran C, Borgstrom M, et al. Racial differences in mortality from severe acute respiratory failure in the United States, 2008–2012. Ann Am Thorac Soc 2016;13(12):2184–9.

38. Kempker JA, Kramer MR, Waller LA, et al. Risk factors for septicemia deaths and disparities in a longitudinal US Cohort. Open Forum Infect Dis 2018;5(12):ofy305.

39. Lippert AM. System failure: the geographic distribution of sepsis-associated death in the USA and factors contributing to the mortality burden of black communities. J Racial Ethn Health Disparities 2022;1–10.

40. Melamed A, Sorvillo FJ. The burden of sepsis-associated mortality in the United States from 1999 to 2005: an analysis of multiple-cause-of-death data. Crit Care 2009;13(1):R28.

41. Danai PA, Moss M, Mannino DM, et al. The epidemiology of sepsis in patients with malignancy. Chest 2006;129(6):1432–40.

42. Chesley CF, Chowdhury M, Small DS, et al. Racial disparities in length of stay among severely ill patients presenting with sepsis and acute respiratory failure. JAMA Netw Open 2023;6(5):e239739.

43. Chang DW, Tseng C-H, Shapiro MF. Rehospitalizations following sepsis: common and costly. Crit Care Med 2015;43(10):2085–93.

44. Lizza BD, Betthauser KD, Juang PH, et al. Racial disparities in readmissions following initial hospitalization for sepsis. Crit Care Med 2021;49(3):e258–68.

45. Galiatsatos P, Follin A, Alghanim F, et al. The association between neighborhood socioeconomic disadvantage and readmissions for patients hospitalized with sepsis. Crit Care Med 2020;48(6):808–14.
46. Fuentes A, Ackermann RR, Athreya S, et al. AAPA statement on race and racism. Am J Phys Anthropol 2019;169(3):400–2.
47. Chaudhary NS, Donnelly JP, Wang HE. Racial differences in sepsis mortality at U.S. Academic medical center-affiliated hospitals. Crit Care Med 2018;46(6):878–83.
48. Moore JX, Donnelly JP, Griffin R, et al. Defining sepsis mortality clusters in the United States. Crit Care Med 2016;44(7):1380–7.
49. Moore JX, Donnelly JP, Griffin R, et al. Community characteristics and regional variations in sepsis. Int J Epidemiol 2017;46(5):1607–17.
50. Wang HE, Devereaux RS, Yealy DM, et al. National variation in United States sepsis mortality: a descriptive study. Int J Health Geogr 2010;9:9.
51. Ogundipe F, Kodadhala V, Ogundipe T, et al. Disparities in sepsis mortality by region, urbanization, and race in the USA: a multiple cause of death analysis. J Racial Ethn Health Disparities 2019;6(3):546–51.
52. Kumar G, Taneja A, Majumdar T, et al. The association of lacking insurance with outcomes of severe sepsis: retrospective analysis of an administrative database. Crit Care Med 2014;42(3):583–91.
53. Degenholtz HB, Thomas SB, Miller MJ. Race and the intensive care unit: disparities and preferences for end-of-life care. Crit Care Med 2003;31(5 Suppl):S373–8.
54. Loggers ET, Maciejewski PK, Paulk E, et al. Racial differences in predictors of intensive end-of-life care in patients with advanced cancer. J Clin Oncol 2009; 27(33):5559–64.
55. Madsen TE, Napoli AM. Analysis of race and time to antibiotics among patients with severe sepsis or septic shock. J Racial Ethn Health Disparities 2017;4(4): 680–6.
56. Taylor SP, Karvetski CH, Templin MA, et al. Hospital differences drive antibiotic delays for black patients compared with white patients with suspected septic shock. Crit Care Med 2018;46(2):e126–31.
57. Chesley CF, Anesi GL, Chowdhury M, et al. Characterizing equity of intensive care unit admissions for sepsis and acute respiratory failure. Ann Am Thorac Soc 2022;19(12):2044–52.
58. Shannon EM, Schnipper JL, Mueller SK. Identifying racial/ethnic disparities in inter-hospital transfer: an observational study. J Gen Intern Med 2020;35(10):2939–46.
59. Tyler PD, Stone DJ, Geisler BP, et al. Racial and geographic disparities in inter-hospital intensive care unit transfers. Crit Care Med 2018;46(1):e76–80.
60. Corl KA, Levy MM, Phillips GS, et al. Racial and ethnic disparities in care following the New York state sepsis initiative. Health affairs (Project Hope) 2019;38(7): 1119–26.
61. Muni S, Engelberg RA, Treece PD, et al. The influence of race/ethnicity and socioeconomic status on end-of-life care in the ICU. Chest 2011;139(5):1025–33.
62. Schulman KA, Berlin JA, Harless W, et al. The effect of race and sex on physicians' recommendations for cardiac catheterization. N Engl J Med 1999;340(8): 618–26.
63. Hoffman KM, Trawalter S, Axt JR, et al. Racial bias in pain assessment and treatment recommendations, and false beliefs about biological differences between blacks and whites. Proc Natl Acad Sci U S A 2016;113(16):4296–301.
64. Linnander EL, Ayedun A, Boatright D, et al. Mitigating structural racism to reduce inequities in sepsis outcomes: a mixed methods, longitudinal intervention study. BMC Health Serv Res 2022;22:975.

65. Scheer CS, Fuchs C, Kuhn S-O, et al. Quality improvement initiative for severe sepsis and septic shock reduces 90-day mortality: a 7.5-year observational study. Crit Care Med 2017;45(2):241.

66. Merdji H, Long MT, Ostermann M, et al. Sex and gender differences in intensive care medicine. Intensive Care Med 2023;49(10):1155–67.

67. Goldstein RH, Walensky RP. Where were the women? gender parity in clinical trials. N Engl J Med 2019;381(26):2491–3.

68. Lat TI, McGraw MK, White HD. Gender differences in critical illness and critical care research. Clin Chest Med 2021;42(3):543–55.

69. Lakbar I, Einav S, Lalevee N, et al. Interactions between gender and sepsis-implications for the future. Microorganisms 2023;11(3).

70. Textoris J, Ban LH, Capo C, et al. Sex-related differences in gene expression following Coxiella burnetii infection in mice: potential role of circadian rhythm. PLoS One 2010;5(8):e12190.

71. Leone M, Honstettre A, Lepidi H, et al. Effect of sex on Coxiella burnetii infection: protective role of 17beta-estradiol. J Infect Dis 2004;189(2):339–45.

72. Weiss SL, Peters MJ, Alhazzani W, et al. Surviving sepsis campaign international guidelines for the management of septic shock and sepsis-associated organ dysfunction in children. Pediatr Crit Care Med 2020;21(2):e52–106.

73. Fleischmann-Struzek C, Goldfarb DM, Schlattmann P, et al. The global burden of paediatric and neonatal sepsis: a systematic review. Lancet Respir Med 2018;6(3):223–30.

74. Dellinger RP, Rhodes A, Evans L, et al. Surviving sepsis campaign. Crit Care Med 2023;51(4):431–44.

75. Raman J, Johnson TJ, Hayes K, et al. Racial differences in sepsis recognition in the emergency department. Pediatrics 2019;144(4).

76. Li E, Ng AP, Williamson CG, et al. Assessment of racial and ethnic disparities in outcomes of pediatric hospitalizations for sepsis across the United States. JAMA Pediatr 2023;177(2):206–8.

77. Mitchell HK, Reddy A, Montoya-Williams D, et al. Hospital outcomes for children with severe sepsis in the USA by race or ethnicity and insurance status: a population-based, retrospective cohort study. Lancet Child Adolesc Health 2021;5(2):103–12.

78. Thavamani A, Umapathi KK, Dhanpalreddy H, et al. Epidemiology, clinical and microbiologic profile and risk factors for inpatient mortality in pediatric severe sepsis in the United States from 2003 to 2014: a Large Population Analysis. Pediatr Infect Dis J 2020;39(9):781–8.

79. Reddy AR, Badolato GM, Chamberlain JM, et al. Disparities associated with sepsis mortality in critically ill children. J Pediatr Intensive Care 2022;11(2):147–52.

80. Bohanon FJ, Nunez Lopez O, Adhikari D, et al. Race, income and insurance status affect neonatal sepsis mortality and healthcare resource utilization. Pediatr Infect Dis J 2018;37(7):e178–84.

81. Mohottige D, Olabisi O, Boulware LE. Use of race in kidney function estimation: lessons learned and the path toward health justice. Annu Rev Med 2023;74:385–400.

82. Fawzy A, Wu TD, Wang K, et al. Clinical outcomes associated with overestimation of oxygen saturation by pulse oximetry in patients hospitalized with COVID-19. JAMA Netw Open 2023;6(8):e2330856.

83. Kingsley M, EcoHealth O. Commentary - climate change, health and green space co-benefits. Health Promot Chronic Dis Prev Can 2019;39(4):131–5.

Racial, Ethnic, and Socioeconomic Differences in Critical Care Near the End of Life: A Narrative Review

Katrina E. Hauschildt, PhD[a], Judith B. Vick, MD, MPH[b,c,d],
Deepshikha Charan Ashana, MD, MBA, MS[e,f],*

KEYWORDS

- Intensive care units • Socioeconomic factors • Racial groups • End of life

KEY POINTS

- Patients from groups that are racially or ethnically minoritized or of low socioeconomic status receive more intensive care near the end of life than others, in part, due to their higher propensity to be admitted to high treatment-intensity hospitals.
- Although individuals from these groups may also prefer more life-sustaining treatments than others, on average, many do not endorse such preferences. System-level and clinician-level factors influence preferences and are the most appropriate targets for intervention.
- Quality of dying among individuals in these groups is worse than others, although contributory mechanisms have not been fully elucidated.

CASE STUDY: INTRODUCTION

Mr Parker, a Black 84 year old man with dementia, was found clammy and lethargic when his daughter visited him at his nursing home. He was admitted to the intensive care unit (ICU) with sepsis. While he improved substantially within a few days, the ICU

Funding sources: NHLBI K23 HL164968 (D.C. Ashana).
[a] Department of Medicine, Johns Hopkins University School of Medicine, 1830 East Monument Street, #520, Baltimore, MD 21205, USA; [b] Durham VA Health Care System; [c] Department of Medicine, Duke University School of Medicine; [d] National Clinician Scholars Program, Duke Clinical and Translational Science Institute, 701 West Main Street, Durham, NC 27701, USA; [e] Duke-Margolis Center for Health Policy, Duke University, Durham, NC, USA; [f] Department of Population Health Sciences, Duke University, Hanes House, 315 Trent Drive, Durham, NC 27705, USA
* Corresponding author. Department of Medicine, Duke-Margolis Center for Health Policy, Duke University, Durham, NC.
E-mail address: deepshikha.ashana@duke.edu

and palliative care teams felt it was important to discuss Mr Parker's goals of care due to his chronic health problems.

Mr Parker's clinicians thought less intensive treatment of recurrent infections might spare Mr Parker what they considered painful interventions and disorienting care transitions given his worsening dementia. Mr Parker's daughter, a nurse, felt a moral obligation to make sure his reversible health problems were addressed. She expressed that he was neglected by nursing home staff, which she suspected contributed to his recurring infections and clinical deterioration. Mr Parker's daughter felt he received better care in the hospital than in his nursing home. Her concerns about reversible problems caused by neglect motivated her to bring her father to the hospital.

(Nonfictional narrative recounted in "Whose Good Death? Valuation and Standardization as Mechanisms of Inequality in Hospitals"[1])

BACKGROUND

ICUs in the United States increasingly provide care to patients nearing the end of life (EOL). Between 2000 and 2015, the proportion of older adults admitted to ICUs in the last month of life increased from 1 in 4 to 1 in 3.[2] The common presumption that this represents low-value care is controversial.[3–5] Certainly, some patients receive ICU care despite their preferences to avoid such care, and still more patients would have preferred to avoid ICU care had they known about their limited survival prognosis. However, other seriously ill patients who prioritize prolonging life or lack structural support for intensive outpatient disease or symptom management may benefit from ICU care, even near the EOL. Clinicians may believe that Black patients and others from structurally marginalized groups have strongly held preferences for "aggressive" care.[6,7] Then, to the extent that the incidence of critical care at the EOL is higher among such patients, this would represent a difference rooted in patient preferences rather than a disparity to be remedied. Yet, research abounds on racial and other disparities in EOL care, suggesting that other modifiable factors contribute to the observed difference.[8–10]

We conducted a narrative review of racial, ethnic, and socioeconomic class differences in access to and quality of ICU care among seriously ill patients at the EOL. Our objectives were to synthesize the literature on this topic, then provide guidance to clinicians and scholars on evaluating the conflicts described earlier.

HEALTH CARE COSTS AND INTENSIVE CARE UNIT UTILIZATION

There are racial and ethnic differences in health care expenditures near the EOL. In nationally representative samples of up to 158,780 decedents, Black and Hispanic older adults accrued approximately 30% and 50% greater health care costs, respectively, than White older adults in the last 6 months of their lives.[11–13] Very little of this racial/ethnic difference was attributable to patient-level factors, such as comorbidities or income; approximately 50% was attributable to geographic variability in EOL treatment intensity while approximately 30% was attributable to greater use of ICUs and high-cost procedures, such as mechanical ventilation, among patients from racial or ethnic minority groups.[11–14]

Additional research has confirmed racial/ethnic and socioeconomic differences in ICU use near the EOL. During 192,705 terminal admissions (ie, during which patients died), Black and Hispanic patients were approximately 30% and 50% more likely to be admitted to ICU, respectively, than non-Hispanic White patients.[15] Among patients with advanced malignancies, those who were underinsured, experiencing financial hardship, or from low-income neighborhoods were also more likely to receive life-sustaining treatment (LST) during a terminal admission.[16-18] Additional studies have confirmed and extended these results, finding comparatively higher rates of ICU use among Asian patients and those living in rural areas.[18-23] As a result, among patients dying in hospital, White patients were most likely to die with limitations on LST, Hispanic patients were most likely to die after withdrawal of LST, and Black patients were most likely to die while receiving LST.[24,25]

It is not definitively known whether observed racial/ethnic differences in EOL ICU use are concordant with patients' preferences for their medical care.[26-28] In one nationally representative sample of 1212 bereaved caregivers, patient race was not significantly associated with caregivers' perceptions of goal-discordant medical care near the EOL.[27] However, 2 analyses of the prospective, multicenter coping with cancer study found Black patients were both less likely than White patients to receive intensive EOL care when they expressed a preference for such care and more likely to receive intensive EOL care when they had comfort-focused preferences or do-not-resuscitate (DNR) orders.[26,28]

In a series of observational studies, Barnato and colleagues identified potential mechanisms underlying racial differences in EOL treatment intensity. First, Black decedents received more LST during terminal hospitalizations than White decedents, while Black survivors received fewer intensive procedures, such as cardiac catheterization and hip replacement, than White survivors.[29] Thus, Black patients were less likely to receive elective, preference-sensitive procedures, but they are more likely to receive urgent, LST in ICU settings where the default is to provide fully restorative care.[30,31] Both may suggest a deficiency in shared decision-making between clinicians and Black patients. Second, although Black patients were more likely than White patients to be admitted to ICU during terminal hospitalizations, this difference was nearly eliminated after adjusting for the hospital where patients received care.[15] Third, however, when comparing Black and White seriously ill patients admitted to the same hospital, Black patients received less intensive treatment than White patients.[32] These studies suggest that higher EOL ICU use among Black patients is largely attributable to hospital practice patterns, although the extent to which practice patterns are influenced by local cultural norms among patients is not known. We did not find similar mechanistic studies that explained differences in ICU utilization for patients of other races or ethnicities or by socioeconomic status.

END OF LIFE TREATMENT PREFERENCES

Many studies in non-ICU care settings have documented racial and ethnic differences in EOL treatment preferences, largely noting that more Black and Hispanic than White respondents express a desire for LST, although heterogeneity is present in all racial/ethnic and socioeconomic groups and the majority of all groups still do not prefer LST in many studies.[26,33-41] Barnato and colleagues found that 24% to 36% of Black respondents, 21% to 29% Hispanic respondents, and 15% to 21% of White respondents expressed preferences for specific LSTs.[36] Although comparatively limited, studies have identified variation among other racial/ethnic groups and varying religious and cultural factors that influence preferences among groups.[37,42,43]

Few studies have directly examined racial, ethnic, or socioeconomic differences in patients' treatment preferences while in the ICU. Studies that examine differences in treatment orders, such as DNR, are often used to infer preferences.[33,44] For example, a national study of 3343 surgical ICU patients found that 13% and 26% of White and Black ICU decedents, respectively, did not have DNR orders at the time of death and that Black patients were less likely to have a change from full code status while in the

ICU.[45] Among 2672 patients with stroke in Texas, early DNR orders were more common among non-Hispanic White patients than Mexican-American and non-Hispanic Black patients (11%, 2%, 7%, respectively), but there were not statistically different rates of late DNR orders (27%–37%).[46] Studies examining treatment preferences among patients from different socioeconomic groups have shown that critically ill individuals with higher incomes or educational attainment are less likely to prefer LST near the EOL than individuals with lower incomes or educational attainment.[34,35]

The specific preferences questions asked and patient populations surveyed have varied substantially, limiting comparison among studies. Martin and colleagues explored 4214 cancer patients' desire for "treatment to extend life as much as possible, even if it meant using up all your financial resources," and a majority of all racial and ethnic groups affirmed they would be willing to use all their financial resources (80% of Black, 72% of Asian, 69% of Hispanic, and 54% of White respondents).[38] However, when Sanders and colleagues queried 2015 Medicare beneficiaries about their desire for LST in the context of severe pain or severe disability, a minority of White, Hispanic, and Black respondents (10%, 31%, and 33%, respectively) stated they would desire such care.[34] These studies suggest preferences are socially and culturally negotiated and vary based on diagnosis and illness severity. Further, substantial variation in the context and specificity of questions challenges efforts to identify, document, and compare preferences.

ADVANCE CARE PLANNING

There are clear racial, ethnic, and socioeconomic differences in advance care planning (ACP), which may then influence preference-concordant use of LST.[39,47–49] Among a national sample of decedents who received intensive care in the last 30 days of life between 2000 and 2015, 36% of non-Hispanic Black versus 16% of non-Hispanic White decedents, and 32% versus 12% of those in the lowest and highest income quartiles, respectively, reported no ACP.[48] Comparisons of ACP between Asian American and White patients are mixed.[50,51] Home ownership and greater net worth predicted both financial and health care planning (eg, wills, living wills, and durable power of health care attorney documentation).[47] Factors contributing to these racial and socioeconomic differences are varied and include clinician comfort in starting ACP conversations,[6,52] patients' religious beliefs,[39,42] low perceived trustworthiness of clinicians,[53,54] patients' preferences,[54,55] and clinicians' stereotypes about treatment preferences that are often inaccurate.[6,7]

SERIOUS ILLNESS AND END OF LIFE COMMUNICATION

ACP is now being reconceptualized as taking different forms across the trajectory of illness with increased recognition of the importance of serious illness communication during hospitalizations when decisions about LST and other aspects of EOL care may be more imminent.[56–59] While some small studies have shown no racial differences in EOL conversations during hospitalizations,[60,61] larger studies have shown that racially or ethnically minoritized groups have fewer goals-of-care conversations while hospitalized[62] and worse perceptions of communication in general at the EOL.[63] Disparities in serious illness communication also exist within the ICU specifically, though this topic is understudied. An examination of 137 ICU family meetings with Black and White families found similar incidence of clinician shared decision-making behaviors, but a lower likelihood of validation of Black families' medical decisions or involvement in care.[64] A high-fidelity simulation study found that ICU clinicians also had worse nonverbal communication scores when interacting with critically ill Black compared to White patients, even while verbal communication scores were similar.[65] Additionally, there is evidence of increased conflict about treatment decisions between ICU clinicians and minoritized patients and families,[66–68] which can lead to longer ICU lengths of stay[69] and psychological distress for patients and families.[70]

QUALITY OF DEATH AND DYING IN THE INTENSIVE CARE UNIT

Bereaved family members of racially/ethnically minoritized patients are less likely than family members of White patients to report quality of EOL care was optimal in many care settings, including the ICU.[9,10,63] Several factors may mediate this association, including not receiving palliative care[71–73] or receiving LST, although the evidence is mixed. One national study of 2.4 million hospital admissions found that critically ill White patients were 6.7 times more likely to receive specialist palliative care consultation than critically ill Black patients.[71] However, single-institution studies have found no racial differences in palliative medicine consultation in the ICU.[74,75] In a study of patients who died in the ICU, lower quality of death ratings were mediated by the absence of a living will and dying with LST.[9] However, among 17,911 veterans who died in all settings (not just the ICU), racially/ethnically minoritized bereaved family members reported lower quality EOL care than White bereaved family members, but this was not mediated by LST.[10] Discrepancies in the mediating role of LST may be explained by differing study designs or practice settings. It is worth nothing that while multiple Veterans Affairs hospital studies have confirmed lower ratings of quality of EOL care,[10,76] they have consistently found no differential use of hospice or palliative care among racial groups,[10,77] differing from most civilian studies.[18,78–81] Processes of care unique to the Veterans Affairs hospital may play a role.[82]

BEREAVED CAREGIVER OUTCOMES

Bereavement outcomes for family members of ICU decedents may differ among racial/ethnic groups, though the evidence is limited and mixed. In one longitudinal study of 30 family members of patients who died in an ICU, non-Hispanic White family members initially had higher levels of depression and posttraumatic stress disorder than Black family members, though this was followed by greater improvements in both in the year after their loved one's death.[83] In a convenience sample of 49 Black bereaved family members, decision regret was significantly higher among family members of decedents who received LST versus those who received comfort-focused care.[84] In a larger, more recent study, however, authors found that a decision to *limit* LST and surrogate Black race were associated with more regret.[85]

A CRITICAL LENS

Understanding disparate patterns of ICU care near the EOL requires careful attention to contextual factors—the nuances of patients' diagnoses and prognoses, preferences of patients and surrogate decision-makers, and patients' and families' available resources in and outside of the ICU. However, studies often fail to address this context, risking obscuring important differences or misleading researchers in the mechanisms that contribute to inequities. Utilization as a quality metric is complicated by studies that show heterogeneity in the EOL treatment patients' desire.[34,36,41,86] As discussed earlier, patient preferences vary both within and between nonmarginalized and marginalized groups. Researchers often fail to account for preferences when making claims about higher and lower quality EOL treatment utilization and "disparities" in treatment utilization.[41,86]

For example, location of death is often justified as a quality metric using studies that show many people report wanting to die at home.[87,88] However, not all Americans report this; there are important differences by race and socioeconomic status, and preferences are context-specific.[35,89,90] When we measure quality of, and disparities in, preference-sensitive outcomes by majority preference, we are most likely to devalue preferences held by marginalized groups. Qualitative studies suggest that devaluing patient and family preferences itself affects perceived quality of care,[1,91] further complicating associations between treatment utilization and quality of care ratings.[9,63]

Further, utilization studies that ignore contextual factors may misrepresent mechanisms contributing to presumed disparities. Location of death simplifies the context in which individuals' deaths take place and the realities of dying patients' care needs. Black, Hispanic, and lower income patients are more likely to disenroll from hospice care; disenrollment often reflects unmet care needs and poorer symptom management among patients with limited access to family caregivers who can supplement the hospice benefit provided through Medicare.[92,93] For these patients, ideal symptom management may not be available outside of the hospital setting, and thus hospice disenrollment, and/or ICU deaths, may reflect an appropriate correction toward a higher quality EOL experience.[94] Poor symptom management during hospice care may also contribute to other families' future hospice preferences.[1]

Efforts to better clarify patient preferences and improve rates of ACP and in-the-moment serious illness communication among Black and other minoritized patients may prove helpful in increasing rates of preference-concordant care; however, they too require contextualization to ensure disparities are appropriately identified and intervened upon. Physicians' biases in what constituted successful ACP, with an emphasis on formal documentation, was one noted barrier to ACP for minoritized patients.[6] Racial and ethnic groups that face more discrimination and decreased access to care may be more reluctant to document context-agnostic treatment limitations, preferring to make decisions when more information is available to themselves or their loved ones.[53,91] Stereotypes about patient preferences based on race/ethnicity, ignorance about contextual factors that shape preferences (eg, family decision-making and fear of discrimination), and overly broad application of comfort-focused preferences all shape access to and the quality of serious illness communication for minoritized groups.[6,7,52,53,95–97] In a similar vein, efforts to ensure patients and families have the information they need and feel supported in decision-making are important endpoints; we should resist efforts to measure successful communication and decision-making by changes in treatment and/or code status.

We have long known that good EOL experiences are subjective, complex, and diverse[98]; this should be acknowledged in all research on EOL care. Further, death and dying are deeply social experiences in addition to biological and clinical phenomena. Recognizing the role of racism and other forms of discrimination in disparities in ICU EOL experiences requires us to look carefully at the questions we ask, the methods we use, and the interpretation of our results.[99,100] We must keep this reality at the forefront of our work to identify and ameliorate disparities and improve EOL care in the ICU.

CASE STUDY REVISITED

Recalling Mr Parker and his daughter, a closer look is needed to identify what issues might create a disparate EOL experience for this family. Racial stereotypes about Black patients' and families' EOL care preferences could overshadow Mr Parker's goals of care and the contextual factors shaping Ms Parker's care decisions. Understanding Ms Parker's worry about suffering related to neglect is essential to thoughtfully navigating conversations about goals of care. Finally, ensuring Mr Parker has adequate symptom management and comfort in dying requires acknowledging the limits of care at his current residence.

SUMMARY

In summary, patients from groups that are racially or ethnically minoritized or of low socioeconomic status accrue greater health care costs than other groups near the EOL, and EOL ICU utilization among these groups may be influenced by a higher propensity to be admitted to high treatment-intensity hospitals. Although individuals from these groups may also prefer more LST than others, on average, many do not endorse such preferences. Many factors can influence treatment preferences, including those at the levels of systems, clinicians, and patients and families. Finally, quality of dying among individuals in these groups may be worse than for others, although the evidence is limited and contributory mechanisms have not been fully elucidated. There is little evidence about outcomes of bereaved caregivers in these groups. Future research should focus on components of care and outcome differences that are driven by societal structures, health care systems, and clinicians, because to the extent that these differences are driven by patient preferences, these may not represent disparities that require remedy.

CLINICS CARE POINTS

- Assess care preferences systematically among all patientsInterrogate personal biases that may influence patient care.
- Evaluate social determinants of health and their influence on end of life care.

ACKNOWLEDGMENTS

The authors thank Steph Hendren, MLIS, AHIP of the Duke University Medical Center Library for her assistance in developing our search strategy. We also thank Connor Fogleman for his assistance with article preparation.

DISCLOSURE

The authors do not have any commercial or financial conflicts of interest.

REFERENCES

1. Hauschildt KE. Whose good death? Valuation and standardization as mechanisms of inequality in hospitals. J Health Soc Behav 2022;002214652211430. https://doi.org/10.1177/00221465221143088.
2. Teno JM, Gozalo P, Trivedi AN, et al. Site of death, place of care, and health care transitions among US Medicare beneficiaries, 2000-2015. JAMA 2018;320(3): 264–71. https://doi.org/10.1001/jama.2018.8981.
3. Hua M, Wunsch H. Placing value on end-of-life care—is it time for a new taxonomy? JAMA Netw Open 2019;2(11):e1914466. https://doi.org/10.1001/jamanetwork open.2019.14466.

4. Rolnick JA, Ersek M, Wachterman MW, et al. The quality of end-of-life care among ICU versus ward decedents. Am J Respir Crit Care Med 2020;201(7): 832–9. https://doi.org/10.1164/rccm.201907-1423OC.

5. Nayfeh A, Yarnell CJ, Dale C, et al. Evaluating satisfaction with the quality and provision of end-of-life care for patients from diverse ethnocultural backgrounds. BMC Palliat Care 2021;20(1):145. https://doi.org/10.1186/s12904-021-00841-z.

6. Ashana DC, D'Arcangelo N, Gazarian PK, et al. "Don't talk to them about goals of care": understanding disparities in advance care planning. J Gerontol A Biol Sci Med Sci 2022;77(2):339–46. https://doi.org/10.1093/gerona/glab091.

7. Barnato AE, Mohan D, Downs J, et al. A randomized trial of the effect of patient race on physicians' intensive care unit and life-sustaining treatment decisions for an acutely unstable elder with end-stage cancer. Crit Care Med 2011; 39(7):1663–9. https://doi.org/10.1097/CCM.0b013e3182186e98.

8. Heitner R, Rogers M, Chambers B, et al. The experience of black patients with serious illness in the United States: a scoping review. J Pain Symptom Manag 2023;66(4):e501–11. https://doi.org/10.1016/j.jpainsymman.2023.07.002.

9. Lee JJ, Long AC, Curtis JR, et al. The influence of race/ethnicity and education on family ratings of the quality of dying in the ICU. J Pain Symptom Manag 2016 2016;51(1):9–16. https://doi.org/10.1016/j.jpainsymman.2015.08.008.

10. Kutney-Lee A, Bellamy SL, Ersek M, et al. Care processes and racial/ethnic differences in family reports of end-of-life care among Veterans: a mediation analysis. J Am Geriatr Soc 2022;70(4):1095–105. https://doi.org/10.1111/jgs.17632.

11. Hanchate A, Kronman AC, Young-Xu Y, et al. Racial and ethnic differences in end-of-life costs: why do minorities cost more than whites? Arch Intern Med 2009;169(5):493–501. https://doi.org/10.1001/archinternmed.2008.616.

12. Kelley AS, Ettner SL, Morrison RS, et al. Determinants of medical expenditures in the last 6 months of life. Ann Intern Med 2011;154(4):235–42. https://doi.org/10.7326/0003-4819-154-4-201102150-00004.

13. Byhoff E, Harris JA, Langa KM, et al. Racial and ethnic differences in end-of-life Medicare expenditures. J Am Geriatr Soc 2016;64(9):1789–97. https://doi.org/10.1111/jgs.14263.

14. Brown CE, Engelberg RA, Sharma R, et al. Race/ethnicity, socioeconomic status, and healthcare intensity at the end of life. J Palliat Med 2018;21(9): 1308–16. https://doi.org/10.1089/jpm.2018.0011.

15. Barnato AE, Berhane Z, Weissfeld LA, et al. Racial variation in end-of-life intensive care use: a race or hospital effect? Health Serv Res 2006;41(6):2219–37. https://doi.org/10.1111/j.1475-6773.2006.00598.x.

16. Deeb S, Chino FL, Diamond LC, et al. Disparities in care management during terminal hospitalization among adults with metastatic cancer from 2010 to 2017. JAMA Netw Open 2021;4(9):e2125328. https://doi.org/10.1001/jamanetworkopen.2021.25328.

17. Tucker-Seeley RD, Abel GA, Uno H, et al. Financial hardship and the intensity of medical care received near death. Psycho Oncol 2015;24(5):572–8. https://doi.org/10.1002/pon.3624.

18. Smith AK, Earle CC, McCarthy EP. Racial and ethnic differences in end-of-life care in fee-for-service Medicare beneficiaries with advanced cancer. J Am Geriatr Soc 2009;57(1):153–8. https://doi.org/10.1111/j.1532-5415.2008.02081.x.

19. Hutchinson RN, Han PKJ, Lucas FL, et al. Rural disparities in end-of-life care for patients with heart failure: are they due to geography or socioeconomic disparity? J Rural Health 2022;38(2):457–63. https://doi.org/10.1111/jrh.12597.

20. Tschirhart EC, Du Q, Kelley AS. Factors influencing the use of intensive proced-ures at the end of life. J Am Geriatr Soc 2014;62(11):2088–94. https://doi.org/10.1111/jgs.13104.
21. Hernandez RA, Hevelone ND, Lopez L, et al. Racial variation in the use of life-sustaining treatments among patients who die after major elective surgery. Am J Surg 2015;210(1):52–8. https://doi.org/10.1016/j.amjsurg.2014.08.025.
22. Miesfeldt S, Murray K, Lucas L, et al. Association of age, gender, and race with intensity of end-of-life care for Medicare beneficiaries with cancer. J Palliat Med 2012;15(5):548–54. https://doi.org/10.1089/jpm.2011.0310.
23. Jia Z, Leiter RE, Sanders JJ, et al. Asian American Medicare beneficiaries disproportionately receive invasive mechanical ventilation when hospitalized at the end-of-life. J Gen Intern Med 2022;37(4):737–44. https://doi.org/10.1007/s11606-021-06794-6.
24. Barnato AE, Johnson GR, Birkmeyer JD, et al. Advance care planning and treat-ment intensity before death among black, hispanic, and white patients hospital-ized with COVID-19. J Gen Intern Med 2022;37(8):1996–2002. https://doi.org/10.1007/s11606-022-07530-4.
25. Rubin MA, Dhar R, Diringer MN. Racial differences in withdrawal of mechanical ventilation do not alter mortality in neurologically injured patients. J Crit Care 2014;29(1):49–53. https://doi.org/10.1016/j.jcrc.2013.08.023.
26. Loggers ET, Maciejewski PK, Paulk E, et al. Racial differences in predictors of intensive end-of-life care in patients with advanced cancer. J Clin Oncol 2009 2009;27(33):5559–64. https://doi.org/10.1200/JCO.2009.22.4733.
27. Khandelwal N, Curtis JR, Freedman VA, et al. How often is end-of-life care in the United States inconsistent with patients' goals of care? J Palliat Med 2017;20(12):1400–4. https://doi.org/10.1089/jpm.2017.0065.
28. Mack JW, Paulk ME, Viswanath K, et al. Racial disparities in the outcomes of communication on medical care received near death. Arch Intern Med 2010;170(17):1533–40. https://doi.org/10.1001/archinternmed.2010.322.
29. Barnato AE, Chang CC, Saynina O, et al. Influence of race on inpatient treatment intensity at the end of life. J Gen Intern Med 2007;22(3):338–45. https://doi.org/10.1007/s11606-006-0088-x.
30. Halpern SD, Ubel PA, Asch DA. Harnessing the power of default options to improve health care. N Engl J Med 2007;357(13):1340–4. https://doi.org/10.1056/NEJMsb071595.
31. Kruser JM, Cox CE, Schwarze ML. Clinical momentum in the intensive care unit. A latent contributor to unwanted care. Ann Am Thorac Soc 2017;14(3):426–31. https://doi.org/10.1513/AnnalsATS.201611-931OI.
32. Barnato AE, Chang CH, Lave JR, et al. The paradox of end-of-life hospital treat-ment intensity among black patients: a retrospective cohort study. J Palliat Med 2018;21(1):69–77. https://doi.org/10.1089/jpm.2016.0557.
33. Johnson RW, Newby LK, Granger CB, et al. Differences in level of care at the end of life according to race. Am J Crit Care 2010;19(4):335–43. https://doi.org/10.4037/ajcc2010161.
34. Sanders JJ, Berrier AI, Nshuti L, et al. Differences by race, religiosity, and mental health in preferences for life-prolonging treatment among Medicare beneficiaries. J Gen Intern Med 2019;1–3. https://doi.org/10.1007/s11606-019-05052-0.
35. Boyce-Fappiano D, Liao K, Miller C, et al. Greater preferences for death in hos-pital and mechanical ventilation at the end of life among non-whites recently diagnosed with cancer. Support Care Cancer 2021;29(11):6555–64. https://doi.org/10.1007/s00520-021-06226-5.

36. Barnato AE, Anthony DL, Skinner J, et al. Racial and ethnic differences in preferences for end-of-life treatment. J Gen Intern Med 2009;24(6):695–701. https://doi.org/10.1007/s11606-009-0952-6.

37. Blackhall LJ, Frank G, Murphy ST, et al. Ethnicity and attitudes towards life sustaining technology. Soc Sci Med 1999 1999;48(12):1779–89. https://doi.org/10.1016/S0277-9536(99)00077-5.

38. Martin MY, Pisu M, Oster RA, et al. Racial variation in willingness to trade financial resources for life-prolonging cancer treatment. Cancer 2011 2011;117(15):3476–84. https://doi.org/10.1002/cncr.25839.

39. Wicher CP, Meeker MA. What influences african American end-of-life preferences? J Health Care Poor Underserved 2012 2012;23(1):28–58. https://doi.org/10.1353/hpu.2012.0027.

40. Ko E, Cho S, Bonilla M. Attitudes toward life-sustaining treatment: the role of race/ethnicity. Geriatr Nurs 2012;33(5):341–9. https://doi.org/10.1016/j.gerinurse.2012.01.009.

41. Pew Research C. Views on end-of-life medical treatments. 2013. Available at: http://www.pewforum.org/2013/11/21/views-on-end-of-life-medical-treatments/.

42. Fang ML, Sixsmith J, Sinclair S, et al. A knowledge synthesis of culturally- and spiritually-sensitive end-of-life care: findings from a scoping review. BMC Geriatr 2016;16:107. https://doi.org/10.1186/s12877-016-0282-6.

43. Kwak J, Haley WE. Current research findings on end-of-life decision making among racially or ethnically diverse groups. Gerontol 2005;45(5):634–41. https://doi.org/10.1093/geront/45.5.634.

44. Hatfield J, Fah M, Girden A, et al. Racial and ethnic differences in the prevalence of do-not-resuscitate orders among older adults with severe traumatic brain injury. J Intensive Care Med 2022;37(12):1641–7. https://doi.org/10.1177/08850666221103780.

45. Purcell LN, Tignanelli CJ, Maine R, et al. Predictors of change in code status from time of admission to death in critically ill surgical patients. Am Surg 2020;86(3):237–44.

46. Bailoor K, Shafie-Khorassani F, Lank RJ, et al. Time trends in race-ethnic differences in do-not-resuscitate orders after stroke. Stroke 2019;50(7):1641–7. https://doi.org/10.1161/STROKEAHA.118.024460.

47. Carr D. The social stratification of older adults' preparations for end-of-life health care. J Health Soc Behav 2012 2012;53(3):297–312. https://doi.org/10.1177/0022146512455427.

48. Block BL, Jeon SY, Sudore RL, et al. Patterns and trends in advance care planning among older adults who received intensive care at the end of life. JAMA Intern Med 2020;180(5):786. https://doi.org/10.1001/jamainternmed.2019.7535.

49. Orlovic M, Smith K, Mossialos E. Racial and ethnic differences in end-of-life care in the United States: evidence from the health and retirement study (HRS). SSM - Population Health 2019;7:100331. https://doi.org/10.1016/j.ssmph.2018.100331.

50. Carr D. Racial and ethnic differences in advance care planning: identifying subgroup patterns and obstacles. J Aging Health 2012;24(6):923–47. https://doi.org/10.1177/0898264312449185.

51. Oh DHW, Conell C, Lyon L, et al. The association of Chinese ethnicity and language preference with advance directive completion among older patients in an integrated health system. J Gen Intern Med 2023;38(5):1137–42. https://doi.org/10.1007/s11606-022-07911-9.

52. Sanders JJ, Johnson KS, Cannady K, et al. From Barriers to Assets: rethinking factors impacting advance care planning for African Americans. Palliat Support Care 2019;17(3):306–13. https://doi.org/10.1017/S147895151800038X.

53. Brown CE, Marshall AR, Snyder CR, et al. Perspectives about racism and patient-clinician communication among black adults with serious illness. JAMA Netw Open 2023;6(7):e2321746. https://doi.org/10.1001/jamanetworkopen.2023.21746.

54. Hong M, Yi E-H, Johnson KJ, et al. Facilitators and barriers for advance care planning among ethnic and racial minorities in the U.S.: a systematic review of the current literature. J Immigrant Minority Health 2018;20(5):1277–87. https://doi.org/10.1007/s10903-017-0670-9.

55. Smith AK, McCarthy EP, Paulk E, et al. Racial and ethnic differences in advance care planning among patients with cancer: impact of terminal illness acknowledgment, religiousness, and treatment preferences. J Clin Oncol 2008;26(25): 4131–7. https://doi.org/10.1200/JCO.2007.14.8452.

56. Jacobsen J, Bernacki R, Paladino J. Shifting to serious illness communication. JAMA 2022;327(4):321–2. https://doi.org/10.1001/jama.2021.23695.

57. Ditto PH, Jacobson JA, Smucker WD, et al. Context changes choices: a prospective study of the effects of hospitalization on life-sustaining treatment preferences. Med Decis Making Jul-Aug 2006;26(4):313–22. https://doi.org/10.1177/0272989X06290494.

58. Lin RJ, Adelman RD, Diamond RR, et al. The sentinel hospitalization and the role of palliative care. J Hosp Med 2014;9(5):320–3. https://doi.org/10.1002/jhm.2160.

59. Hickman SE, Lum HD, Walling AM, et al. The care planning umbrella: the evolution of advance care planning. J Am Geriatr Soc 2023;71(7):2350–6. https://doi.org/10.1111/jgs.18287.

60. Coats H, Downey L, Sharma RK, et al. Quality of communication and trust in patients with serious illness: an exploratory study of the relationships of race/ethnicity, socioeconomic status, and religiosity. J Pain Symptom Manag 2018; 56(4):530–540 e6. https://doi.org/10.1016/j.jpainsymman.2018.07.005.

61. Chuang E, Fiter RJ, Sanon OC, et al. Race and ethnicity and satisfaction with communication in the intensive care unit. Am J Hosp Palliat Care 2020;37(10): 823–9. https://doi.org/10.1177/1049909120916126.

62. Uyeda AM, Lee RY, Pollack LR, et al. Predictors of documented goals-of-care discussion for hospitalized patients with chronic illness. J Pain Symptom Manag 2023;65(3):233–41. https://doi.org/10.1016/j.jpainsymman.2022.11.012.

63. Welch LC, Teno JM, Mor V. End-of-life care in black and white: race matters for medical care of dying patients and their families. J Am Geriatr Soc 2005 2005; 53(7):1145–53. https://doi.org/10.1111/j.1532-5415.2005.53357.x.

64. You H, Ma JE, Haverfield MC, et al. Racial differences in physicians' shared decision-making behaviors during intensive care unit family meetings. Ann Am Thorac Soc 2023. https://doi.org/10.1513/AnnalsATS.202212-997RL.

65. Elliott AM, Alexander SC, Mescher CA, et al. Differences in physicians' verbal and nonverbal communication with black and white patients at the end of life. J Pain Symptom Manag 2016;51(1):1–8. https://doi.org/10.1016/j.jpainsymman.2015.07.008.

66. Muni S, Engelberg RA, Treece PD, et al. The influence of race/ethnicity and socioeconomic status on end-of-life care in the ICU. Chest 2011;139(5):1025–33. https://doi.org/10.1378/chest.10-3011.

67. Schuster RA, Hong SY, Arnold RM, et al. Investigating conflict in ICUs-is the clinicians' perspective enough? Crit Care Med 2014;42(2):328–35. https://doi.org/10.1097/CCM.0b013e3182a27598.

68. Ashana DC, Jan A, Parish A, et al. Interpersonal perception: family- and physician-reported conflict in the intensive care unit. Ann Am Thorac Soc 2022;19(11):1937–42. https://doi.org/10.1513/AnnalsATS.202202-147RL.

69. Gruenberg DA, Shelton W, Rose SL, et al. Factors influencing length of stay in the intensive care unit. Am J Crit Care 2006;15(5):502–9.

70. Wendlandt B, Ceppe A, Choudhury S, et al. Modifiable elements of ICU supportive care and communication are associated with surrogates' PTSD symptoms. Intensive Care Med 2019;45(5):619–26. https://doi.org/10.1007/s00134-019-05550-z.

71. Ali H, Pamarthy R, Bolick NL, et al. Inpatient outcomes and racial disparities of palliative care consults in mechanically ventilated patients in the United States. SAVE Proc 2022;35(6):762–7. https://doi.org/10.1080/08998280.2022.2106537.

72. Wiskar KJ, Celi LA, McDermid RC, et al. Patterns of palliative care referral in patients admitted with heart failure requiring mechanical ventilation. Am J Hosp Palliat Care 2018;35(4):620–6. https://doi.org/10.1177/1049909117727455.

73. Chatterjee K, Goyal A, Kakkera K, et al. National trends (2009-2013) for palliative care utilization for patients receiving prolonged mechanical ventilation. Crit Care Med 2018;46(8):1230–7. https://doi.org/10.1097/ccm.0000000000003182.

74. Fassas S, King D, Shay M, et al. Palliative medicine and end of life care between races in an academic intensive care unit. J Intensive Care Med 2023;8850666231200383. https://doi.org/10.1177/08850666231200383.

75. Gutierrez C, Hsu W, Ouyang Q, et al. Palliative care intervention in the intensive care unit: comparing outcomes among seriously ill Asian patients and those of other ethnicities. J Palliat Care. Autumn 2014;30(3):151–7.

76. Kutney-Lee A, Smith D, Thorpe J, et al. Race/ethnicity and end-of-life care among veterans. Med Care 2017;55(4):342–51. https://doi.org/10.1097/MLR.0000000000000637.

77. Burgio KL, Williams BR, Dionne-Odom JN, et al. Racial differences in processes of care at end of life in VA medical centers: planned secondary analysis of data from the BEACON trial. J Palliat Med 2016 2016;19(2):157–63. https://doi.org/10.1089/jpm.2015.0311.

78. Johnson KS, Kuchibhatla M, Payne R, et al. Race and residence: intercounty variation in black-white differences in hospice use. J Pain Symptom Manag 2013;46(5):681–90. https://doi.org/10.1016/j.jpainsymman.2012.12.006.

79. Samuel-Ryals CA, Mbah OM, Hinton SP, et al. Evaluating the contribution of patient-provider communication and cancer diagnosis to racial disparities in end-of-life care among Medicare beneficiaries. J Gen Intern Med 2021;36(11):3311–20. https://doi.org/10.1007/s11606-021-06778-6.

80. Ornstein KA, Roth DL, Huang J, et al. Evaluation of racial disparities in hospice use and end-of-life treatment intensity in the REGARDS cohort. JAMA Netw Open 2020;3(8):e2014639. https://doi.org/10.1001/jamanetworkopen.2020.14639.

81. Faigle R, Ziai WC, Urrutia VC, et al. Racial differences in palliative care use after stroke in majority-white, minority-serving, and racially integrated U.S. Hospitals. Crit Care Med 2017;45(12):2046–54. https://doi.org/10.1097/CCM.0000000000002762.

82. Sullivan DR, Teno JM, Reinke LF. Evolution of palliative care in the department of veterans affairs: lessons from an integrated health care model. J Palliat Med 2022;25(1):15–20. https://doi.org/10.1089/jpm.2021.0246.

83. La IS, Scharf B, Zhu S, et al. Family bereavement adaptation after death of a loved one in an intensive care unit: impact of race/ethnicity. J Hosp Palliat Nurs 2020;22(6):512–22. https://doi.org/10.1097/njh.0000000000000705.

84. Smith-Howell ER, Hickman SE, Meghani SH, et al. End-of-Life decision making and communication of bereaved family members of african Americans with serious illness. J Palliat Med 2016;19(2):174–82. https://doi.org/10.1089/jpm.2015.0314.

85. Andersen SK, Butler RA, Chang CH, et al. Prevalence of long-term decision regret and associated risk factors in a large cohort of ICU surrogate decision makers. Crit Care 2023;27(1):61. https://doi.org/10.1186/s13054-023-04332-w.

86. Walkey AJ, Barnato AE, Wiener RS, et al. Accounting for patient preferences regarding life-sustaining treatment in evaluations of medical effectiveness and quality. Am J Respir Crit Care Med 2017;196(8):958–63. https://doi.org/10.1164/rccm.201701-0165CP.

87. Pennec S, Gaymu J, Riou F, et al. Dying at home: a majority wish but an uncommon situation. Popul Soc 2015;524(7):1–4. https://doi.org/10.3917/popsoc.524.0001.

88. Chino F, Kamal AH, Leblanc TW, et al. Place of death for patients with cancer in the United States, 1999 through 2015: racial, age, and geographic disparities. Cancer 2018;124(22):4408–19. https://doi.org/10.1002/cncr.31737.

89. Steinhauser KE, Christakis NA, Clipp EC, et al. Factors considered important at the end of life by patients, family, physicians, and other care providers. JAMA 2000;284(19):2476–82. https://doi.org/10.1001/jama.284.19.2476.

90. Gomes B, Calanzani N, Gysels M, et al. Heterogeneity and changes in preferences for dying at home: a systematic review. BMC Palliat Care 2013;12:7. https://doi.org/10.1186/1472-684X-12-7.

91. McCleskey SG, Cain CL. Improving end-of-life care for diverse populations: communication, competency, and system supports. Am J Hosp Palliat Care 2019;36(6):453–9. https://doi.org/10.1177/1049909119827933.

92. Russell D, Diamond EL, Lauder B, et al. Frequency and risk factors for live discharge from hospice. J Am Geriatr Soc 2017;65(8):1726–32. https://doi.org/10.1111/jgs.14859.

93. Hunt LJ, Gan S, Smith AK, et al. Hospice quality, race, and disenrollment in hospice enrollees with dementia. J Palliat Med 2023;26(8):1100–8. https://doi.org/10.1089/jpm.2023.0011.

94. Wachterman MW, Luth EA, Semco RS, et al. Where Americans die - is there really "No place like home"? N Engl J Med 2022;386(11):1008–10. https://doi.org/10.1056/NEJMp2112297.

95. Kagawa-Singer M, Blackhall LJ. Negotiating cross-cultural issues at the end of life. JAMA 2001 2001;286(23):2993. https://doi.org/10.1001/jama.286.23.2993.

96. Stevenson EK, Mehter HM, Walkey AJ, et al. Association between do not resuscitate/do not intubate status and resident physician decision-making. A national survey. Ann Am Thorac Soc 2017;14(4):536–42. https://doi.org/10.1513/AnnalsATS.201610-798OC.

97. Neufeld MY, Sarkar B, Wiener RS, et al. The effect of patient code status on surgical resident decision making: a national survey of general surgery residents. Surgery 2020;167(2):292–7. https://doi.org/10.1016/j.surg.2019.07.002.

98. Steinhauser KE, Clipp EC, McNeilly M, et al. In search of a good death: observations of patients, families, and providers. Ann Intern Med 2000 2000;132(10): 825–32. https://doi.org/10.7326/0003-4819-132-10-200005160-00011.
99. Hardeman RR, Karbeah JM. Examining racism in health services research: a disciplinary self-critique. Health Serv Res 2020;55(Suppl 2):777–80. https://doi.org/10.1111/1475-6773.13558.
100. Brown CE, Curtis JR. Time for a new approach investigating and eliminating racial inequities in the ICU. Crit Care Med 2022;50(1):144–7. https://doi.org/10.1097/CCM.0000000000005280.

Workforce Diversity and Equity Among Critical Care Physicians

Sherie A. Gause, MD[a], Kelly C. Vranas, MD, MCR[a,b,*]

KEYWORDS

- Women underrepresented in medicine • Minoritized populations
- Health care disparities • Critical care physician workforce • Diversity and equity

KEY POINTS

- Health disparities persist among minoritized populations; the coronavirus 2019 disease pandemic exposed and exacerbated these disparities in access to care and outcomes.
- A diverse physician workforce helps to improve and reduce health disparities and patient outcomes.
- However, gender, racial, and ethnic diversity are lacking among the critical care physician workforce.
- The leaky pipeline and vicious cycle of academic medicine contribute to low representation of women and individuals underrepresented in medicine within the field of critical care.
- To improve health care disparities in the critically ill, the authors must increase physician representation of diverse backgrounds through a variety of individual, institutional, and systematic approaches.

INTRODUCTION

Health outcomes for patients with a variety of conditions common in the intensive care unit (ICU) (eg, sepsis, respiratory failure) have improved over time, in part due to advances in medical therapies and technologies.[1–3] Yet, particularly in the Unites States (U.S.), health disparities persist among persons with characteristics historically linked to discrimination or exclusion (eg, race, ethnicity, sexual identity, or orientation).[4–8] For example, a recent study found that Black and Hispanic patients were 42% and 21% more likely to die within 30 days of surgery compared to White patients, respectively.[9]

[a] Division of Pulmonary, Allergy, and Critical Care Medicine, Department of Medicine, Oregon Health & Science University, 3181 Southwest Sam Jackson Park Road, Portland, OR 97239, USA;
[b] Center to Improve Veteran Involvement in Care (CIVIC), VA Portland Health Care System, 3710 Southwest US Veterans Hospital Road, Portland, OR 97239, USA
* Corresponding author.
E-mail address: vranas@ohsu.edu

Crit Care Clin 40 (2024) 767–787
https://doi.org/10.1016/j.ccc.2024.05.008
0749-0704/24/Published by Elsevier Inc.

criticalcare.theclinics.com

Additionally, there is a growing evidence base demonstrating persistent disparities in maternal mortality, with one recent study showing that, during childbirth, Black women die at a rate 2.6 times that of White women.[10]

The coronavirus 2019 disease (COVID-19) pandemic further exacerbated these disparities, with multiple studies demonstrating that racial and ethnic minorities were at increased risk of infection, hospitalization, and death related to COVID-19.[11] Causes of these disparities are multifactorial and include increased exposure to environmental risk factors (eg, air pollution, occupational hazards, obesity, and tobacco use) among minoritized populations over time, in part due to structural racism.[8,12] In addition, social determinants of health (eg, access to transportation, health insurance, stable housing, quality education, and economic stability), are less common among American Indian or Alaska Native, Asian or Pacific Islander, Latino, and Black populations, impacting their ability to access high-quality medical care.[11,13] Addressing and eliminating such disparities is a crucial component of efforts to attain health equality across populations–a goal that is both cost-effective and morally imperative.[14]

Fostering a diverse and inclusive workforce is a key factor in improving access to high-quality care and reducing health disparities among underserved populations. For example, there is evidence that patient-clinician concordance (defined as shared characteristics like gender, race and ethnicity, or socioeconomic status) improves outcomes among general medical populations. Specifically, patient-clinician concordance has been associated with greater satisfaction with care among patients[15–19]; improved medication adherence and continuity of care[20–22]; and more effective therapeutic relationships,[23] potentially through mechanism of increased trust.[24–26] Trust between patients and clinicians is particularly important when eliciting goals of care and treatment preferences among patients with serious illness, as this process requires high-quality communication and shared-decision making between clinicians, patients, and families.[27]

From the perspective of the health care system, patient-clinician concordance has also been associated with lower emergency department use and reduced health care expenditures.[23] Additionally, clinicians from populations under-represented in medicine (URiM)[28] – defined as those who identify as Black, Hispanic, and Indigenous[29] – are more likely to work in underserved areas and include minoritized populations in research studies, reiterating the importance of training a diverse workforce as part of efforts to reduce health disparities.[8,30,31]

Yet, the general physician workforce in the U.S. remains predominantly male and White (**Table 1**). Women comprise approximately 37% of active physicians, despite making up at least 50% of medical school matriculants since 2017.[32,33] Furthermore, 63.9% of active physicians identify as White, 20.6% as Asian, 5.7% as Black, 6.9% as Hispanic, and 0.3% as American Indian or Alaska Native.[34] Within critical care medicine specifically, disparities in gender, race, and ethnicity persist: approximately 27.3% of critical care physicians are women, 4.1% are Black, 7.5% Hispanic, and 0.1% as American Indian or Alaska native[34]; data on physicians in critical care who identify as LGBTQIA + are wholly lacking.[35] Moreover, the number of Black male physicians in the U.S. – currently at 2.7% –actually decreased between 1978 and 2014.[36] Unfortunately, this lack of representation among women and minoritized populations within critical care medicine is unlikely to improve in the near future, as the proportion of URiM fellows training in the field remains low and essentially unchanged between 2005 (10.5%) and 2018 (10.3%).[8,37]

In this commentary, the authors will first review the systemic reasons underlying the lack of representation of minoritized populations among the critical care physician workforce. To do so, the authors will utilize the conceptual model of the "leaky

Table 1
Proportion of critical care physicians by gender,[a] race, and ethnicity in 2021

Specialty	Total No. Active Physicians	Female N (%)	White N (%)	Black or African American N (%)	Asian N (%)	American Indian or Alaska Native N (%)	Native Hawaiian or Pacific Islander N (%)	Hispanic N (%)
All	946,790	351,117 (37.1)	537,351 (63.9)	48,248 (5.7)	173,283 (20.6)	2,583 (0.3)	961 (0.1)	58,395 (6.9)
Critical Care Medicine	14,142	3,861 (27.3)	7,411 (54.4)	564 (4.1)	4,057 (29.8)	19 (0.1)	17 (0.1)	1,015 (7.5)

[a] AMA Physician Dataset defines gender as "male" or "female" only.
American Medical Association. AMA Physician Masterfile (Dec. 31, 2021).

pipeline"– a framework that conceptualizes low representation within academic medicine based on "leaks" resulting from systemic barriers across the education and training continuum[38,39] – to better understand the reasons behind such disparities among ICU physicians (**Fig. 1**). Next, the authors will review challenges to retaining and sustaining a diverse critical care workforce, including discussion of how the "vicious cycle" of bias in academic medicine may reinforce the lack of diversity observed within the critical care physician workforce (**Fig. 2**)[40,41]; the authors will then finish by describing interventions aimed at increasing representation and fostering an environment within medicine that prioritizes equity and inclusion among ICU physicians.

Of note, little is known about critical care physicians who identify as LGBTQIA+; for this reason, the authors chose to focus this narrative review on women and URiM individuals based on the available data. However, the authors acknowledge that LGBTQIA + individuals are underrepresented in the physician workforce (comprising approximately 6.3% of graduating medical students)[42] and that more work is needed to better understand their experiences through medical training and as part of efforts to create a diverse and inclusive critical care workforce.

THE ORIGINS AND CONSEQUENCES OF THE LEAKY PIPELINE
Primary Education

As described earlier, the "leaky pipeline" framework conceptualizes low representation within academic medicine based on "leaks" resulting from systemic barriers faced by women and those identified as URiM (see **Fig. 1**; **Fig. 3**). Particularly for URiM individuals, the leaky pipeline begins as early as elementary school.[38,39] Indeed, there is evidence that Black and Hispanic children in the U.S. have worse academic performance and standardized test scores compared to White children.[43–45] Reasons for this are multifactorial, driven in part to the history of racial segregation in schools,[45] as well as historic redlining (ie, government homeownership programs created as part of the 1930s-era New Deal, in which neighborhoods predominantly inhabited by Black residents were deemed risky for investment.)[46] As a result, school districts within historically redlined neighborhoods have had less funding and resources

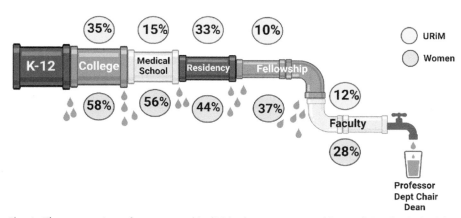

Fig. 1. The proprotion of women and individuals unrepresented in medicine (URiM) within the critical care workforce at each stage of the critical care medicine pipeline. (Created with BioRender.com.)

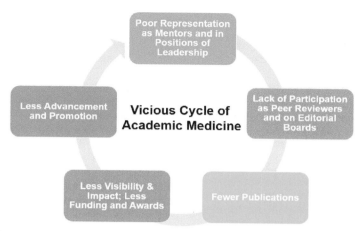

Fig. 2. The Vicious cycle of academic medicine. (*Reprinted with permission from* Elsevier. The Lancet, February 2019, 393 (10171), 508-510.)

compared to predominantly white schools[47]; over the time, the cumulative impact of these policies has resulted in lower quality education and reduced opportunities offered to children of color who predominately attend those schools.[47]

Additionally, unconscious bias may impact recognition of students of color for academic opportunities early on in their academic journeys. For example, a 2016 study found that Black elementary school students were less likely to be seen as "gifted"

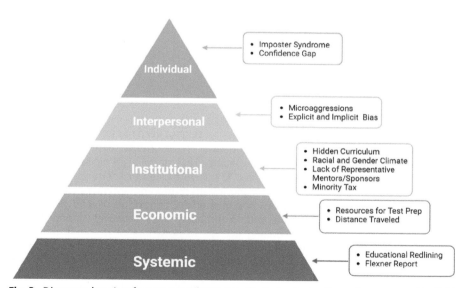

Fig. 3. Diagram showing factors contributing to the lack of retention of women and individuals underrepresented in medicine within the critical care workforce. (Created with BioRender.com.)

relative to White students, and were therefore overlooked for placement into advanced programs, even after controlling for test scores.[48] This gap is further widened by socioeconomic status and parental education attainment where students with parents who did not obtain a bachelor's degree also tend to have worse academic performance.[49]

Premedical Experiences

Gaps in educational opportunity persist for female, Black, and Hispanic students through secondary school. For example, a 2014 study performed by the Association of American Medical Colleges found that, among sophomore students aspiring to enter medical school, 74% were female, 18% were Black, and 48% White. However, women comprised only 50% of medical school applicants and matriculants; Black students comprised only 7% of medical school applicants and 6% of matriculants, whereas White students comprised approximately 60% of applicants and matriculants.[50] Barriers to attending medical school disproportionately experienced by Black and Hispanic students include the financial burden of pre-medical school testing and admissions processes, lack of guidance and social support, and belief that they are not strong enough as candidates to be accepted.[51] In fact, URiM applicants to medical school are disproportionately from low-income households and overrepresented in the lowest strata of the Association of American Medical College's parental education and occupational indicator compared to non-URiM applicants.[29,52] These barriers–financial and otherwise–can be further exacerbated by individual bias among students' advisors, resulting in non-White students being discouraged from applying to medical school more often than White students.[53]

Furthermore, there is evidence that admission tests to medical school may perpetuate the effects of structural racism on non-White applicants. One study found that URiM applicants have lower scores on the Medical College Admission Test (MCAT) compared to non-URiM applicants,[54] in part due to reasons described earlier; another study found that socioeconomic status is a strong predictor of MCAT performance.[55] Yet, despite evidence that applicants with mid-range MCAT scores are successful in medical school, many programs often overlook applicants whose scores do not meet a specific cut-off as part of the admissions process.[29,56] For this reason, it is important for medical schools to reexamine the use of MCAT scores in admission processes as part of efforts to diversify the physician workforce.[56]

In addition to these structural disadvantages, URiM students in particular are often missing a key component to the graduate school admissions process: access to the hidden curriculum.[57] The concept of the hidden curriculum has been defined as "the method by which the values, skills, and attitudes of a group being joined are adopted."[58] Within medicine, the hidden curriculum is distinct from the formal coursework, and instead represents lessons that are embedded in the organizational structure and culture of an institution, which are not explicitly presented.[57] The hidden curriculum can include the social connections required to cultivate clinical experiences and pertinent extracurricular activities, obtain strong letters of recommendation, and acquire guidance on how to be successful through medical school admission processes and beyond. Less familiarity with the hidden curriculum may negatively impact career development opportunities by reducing access to networks of potential mentors, diminishing a sense of belonging within one's field and institution, and limiting knowledge of how to navigate the complex system of influences within medicine more broadly.[29,57]

Finally, URiM individuals in particular often face challenges in the journey to medical school related to underlying systemic barriers as described earlier. This concept–known as the "distance traveled" – is defined as differences between individuals in the path to their present position.[59] For some, achieving admission to medical school entails "traveling" a greater distance than for others (eg, having to work during undergraduate years to help meet financial obligations at home).[59] Recognizing the distance traveled by individuals, especially among URiM applicants, is a crucial part of efforts to achieve equitable opportunities for career development and ultimately a diverse and proficient critical care workforce.

Medical School and Residency

The underrepresentation of Black physicians in particular can be traced back to the release of the Flexner report in 1910, which examined medical education and suggested reform for medical colleges (including increasing standards, partnering with hospitals for clinical training, and closing schools that could not afford to update and maintain facilities.)[60]

The Flexner report, which was initiated by the American Medical Association's Council on Medical Education, drastically changed medical education and led to the closing of more than half of all medical schools in the U.S. and Canada, including the majority of Black medical schools. Only 2 medical schools remained as options for Black applicants: Howard University College of Medicine in Washington, D.C., and Meharry Medical College in Nashville, Tennessee, both of which remain today.[60]

In practice, the Flexner report all but eliminated medical education for Black individuals, and its effects on health care inequality continue to persist.[61]

In 2008, nearly a century after the Flexner report was published, the American Medical Association issued an apology for its "history of racial inequality toward African-American physicians."[61,62] Since then, societies such as the American Academy of Medical Colleges have urged medical schools to adopt anti-racist and inclusive practices.[63] Despite these efforts, medical school can be a challenging environment for URiM students. For example, in a nationwide sample of approximately 3800 medical students, 64% reported a hostile racial climate, while 81% and 94%, respectively, reported witnessing discrimination toward students and negative role modeling (eg, physicians speaking negatively about Black patients).[29,64] Microaggressions–defined as commonplace interactions that communicate bias against an individual or group–are also commonly experienced by both URiM and female trainees, are associated with increased odds of reporting depressive symptoms,[65] and contribute to an overall negative racial climate.[29] Perhaps not surprisingly, then, there is a disproportionately high attrition rate among URiM medical students.[66]

These trends likely continue throughout medical training as well. A 2021 study describing trends in racial and ethnic diversity in internal medicine subspecialty fellowships between 2006 and 2018 found that no specialties reflected the diversity of the U.S. population. Furthermore, authors found that the subspecialties with the lowest percentage of URiM fellows (including pulmonary and critical care medicine) were also the largest fellowships and the more procedural specialties; these findings raise the possibility that systemic factors are affecting career choices for URiM residents.[37] Even more concerning were findings from a complementary study focusing on the pipeline for pulmonary and critical care medicine specifically. Authors found that less than 33% of all pulmonary or critical care fellows are women, and less than 12% of fellows in the field are URiM. Over the last decade, the percentage of female fellows in pulmonary and critical care fellowship programs has remained unchanged, while the percentage of URiM pulmonary and critical care fellows has decreased. Additionally, authors identified a discrepancy between the number of URiM residents who apply for fellowship in pulmonary and critical care, and the number who match successfully, suggesting that URiM applicants are matching to these fellowships at a disproportionately low rate.[67] Such persistent disparities in the pipeline must be addressed as part of efforts to grow and sustain a diverse critical care workforce.

CHALLENGES TO RETAINING AND SUSTAINING A DIVERSE CRITICAL CARE WORKFORCE
Disparities in Academic Publishing Within Pulmonary or Critical Care Literature

Even if individuals are able to overcome the multiple structural, institutional, and economic barriers to become critical care physicians described earlier, there is a myriad of challenges to retain and sustain a diverse ICU workforce that persist, particularly within academic medicine. For example, female and URiM physicians remain underrepresented in scholarly critical care activities (eg, academic publishing) that are considered essential for hiring and promotion.[8,14,35,68–71] A recent study found that women comprise less than one-third of first authors and less than one-fourth of senior authors of critical care original research, with minimal increase over the past decade.[70] Additionally, female first authors of critical care literature are also more likely to publish in lower-impact journals compared to men,[70] while female senior authors of original pulmonary and critical care research have lower odds of acceptance compared with articles by male senior authors.[72] Regarding URiM representation in academic publishing, a 2022 study focused on the diversity of authors of publications from the Canadian Critical Care Trials Group found that of among 1,205 unique authors, approximately 15% of first authors and 10% of senior authors were members of a visible minority group.[73]

With these findings in mind–that female and URiM physician and scientists are underrepresented as authors, and are more likely to have their research published in lower impact journals or not published at all–it is not surprising that their expertize might be overlooked, as demonstrated by their underrepresentation on guideline panels and editorial boards, and as speakers or chairs at critical care conferences.[69,70,74–79] For example, women were notably absent from the development of prominent critical care consensus statements and clinical practice guidelines, including the recent Berlin acute respiratory distress syndrome and Sepsis-3 definitions.[69,80–83] Women also comprised between 5% and 26% of speakers across 5 international critical care conferences between 2010 and 2016, despite comprising between 20% and 40% of the critical care workforce globally.[68,84]

The "Vicious Cycle" of Academic Medicine

Taken together, these data reveal possible mechanisms contributing to the "vicious cycle" in academic medicine in which less representation as authors and reviewers may lead to fewer publications and speaking opportunities, less funding and awards, and ultimately less career advancement (see **Fig. 2**).[40,41,70] This "vicious cycle" may, in turn, explain the persistence of the glass ceiling as demonstrated by the underrepresentation of women and URiM in positions of leadership within academic medicine.[40] Specifically, women comprise only 24% of all Division Chiefs, 24% of Vice Chairs, 15% of Department Chairs, and 16% of all medical school Deans.[85] A 2014 study by Jena and colleagues found that, among 90,000 faculties at U.S. medical schools, women were less likely than men to achieve full professor status, even after adjusting for age, specialty, productivity, and experience.[70,86] Similarly, a 2013 study found that only 8% of faculty in U.S. medical schools were URiM.[87] More recently, the data from the Association of American Medical Colleges Medical Association found that in 2022, URiM faculty comprised 13% of interim or permanent Deans at U.S. medical schools compared to 7% in 1993.[88]

Additionally, there are a variety of other factors that likely contribute to the vicious cycle within academic medicine. First, within academic publishing, female and URiM physicians and scientists comprise a minority of journal editors and editorial board members, which may adversely impact their success in publishing their research in a particular journal.[70,76,77,84] Furthermore, most journals do not conduct double-blind review of submitted articles, despite evidence that it may help overcome unconscious biases and gender stereotypes that contribute to underrepresentation of women and URiM as authors.[70,89–91]

Second, the "confidence gap" between men and women that has been observed across a variety of industries may contribute to a reluctance of individuals from underrepresented groups to submit their research to high-impact journals or seek other career advancement opportunities.[70] For example, the journal Science performed an audit of the gender of its published authors and found that the journal received one-third fewer articles from female authors than would be expected based on the number of women in their respective fields.[70,92] Similarly, there is evidence that fewer women apply for National Institute of Health grant applications than men, but with similar success rates.[89,92] Female and URiM physicians may also experience the related but distinct concept of imposter syndrome, defined as the perception that the individual did not earn the position that they are occupying.[93] Overcoming both the confidence gap and imposter syndrome are crucial for individuals to achieve psychologic safety and enable career development and advancement within academic medicine.[94,95]

Third, the institutional climate surrounding diversity, equity, and inclusion within the critical care workforce (eg, implicit bias; funding opportunities; compensation; consideration for leadership, academic, and networking opportunities; sponsorship and mentorship practices; and processes for promotion and tenure) may contribute to lack of representation and attrition among women and URiM faculty.[96] For example, one study found that 70% of female career development award recipients perceived gender bias compared to 22% of male award recipients.[97] Gender bias has been shown to exist in student evaluations of faculty members, as well as hiring practices.[96,98,99] There is also evidence that female physicians are disproportionately responsible for caregiving and family responsibilities, which may impact their productivity over time, as well as job satisfaction, mental health, and burnout.[96]

Finally, faculties from underrepresented groups are often subject to additional responsibilities and expectations in order to "represent" diversity in multiple clinical and administrative roles–a phenomenon described as the "minority tax."[59] Such a tax results in women and URiM faculties being more isolated amongst their peers with less access to faculty development and mentorship, less time to dedicate toward academic pursuits, lower job satisfaction and work performance, and ultimately less career advancement.[59]

STRATEGIES TO IMPROVE DIVERSITY AND EQUITY WITHIN THE PHYSICIAN WORKFORCE
Improving the Pipeline for Women and Underrepresented in Medicine in the Critical Care Physician Workforce

Improving the diversity and equity of the critical care workforce requires interventions far upstream of the faculty hiring process. A 2018 scoping review found that pipeline and pathway programs are the most frequently used approaches to increase representation of women and URiM in the medical workforce.[100] Such programs may start as early as elementary school and include efforts to identify and support future medical students from diverse backgrounds through outreach programs, shadowing opportunities, guidance on admissions testing, education on financing medical school, and mentorship more broadly.[101] Additionally, combined college-to-medical school pathways (such as the Mount Sinai School of Medicine Humanities and Medicine Program)[102] offer early admissions to medical school that may not require MCAT test scores, thus, removing 1 barrier of acceptance to medical school. Post-baccalaureate pathway programs also represent important strategies for increasing diversity among medical school matriculants.[100] Specifically, post-baccalaureate programs can help URiM overcome known barriers to medical school admission (eg, lower MCAT scores, fewer premedical clinical opportunities) through curricula that emphasize basic science skills required for admission testing, academic enrichment skills, and research options.[100,103] Finally, formal collaborations between historically Black colleges and universities, as well as collaborations between minority medical student organizations (such as the American Medical Women's Association and the Student National Medical Association) and medical school admissions offices, represent potentially underutilized opportunities to facilitate the recruitment of women and URiM students into the physician workforce.[104]

Holistic review of applicants throughout medical school, residency, and fellowship admission processes represents another promising intervention that can be implemented to improve the diversity of the critical care physician workforce. Holistic review is defined as a "flexible, individualized way of assessing an applicant's capabilities, by which balanced consideration is given to experiences, attributes, competencies, and academic or scholarly metrics, and when considered in combination, how the individual might contribute value to the institution's mission."[105] Practically speaking, holistic review seeks to evaluate applicants as a whole rather than as a sum of their parts, taking into account the distances traveled by individuals as part of efforts to create a more diverse physician workforce. It typically involves the use of a set of standardized interview questions and rank system to help reduce bias in the selection process.[105] This technique is being increasingly applied nationwide at the level of undergraduate admissions, as well as for medical school and residency selection processes.[106] A growing body of evidence has shown that holistic review improved the representation of women and URiM among medical school and residency applicants invited for interview, as well as the proportion of URiM matriculants in residency programs.[106,107] It stands to reason that this strategy could be particularly helpful in the field of critical care–a field in which disparities persist and have been slow to improve.[34] However, given the recent Supreme Court decision eliminating race-conscious admissions programs,[108] the future of holistic review in medical school, residency, and fellowship application processes is uncertain.

Additionally, some institutions have implemented academic coaching programs for individuals from underrepresented settings who matriculate into medical training programs. Academic coaching has been defined as a process in which an individual learner meets regularly over time with a faculty coach to create goals, identify strategies to manage challenges, improve the learning environment experienced by URiM trainees, and reach the learner's highest potential.[109,110] It is distinct from mentoring insofar as academic coaching is learner and task driven, emphasizes an individual's goals, and creates space for that individual to determine their own path toward achieving those goals; in contrast, mentoring is a relationship-driven advisory process designed to guide and support a person for their career development.[109]

A recent mixed-methods study of an academic coaching program at a single academic medical institution revealed that URiM trainees reported having distinct needs compared to White students. Specifically, URiM students experienced more pressure to perform, felt more anxious about showing vulnerability during their coaching sessions, and desired a coach who exhibited cultural humility; however, these differences between URiM and White trainees were largely unrecognized by their coaches.[109] Following this study, a group of faculty advisors called "Diversity Navigators" were formed under the School of Medicine at that institution to improve the URiM experience in medical school, foster community, and support underrepresented medical students through specific challenges that they might face as members of minoritized populations.[111,112] Although the impact of this intervention requires further study, it represents a potential mechanism to enhance the pipeline of URiM individuals within the critical care physician workforce more broadly.

Breaking the Vicious Cycle of Academic Medicine

Within academic medicine, several strategies exist to help break the vicious cycle that has served to perpetuate disparities for women and URiM in the critical care workforce. To begin, journals play a central role in the transmission of scientific knowledge and the validation of academic achievement.[41] Therefore, it is imperative that journals address imbalances among women and URiM in academic publishing through a variety of mechanisms, including: (1) implementing double-blind review of submitted articles, which has been shown to favor increased representation of female authors by overcoming unconscious biases and gender stereotypes;[70,89–91] (2) training journals on diversity initiative and unconscious bias; (3) collecting and publishing data on journals' internal processes, including their proportion of editorial staff and peer reviewers who are women or URiM; and (4) setting diversity targets for commissioned content, peer reviewers, and editorial roles with frequent audits of journals' performance in these areas.[41,113,114] Similar goals could be set for Critical Care Societies as well, including establishing diversity policies for populating panels they commission, as well as tracking and publicly reporting representation of women and URiM individuals on panels for definition documents, consensus statements, and practice guidelines.[69]

At the institutional level, enhancing opportunities for mentorship is a crucial component of strategies to recruit and retain a diverse critical care physician workforce. Mentorship has been associated with increased career satisfaction, faculty retention, research productivity (eg, publication and grant success), and overall career advancement.[70,115] The benefits of mentorship were exemplified in a recent study evaluating gender differences in authorship of critical are literature. In this study, authors found that female senior authors were significantly more likely than male senior authors to publish with female first and middle authors, suggesting that women may mentor and collaborate with other women more often than men do.[70] Yet, prior literature has shown that women are less likely than their male colleagues to have a mentor across varying levels of training.[116–118] There is also an evidence that URiM physicians are less likely to have effective mentorship and apply for awards and grant support compared to non-URiM physicians.[119] Taken together, these findings highlight the value of efforts to increase the pool of women and URiM in senior academic positions who are available to serve as mentors for junior faculty, who are particularly vulnerable to attrition from academic medicine.[70,116]

In addition to mentorship, sponsorship is a necessary component to help break the vicious cycle of academic medicine and help advance women and URiM physicians to positions of leadership within critical care. Sponsors differ from mentors—in that sponsors are in a position of power within an institution, and are therefore, able to advocate publicly for the advancement of nascent talent within an institution.[70,118] Sponsorship programs–which are being increasingly used in the corporate world to raise the visibility of women and help advance them into positions of leadership[120,121]

– represent an additional tool to help address disparities that persist within the field of critical care.

Furthermore, it is important that institutions deliberately implement interventions to enable women and URiM physicians to overcome systemic barriers to career advancement. For example, the University of California, Davis School of Medicine established the Women in Medicine and Health Science program to help women advance to positions of leadership within their institution through explicit advocacy.[122] Notably, the percentage of female faculty doubled from 18% to 36% in the first 10 years of the program, with a concomitant increase in the number of female full professors and department chairs.[70,122] As part of these initiatives, however, it is imperative that institutions collect data (including promotion and tenure decisions) with a commitment to transparency and accountability as part of efforts to inform institutional actions and effect necessary change.

A recent perspective piece by Chesley and colleagues described an approach by which academic institutions can promote equity and address structural racism, anchored by 4 pillars: (1) promoting education on social justice topics (eg, implicit bias, anti-racism); (2) improving community outreach (eg, pipeline development activities, access to voting); (3) restructuring clinical practices to promote anti-racism (eg, establishing racial disparities in critical care outcomes as a quality target); and (4) fostering an anti-racist workplace climate (eg, training faculty on implicit bias; increasing recruitment of URiM candidates).[123] Importantly, authors note that these initiatives must not rest disproportionately on underrepresented members (ie, the "minority tax"), but instead requires collective action from the entire institution and broader community.[123]

Finally, at a national level, several opportunities exist to enhance and sustain a more diverse critical care physician workforce.[8] For example, the American Thoracic Society (ATS) offers Minority Trainee Development Scholarship to support travel for URiM trainees to attend the ATS International Conference, where they can present their work and be exposed to networking opportunities as part of their career development.[124] The Harold Amos Medical Faculty Development Program has also partnered with multiple professional societies, including the ATS, American Lung Association, and American College of Chest Physicians, to address the shortages of scholars with academic and research appointments in the field of pulmonary and critical care medicine who come from historically marginalized backgrounds.[125] In addition, the U.S. National Institutes of Health Office of Research on Women's Health implemented several initiatives to promote the career of women in biomedical scientists; these include the creation of a working group that assists with mentoring and networking opportunities, as well as programming to support researchers returning to workforce after a qualifying hiatus.[126] These efforts are crucial to build and sustain a diverse critical care physician workforce that will ultimately lead to more equitable and higher-quality care for our patients.

SUMMARY

Health disparities persist among minoritized populations; the COVID-19 pandemic exposed and exacerbated these disparities in access to high-quality care and outcomes. A diverse physician workforce helps reduce health disparities and improve patient outcomes. Yet, gender, racial, and ethnic diversity are lacking among the critical care physicians due to a variety of historic and current factors that contribute to the lack of retention (a.k.a. the "leaky pipeline") of women and URiM in the workforce and the vicious cycle of academic medicine. To improve health care disparities in the critically ill, the authors must increase physician representation of diverse backgrounds through a variety of individual, institutional, systematic, and societal approaches that combat gender bias and structural racism. These efforts should first focus on stabilizing the pipeline to critical care medicine by adopting practices such as pipeline programs, holistic admissions, and academic coaching. Additionally, targeted efforts by journals, professional societies, and academic institutions are necessary to break the vicious cycle of academic medicine in ways that minimize the minority tax. Strategies can include implementation of double-blind peer review of submitted articles; setting diversity targets (eg, representation of women and URiM on editorial boards, guideline committees, promotion and tenure decisions, and in positions of academic leadership); and collecting and publishing data on internal processes and decisions to ensure transparency and accountability. Lastly, both mentorship and sponsorship of women and URiM critical care physicians are vital for career advancement. With increased representation, health care outcomes such as access to high-quality critical care and therapeutic relationships will likely improve.

CLINICS CARE POINTS

Pitfalls
- Beware of unconscious bias, confidence gap, distance traveled, imposter syndrome, and minority tax, which all contribute to and perpetuate lower representation of URiM and women in the critical care physician workforce.
- There is a discrepancy between the number of URiM applicants who apply for fellowship in pulmonary and critical care, and the number who match successfully, suggesting that URiM applicants are matching to these fellowships at a disproportionately low rate.
- Persistent disparities in the pipeline must be addressed in order to grow and sustain a diverse critical care workforce.

Pearls
- Holistic review improves representation of women and URiM throughout stages of medical training.
- Targeted efforts by journals, professional societies, and academic institutions are necessary to break the vicious cycle of academic medicine; strategies can include implementation of double-blind peer review of submitted articles; setting diversity targets (eg, representation of women and URiM on editorial boards, guideline committees, promotion and tenure decisions, and in positions of academic leadership); and collecting and publishing data on internal processes and decisions to ensure transparency and accountability.
- Mentorship and sponsorship of women and URiM critical care physicians are vital to their career advancement.

DISCLOSURE

The authors have nothing to disclose.

FUNDING

Dr Vranas is supported by resources from the VA Portland Health Care System.

The Department of Veterans Affairs did not have a role in the conduct of the study; in the collection, management, analysis, or interpretation of data; or in the preparation of the manuscript. The views expressed in this article are those of the authors and do not necessarily represent the views of the Department of Veterans Affairs or the U.S. government.

REFERENCES

1. Ramirez M, Kamal R, Cox C. How has the quality of the U.S. healthcare system changed over time?. 2019. Available at: https://www.healthsystemtracker.org/chart-collection/how-has-the-quality-of-the-u-s-healthcare-system-changed-over-time/#Age-standardized%20years%20of%20life%20lost%20(YLL)%20rate%20per%20100,000%20population,%201990-2017. [Accessed 1 November 2023].
2. Kaukonen K-M, Bailey M, Suzuki S, et al. Mortality related to severe sepsis and septic shock among critically ill patients in Australia and New Zealand, 2000-2012. JAMA 2014;311(13):1308–16.
3. Palakshappa JA, Krall JTW, Belfield LT, et al. Long-term outcomes in acute respiratory distress syndrome: epidemiology, mechanisms, and patient evaluation. Crit Care Clin 2021;37(4):895–911.
4. Ku L, Vichare A. The association of racial and ethnic concordance in primary care with patient satisfaction and experience of care. J Gen Intern Med 2023;38(3):727–32.
5. Bailey ZD, Krieger N, Agénor M, et al. Structural racism and health inequities in the USA: evidence and interventions. Lancet 2017;389(10077):1453–63.
6. Manuel JI. Racial/ethnic and gender disparities in health care use and access. Health Serv Res 2018;53(3):1407–29.
7. National healthcare quality and disparities report. Content last reviewed july 2023. Rockville, MD: Agency for Healthcare Research and Quality; 2021. Available at: https://www.ahrq.gov/research/findings/nhqrdr/nhqdr21/index.html. [Accessed 2 November 2023].
8. Celedón JC. Building a diverse workforce in pulmonary, critical care, and sleep medicine. ATS scholar 2021;2(2):145–8.
9. Reports and Proceedings American Society of Anesthesiologists. Black and Hispanic patients much more likely to die after surgery than white patients. Published October 15, 2023. Available at: https://www.asahq.org/about-asa/newsroom/news-releases/2023/10/black-and-hispanic-patients. Accessed November 1, 2023.
10. Harris E. US maternal mortality continues to worsen. JAMA 2023;329(15):1248.
11. Acosta AM, Garg S, Pham H, et al. Racial and ethnic disparities in rates of COVID-19-associated hospitalization, intensive care unit admission, and in-hospital death in the United States from march 2020 to february 2021. JAMA Netw Open 2021;4(10):e2130479.
12. Paradies Y, Priest N, Ben J, et al. Racism as a determinant of health: a protocol for conducting a systematic review and meta-analysis. Syst Rev 2013;2:85.
13. Raine S, Liu A, Mintz J, et al. Racial and ethnic disparities in COVID-19 outcomes: social determination of health. Int J Environ Res Public Health 2020;17(21):8115.
14. Celedón JC, Burchard EG, Schraufnagel D, et al. An American thoracic society/national heart, Lung, and blood institute workshop report: addressing respiratory health equality in the United States. Annals of the American Thoracic Society 2017;14(5):814–26.
15. Laveist TA, Nuru-Jeter A. Is doctor-patient race concordance associated with greater satisfaction with care? J Health Soc Behav 2002;43(3):296–306.
16. Saha S, Komaromy M, Koepsell TD, et al. Patient-physician racial concordance and the perceived quality and use of health care. Arch Intern Med 1999;159(9):997–1004.

17. Cooper LA, Roter DL, Johnson RL, et al. Patient-centered communication, ratings of care, and concordance of patient and physician race. Ann Intern Med 2003;139(11):907–15.

18. Derose KP, Hays RD, McCaffrey DF, et al. Does physician gender affect satisfaction of men and women visiting the emergency department? J Gen Intern Med 2001;16(4):218–26.

19. Takeshita J, Wang S, Loren AW, et al. Association of racial/ethnic and gender concordance between patients and physicians with patient experience ratings. JAMA Netw Open 2020;3(11):e2024583.

20. Traylor AH, Schmittdiel JA, Uratsu CS, et al. Adherence to cardiovascular disease medications: does patient-provider race/ethnicity and language concordance matter? J Gen Intern Med 2010;25(11):1172–7.

21. Konrad TR, Howard DL, Edwards LJ, et al. Physician-patient racial concordance, continuity of care, and patterns of care for hypertension. Am J Publ Health 2005;95(12):2186–90.

22. Waibel S, Wong ST, Katz A, et al. The influence of patient-clinician ethnocultural and language concordance on continuity and quality of care: a cross-sectional analysis. CMAJ open 2018;6(3):E276–84.

23. Jetty A, Jabbarpour Y, Pollack J, et al. Patient-physician racial concordance associated with improved healthcare use and lower healthcare expenditures in minority populations. Journal of racial and ethnic health disparities 2022; 9(1):68–81.

24. Tajfel H. The social psychology of intergroup relations. Annu Rev Psychol 1982; 33(1):1–39.

25. Anderson SR, Gianola M, Perry JM, et al. Clinician-patient racial/ethnic concordance influences racial/ethnic minority pain: evidence from simulated clinical interactions. Pain Med 2020;21(11):3109–25.

26. Doescher MP, Saver BG, Franks P, et al. Racial and ethnic disparities in perceptions of physician style and trust. Arch Fam Med 2000;9(10):1156–63.

27. Zapata C, Poore T, O'Riordan D, et al. Hispanic/latinx and Spanish language concordance among palliative care clinicians and patients in hospital settings in California. Am J Hosp Palliat Care 2023. 10499091231171337.

28. Association of American Medical Colleges. Underrepresented in medicine definition. 2004. Available at: https://www.aamc.org/what-we-do/equity-diversity-inclusion/underrepresented-in-medicine. [Accessed 1 November 2023].

29. Nguemeni Tiako MJ, Ray V, South EC. Medical schools as racialized organizations: how race-neutral structures sustain racial inequality in medical education-a narrative review. J Gen Intern Med 2022;37(9):2259–66.

30. Burchard EG, Oh SS, Foreman MG, et al. Moving toward true inclusion of racial/ethnic minorities in federally funded studies. A key step for achieving respiratory health equality in the United States. Am J Respir Crit Care Med 2015;191(5): 514–21.

31. Marrast LM, Zallman L, Woolhandler S, et al. Minority physicians' role in the care of underserved patients: diversifying the physician workforce may be key in addressing health disparities. JAMA Intern Med 2014;174(2):289–91.

32. Association of American Medical Colleges. Physician specialty data report: active physicians by sex and specialty. 2021. Available at: https://www.aamc.org/data-reports/workforce/data/active-physicians-sex-specialty-2021. [Accessed 1 November 2023].

33. Association of American Medical Colleges. Applicants, matriculants, enrollment, graduates, MD-PHD, and residency applicants data. 2019. Available at: https://

www.aamc.org/data-reports/students-residents/report/facts. [Accessed 1 November 2023].

34. Association of American Medical Colleges. Physician specialty data report. 2022. Available at: https://www.aamc.org/data-reports/workforce/report/physician-specialty-data-report. [Accessed 1 November 2023].

35. Tjoeng YL, Myers C, Irving SY, et al. The current state of workforce diversity and inclusion in pediatric critical care. Crit Care Clin 2023;39(2):327–40.

36. Ly DP. Historical trends in the representativeness and incomes of Black physicians, 1900-2018. J Gen Intern Med 2022;37(5):1310–2.

37. Santhosh L, Babik JM. Trends in racial and ethnic diversity in internal medicine subspecialty fellowships from 2006 to 2018. JAMA Netw Open 2020;3(2): e1920482.

38. Sarraju A, Ngo S, Rodriguez F. The leaky pipeline of diverse race and ethnicity representation in academic science and technology training in the United States, 2003-2019. PLoS One 2023;18(4):e0284945.

39. Carr PL, Gunn CM, Kaplan SA, et al. Inadequate progress for women in academic medicine: findings from the National Faculty Study. Journal of Women's Health (2002) 2015;24(3):190–9.

40. van den Besselaar P, Sandström U. Vicious circles of gender bias, lower positions, and lower performance: gender differences in scholarly productivity and impact. PLoS One 2017;12(8):e0183301.

41. Clark J, Horton R. What is the Lancet doing about gender and diversity? Lancet 2019;393(10171):508–10.

42. Mori WS, Gao Y, Linos E, et al. Sexual orientation diversity and specialty choice among graduating allopathic medical students in the United States. JAMA Netw Open 2021;4(9):e2126983.

43. Hemphill FC, Vanneman A. Achievement gaps: how hispanic and white students in public schools perform. In: Mathematics and reading on the national assessment of educational progress (NCES 2011-459). Washington, DC: National Center for Education Statistics, Institute of Education Sciences, U.S. Department of Education; 2011.

44. LoGerfo L, Nichols A, Reardon SF. Achievement gains in elementary and high school. Washington, DC: The Urban Institute; 2006.

45. Reardon SF, Kalogrides D, Shores K. The geography of racial/ethnic test score gaps. Am J Sociol 2019;124(4).

46. Jackson C. What is redlining?. 2021. Available at: https://www.nytimes.com/2021/08/17/realestate/what-is-redlining.html. [Accessed 1 November 2023].

47. Lukes D. and Cleveland C. The Lingering Legacy of Redlining on School Funding, Diversity, and Performance. 2021. (EdWorkingPaper: 21-363). Retrieved from Annenberg Institute at Brown University: work-in-progress publications. https://doi.org/10.26300/qeer-8c25.

48. Grissom JA, Redding C. Discretion and disproportionality:explaining the under-representation of high-achieving students of color in gifted programs. AERA Open 2016;2(1). 2332858415622175.

49. Hung M, Smith WA, Voss MW, et al. Exploring student achievement gaps in school districts across the United States. Educ Urban Soc 2020;52(2):175–93.

50. Morrison E, Cort DA. An analysis of the medical school pipeline: a high school aspirant to applicant and enrollment view. AAMC Analysis in Brief 2014; 14(3):1–2.

51. Hadinger MA. Underrepresented minorities in medical school admissions: a qualitative study. Teach Learn Med 2017;29(1):31–41.

52. Association of American Medical Colleges. An updated look at the economic diversity of U.S. medical students. 2018. Available at: https://www.aamc.org/data-reports/analysis-brief/report/updated-look-economic-diversity-us-medical-students. [Accessed 1 November 2023].

53. Faiz J, Essien UR, Washington DL, et al. Racial and ethnic differences in barriers faced by medical college admission test examinees and their association with medical school application and matriculation. JAMA health forum 2023;4(4): e230498.

54. Girotti JA, Chanatry JA, Clinchot DM, et al. Investigating group differences in examinees' preparation for and performance on the new MCAT exam. Acad Med 2020;95(3):365–74.

55. Grbic D, Jones DJ, Case ST. The role of socioeconomic status in medical school admissions: validation of a socioeconomic indicator for use in medical school admissions. Acad Med 2015;90(7):953–60.

56. Terregino CA, Saguil A, Price-Johnson T, et al. The diversity and success of medical school applicants with scores in the middle third of the MCAT score scale. Acad Med 2020;95(3):344–50.

57. Lehmann LS, Sulmasy LS, Desai S. Hidden curricula, ethics, and professionalism: optimizing clinical learning environments in becoming and being a physician: a position paper of the American college of physicians. Ann Intern Med 2018;168(7):506–8.

58. Jackson PW. Life in Classrooms. New York.: Holt, Rinehart, and Winston; 1968. https://openlibrary.org/books/OL9227181M/Life_in_Classrooms.

59. Campbell KM, Hudson BD, Tumin D. Releasing the net to promote minority faculty success in academic medicine. Journal of racial and ethnic health disparities 2020;7(2):202–6.

60. Perspectives of Change. Harvard medical school. The flexner report. Available at: https://perspectivesofchange.hms.harvard.edu/node/99. [Accessed 1 November 2023].

61. Wright-Mendoza J. The 1910 report that disadvantaged minority doctors. 2019. Available at: https://daily.jstor.org/the-1910-report-that-unintentionally-disadvantaged-minority-doctors/. [Accessed 1 November 2023].

62. Washington H. Apology shines light on racial schism in medicine. 2008. Available at: https://www.nytimes.com/2008/07/29/health/views/29essa.html. [Accessed 26 October 2023].

63. Skorton DJ, Acosta DA. AAMC statement on police brutality and racism in America and their impact on health. Association of American medical colleges website. 2020. Available at: https://www.aamc.org/news-insights/press-releases/aamc-statement-police-brutality-and-racism-america-and-their-impact-health. [Accessed 24 October 2023].

64. Hardeman RR, Przedworski JM, Burke S, et al. Association between perceived medical school diversity climate and change in depressive symptoms among medical students: a report from the medical student change study. J Natl Med Assoc 2016;108(4):225–35.

65. Anderson N, Lett E, Asabor EN, et al. The association of Microaggressions with depressive symptoms and institutional satisfaction among a national cohort of medical students. J Gen Intern Med 2022;37(2):298–307.

66. Nguyen M, Chaudhry SI, Desai MM, et al. Association of sociodemographic characteristics with US medical student attrition. JAMA Intern Med 2022; 182(9):917–24.

67. Santhosh L, Babik JM. Diversity in the pulmonary and critical care medicine pipeline. Trends in gender, race, and ethnicity among applicants and fellows. ATS scholar 2020;1(2):152–60.
68. Venkatesh B, Mehta S, Angus DC, et al. Women in Intensive Care study: a preliminary assessment of international data on female representation in the ICU physician workforce, leadership and academic positions. Crit Care 2018;22(1):211.
69. Mehta S, Burns KEA, Machado FR, et al. Gender parity in critical care medicine. Am J Respir Crit Care Med 2017;196(4):425–9.
70. Vranas KC, Ouyang D, Lin AL, et al. Gender differences in authorship of critical care literature. Am J Respir Crit Care Med 2020;201(7):840–7.
71. Nivet MATV, Butts GC, Strelnick AH, et al. Diversity in Academic Medicine no. 1 case for minority faculty development today. Mt. Sinai J Med 2008;75(6):491–8.
72. Gershengorn HB, Vranas KC, Ouyang D, et al. Influence of the COVID-19 pandemic on author sex and manuscript acceptance rates among pulmonary and critical care journals. Annals of the American Thoracic Society 2023; 20(2):215–25.
73. Mehta S, Ahluwalia N, Heybati K, et al. Diversity of authors of publications from the Canadian critical care Trials group. Crit Care Med 2022;50(4):535–42.
74. Metaxa V. Is this (still) a man's world? Crit Care 2013;17(1):112.
75. Weinacker A, Stapleton RD. Still a man's world, but why? Crit Care 2013; 17(1):113.
76. Morton MJ, Sonnad SS. Women on professional society and journal editorial boards. J Natl Med Assoc 2007;99(7):764–71.
77. Amrein K, Langmann A, Fahrleitner-Pammer A, et al. Women underrepresented on editorial boards of 60 major medical journals. Gend Med 2011;8(6):378–87.
78. Erren TC, Gross JV, Shaw DM, et al. Representation of women as authors, reviewers, editors in chief, and editorial board members at 6 general medical journals in 2010 and 2011. JAMA Intern Med 2014;174(4):633–5.
79. Wehner MR, Nead KT, Linos K, et al. Plenty of moustaches but not enough women: cross sectional study of medical leaders. BMJ 2015;351:h6311.
80. Singer M, Deutschman CS, Seymour CW, et al. The third international consensus definitions for sepsis and septic shock (Sepsis-3). JAMA 2016;315(8):801–10.
81. Brochard L, Abroug F, Brenner M, et al. An official ATS/ERS/ESICM/SCCM/SRLF statement: prevention and management of acute renal failure in the ICU patient: an international consensus conference in intensive care medicine. Am J Respir Crit Care Med 2010;181(10):1128–55.
82. Cecconi M, De Backer D, Antonelli M, et al. Consensus on circulatory shock and hemodynamic monitoring. Task force of the European Society of Intensive Care Medicine. Intensive Care Med 2014;40(12):1795–815.
83. Ranieri VM, Rubenfeld GD, Thompson BT, et al. Acute respiratory distress syndrome: the Berlin Definition. JAMA 2012;307(23):2526–33.
84. Mehta S, Rose L, Cook D, et al. The speaker gender gap at critical care conferences. Crit Care Med 2018;46(6):991–6.
85. Association of American Medical Colleges. The state of women in academic medicine: the pipeline and pathways to leaderhip -aNAfh. Available at: https://www.aamc.org/data-reports/faculty-institutions/report/state-women-academic-medicine. (Accessed 1 November 2023).
86. Jena AB, Khullar D, Ho O, et al. Sex differences in academic rank in US medical schools in 2014. JAMA 2015;314(11):1149–58.

87. Guevara JP, Adanga E, Avakame E, et al. Minority faculty development programs and underrepresented minority faculty representation at US medical schools. JAMA 2013;310(21):2297–304.

88. Association of American Medical Colleges. Faculty roster: U.S. Medical school faculty report 2022. U.S. Medical School Deans by Dean Type and Race/Ethnicity (URiM vs. non-URiM). Available at: https://www.aamc.org/data-reports/faculty-institutions/data/us-medical-school-deans-trends-type-and-race-ethnicity. [Accessed 1 November 2023].

89. Filardo G, da Graca B, Sass DM, et al. Trends and comparison of female first authorship in high impact medical journals: observational study (1994-2014). BMJ 2016;352:i847.

90. Budden AE, Tregenza T, Aarssen LW, et al. Double-blind review favours increased representation of female authors. Trends Ecol Evol 2008;23(1):4–6.

91. Kaatz A, Gutierrez B, Carnes M. Threats to objectivity in peer review: the case of gender. Trends Pharmacol Sci 2014;35(8):371–3.

92. Berg J. Looking inward at gender issues. Science 2017;355(6323):329.

93. LaDonna KA, Ginsburg S, Watling C. "Rising to the level of your incompetence": what physicians' self-assessment of their performance reveals about the imposter syndrome in medicine. Acad Med 2018;93(5):763–8.

94. Tsuei S.H., Lee D., Ho C., et al., Exploring the Construct of Psychological Safety in Medical Education. Acad Med. 2019;94(11S Association of American Medical Colleges Learn Serve Lead: Proceedings of the 58th Annual Research in Medical Education Sessions; Phoenix, AZ, November 8-12, 2019):S28-s35.

95. Russell R. On overcoming imposter syndrome. Acad Med 2017;92(8):1070.

96. Thomson CC, Riekert KA, Bates CK, et al. Addressing gender inequality in our disciplines: report from the association of pulmonary, critical care, and sleep division Chiefs. Annals of the American Thoracic Society 2018;15(12):1382–90.

97. Jagsi R, Griffith KA, Jones RD, et al. Factors associated with success of clinician-researchers receiving career development awards from the national Institutes of health: a longitudinal cohort study. Acad Med 2017;92(10):1429–39.

98. Fan Y, Shepherd LJ, Slavich E, et al. Gender and cultural bias in student evaluations: why representation matters. PLoS One 2019;14(2):e0209749.

99. Moss-Racusin CA, Dovidio JF, Brescoll VL, et al. Science faculty's subtle gender biases favor male students. Proc Natl Acad Sci U S A 2012;109(41):16474–9.

100. Kelly-Blake K, Garrison NA, Fletcher FE, et al. Rationales for expanding minority physician representation in the workforce: a scoping review. Med Educ 2018.

101. Parsons M, Caldwell MT, Alvarez A, et al. Physician pipeline and pathway programs: an evidence-based guide to best practices for diversity, equity, and inclusion from the Council of residency directors in emergency medicine. West J Emerg Med 2022;23(4):514–24.

102. Butts GC, Hurd Y, Palermo AGS, et al. Mount Sinai journal of medicine: a journal of translational and personalized medicine. 2022. Available at: https://onlinelibrary.wiley.com/doi/abs/10.1002/msj.21323. [Accessed 1 November 2023].

103. Metz AM. Medical school outcomes, primary care specialty choice, and practice in medically underserved areas by physician alumni of MEDPREP, a

postbaccalaureate premedical program for underrepresented and disadvantaged students. Teach Learn Med 2017;29(3):351–9.

104. Rumala BB, Cason FD. Recruitment of underrepresented minority students to medical school: minority medical student organizations, an untapped resource. J Natl Med Assoc 2007;99(9):1000–9.

105. Association of American Medical Colleges. Holistic review. Available at: https://www.aamc.org/services/member-capacity-building/holistic-review. [Accessed 1 November 2023].

106. Aibana O, Swails JL, Flores RJ, et al. Bridging the gap: holistic review to increase diversity in graduate medical education. Acad Med 2019;94(8):1137–41.

107. Grabowski CJ. Impact of holistic review on student interview pool diversity. Adv Health Sci Educ : Theor Pract 2018;23(3):487–98.

108. Totenberg N. Supreme Court guts affirmative action, effectively ending race-conscious admissions. 2023. Available at: https://www.npr.org/2023/06/29/1181138066/affirmative-action-supreme-court-decision. [Accessed 1 November 2023].

109. Najibi S, Carney PA, Thayer EK, Deiorio NM. Differences in Coaching Needs Among Underrepresented Minority Medical Students. Fam Med 2019;51(6):516–22.

110. Deiorio NM, Carney PA, Kahl LE, et al. Coaching: a new model for academic and career achievement. Med Educ Online 2016;21(1):33480.

111. Gause S. Personal communication 2023.

112. Bonifacino E, Ufomata EO, Farkas AH, et al. Mentorship of underrepresented physicians and trainees in academic medicine: a systematic review. J Gen Intern Med 2021;36(4):1023–34.

113. Lundine J, Bourgeault IL, Clark J, et al. The gendered system of academic publishing. Lancet 2018;391(10132):1754–6.

114. Berg J. Measuring and managing bias. Science 2017;357(6354):849.

115. Sambunjak D, Straus SE, Marusic A. Mentoring in academic medicine: a systematic review. JAMA 2006;296(9):1103–15.

116. Farkas AH, Bonifacino E, Turner R, et al. Mentorship of women in academic medicine: a systematic review. J Gen Intern Med 2019;34(7):1322–9.

117. Osborn EH, Ernster VL, Martin JB. Women's attitudes toward careers in academic medicine at the University of California, San Francisco. Acad Med 1992;67(1):59–62.

118. DeCastro R, Griffith KA, Ubel PA, et al. Mentoring and the career satisfaction of male and female academic medical faculty. Acad Med: Journal of the Association of American Medical Colleges 2014;89(2):301–11.

119. Idossa D, Velazquez AI, Horiguchi M, et al. Mentorship experiences are not all the same: a survey study of oncology trainees and early-career faculty. JCO oncology practice 2023;19(9):808–18.

120. Travis EL, Doty L, Helitzer DL. Sponsorship: a path to the academic medicine C-suite for women faculty? Acad Med 2013;88(10):1414–7.

121. Hewlett SAPK, Sherbin L, Sumberg K. The sponsor effect: breaking through the last glass ceiling. Boston, Mass: Harvard Business Review; 2011.

122. Bauman MD, Howell LP, Villablanca AC. The women in medicine and health science program: an innovative initiative to support female faculty at the university of California Davis school of medicine. Acad Med 2014;89(11):1462–6.

123. Chesley C, Lee JT, Clancy CB. A framework for commitment to social justice and antiracism in academic medicine. ATS scholar 2021;2(2):159–62.

124. Suber TL, Neptune ER, Lee JS. Inclusion in the pulmonary, critical care, and sleep medicine physician-scientist workforce. Building with intention. ATS scholar 2020; 1(4):353–63.

125. Harold Amos medical faculty development program partners. Available at: https://www.amfdp.org/about/partners. [Accessed 4 December 2023].

126. Plank-Bazinet JL, Bunker Whittington K, Cassidy SK, et al. Programmatic efforts at the national Institutes of health to promote and support the careers of women in biomedical science. Acad Med 2016;91(8):1057–64.

Cultivating Diversity, Equity, and Inclusion in Pulmonary and Critical Care Training: A Path Toward Health Care Excellence

Daniel Colon Hidalgo, MD, MPH[a], Kara Calhoun, MD, MPH[a],
Anna Neumeier, MD[a,b],*

KEYWORDS

- Diversity • Equity • Critical care • Fellowship • Training

KEY POINTS

- Despite growing numbers of applicants to the field of pulmonary and critical care medicine, the rate of matriculation is stagnant; our current workforce does not reflect the patients for whom we care.
- Racial and gender inequities and impacts of bias are experienced by underrepresented in medicine trainees at every stage of the continuum of learning.
- There is value in diversifying the pulmonary and critical care workforce at the physician, patient, and population level as diverse workforces enhance trust, innovation, and improve patient outcomes.
- Expansion of diversity and promotion of equity and inclusion within Pulmonary and Critical Care Medicine must occur across the training continuum and includes bias mitigation strategies as they relate to learner assessment, applicant selection, the learning environment, and faculty recruitment and retention.

INTRODUCTION

Pulmonary and Critical Care Medicine (PCCM) fellowship training has become increasingly competitive with increasing interest and number of applicants to this field. In the setting of this growth, there is heightened awareness that many PCCM training programs and their faculty still do not reflect the diversity of populations they serve.

[a] Division of Pulmonary Sciences and Critical Care Medicine, University of Colorado, 12700 East 19th Avenue, 9C03, Aurora, CO 80045, USA; [b] Denver Health Pulmonary, Critical Care and Sleep Medicine Division, 777 Bannock Street, Denver, CO 80204, USA
* Corresponding author. University of Colorad Division of Pulmonary Sciences and Critical Care Medicine, 12700 E 19th Avenue, 9C03, Aurora, CO 80045.
E-mail address: anna.neumeier@cuanschutz.edu

Crit Care Clin 40 (2024) 789–803
https://doi.org/10.1016/j.ccc.2024.05.009 criticalcare.theclinics.com
0749-0704/24/© 2024 Elsevier Inc. All rights reserved, including those for text and data mining, AI training, and similar technologies.

Moreover, the lack of diversity in PCCM training programs is worsening.[1] As a diverse workforce is an important aspect to address health disparities and minimize bias against patients, implementation of structured programs that expand diversity are needed.[2,3] The lack of diversity in this space negatively impacts our trainees, our practitioners, and our patients. It is imperative that we identify and use sustainable solutions to establish a clear path toward achieving diversity, equity, and inclusion in PCCM.

THE CURRENT STATE OF DIVERSITY AMONG PULMONARY CRITICAL CARE PHYSICIANS TRAINING PROGRAMS

According to US Census Data, the US population continues to become more diverse over time. From 2010 to 2020, the largest race or ethnicity group, non-Hispanic White, decreased by 8.6% and the fastest growing ethnic group, Hispanic or Latino, grew by 23%.[4] **Fig. 1**A shows the 2022 self-identified race and ethnicity US census data. Non-Hispanic White people comprise the majority of the population with 58.9%. However, per 2021 Association of American Medical Colleges (AAMC) active physician data, non-Hispanic White physicians make up 75.8% of active PCCM attending physicians (**Fig. 1**B).[5] In comparison, Hispanic or Latino people comprise 19.1% of the US population but represent only 6.7% of active PCCM physicians. African Americans comprise 13.6% of the general population but only 3.2% of active attending physicians per 2021

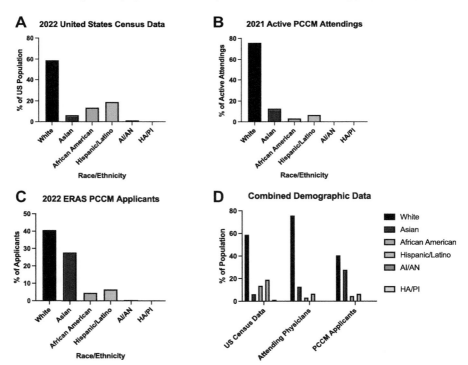

Fig. 1. (A) 2022 US Census data by race or ethnicity. (B) 2021 AAMC Active PCCM attending data by race or ethnicity. (C) 2022 ERAS PCCM applicant data by race or ethnicity. (D) Combined demographic data from US Census, Active PCCM attendings, and ERAS PCCM applicants. AI/AN, American Indian/Alaskan Native; HA/PI, Hawaiian/Pacific Islander. (Figure created using GraphPad Prism 9.)

AAMC data (see **Fig. 1**A, B).[6,7] Overall non-Hispanic White and Asian American physicians are overrepresented in the PCCM subspeciality while African American, Hispanic or Latino, American Indian/Alaska Native, and Hawaiian/Pacific Islander physicians are significantly underrepresented. This trend is also reflected in the 2022 AAMC Electronic Residency Application Service (ERAS) PCCM applicant data. Non-Hispanic White and Asian American residents make up a majority of AAMC ERAS PCCM applicants (**Fig. 1**C).[8] **Fig. 1**D shows all these data combined and visually illustrates that there clearly is a significant mismatch in the representation of our workforce.

Previous studies of application trends over prior decades suggest that a "leaky pipeline" is responsible for underrepresentation in PCCM.[1] However, based on more recent data in the past 3 years, the pipeline has expanded. Yet, this has not resulted in a change in actively practicing PCCM physicians as the number of matriculating PCCM underrepresented in medicine (UIM) applicants remains low, suggesting that UIM applicants are matching at a disproportionately lower rate. Based on 2022 AAMC ERAS self-reported data, non-Hispanic White and Asian American residents make up the majority of PCCM applicants (40.6% and 27.8%, respectively—see **Fig. 1**C).[8] When plotted over time, the number of non-Hispanic White and Asian American applicants appears to have steadily increased over time while all other race or ethnicities have remained relatively stagnant (**Fig. 2**A). However, when plotted as a

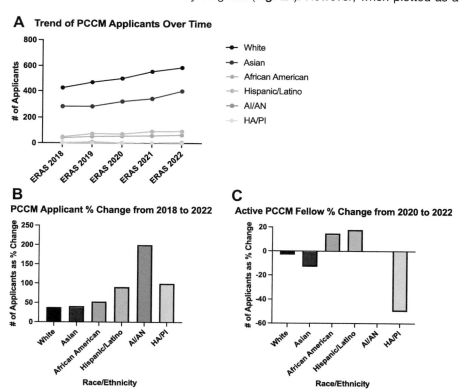

Fig. 2. (*A*) Trend in the number of PCCM applicants by race from 2018 to 2022 according to AAMC ERAS data. (*B*) Percent change in the number of PCCM applicants by race from 2018 to 2022 according to AAMC ERAS data. (*C*) Percent change in the number of active PCCM fellows from 2020 to 2022 based on AAMC data. AI/AN, American Indian/Alaskan Native; HA/PI, Hawaiian/Pacific Islander. (Figure created using GraphPad Prism 9.)

percent change, from 2018 to 2022, African American and Hispanic applicants have increased by 53% and 91%, respectively, compared to a 38% increase in non-Hispanic White and 41% increase in Asian American applicants (**Fig. 2**B). Unfortunately, this increase in applicants is not reflected in the active PCCM fellows' data. The percent change in the number of African American fellows increased by only 15% from 2020 to 2022 and Hispanic or Latino by 18% (**Fig. 2**C) per AAMC data.[9] Additionally, African American residents are applying on average to 53.6 programs per applicant compared to non-Hispanic White residents applying to 40.7 programs per applicant.[9] These data imply that more African American medical residents are applying to PCCM, and to a myriad of programs, but they are not actually matriculating into programs further exacerbating the disparities in our workforce.

Although the total number of PCCM applicants from UIM backgrounds is slowly increasing, the percentage compared to national demographics remains low. This is consistent with prior study demonstrating that absolute numbers of physicians from underrepresented minorities have increased over time yet still do not reflect our overall population.[10] The multifactorial causes arise from the structural inequities that exist in our society. Systemic and structural racism leads to social and financial disadvantages. Acknowledging these disadvantages will inform system design to dismantle inequity and guide meaningful change.

THE LEARNING DISADVANTAGES AND EXPERIENCES OF UNDERREPRESENTED IN MEDICINE TRAINEES

The medical school and graduate training environments perpetuate racial and gender inequities. The impacts of bias are experienced by UIM trainees at every stage of the continuum of learning (**Fig. 3**).[11]

Admission to Medical School

Students from UIM backgrounds face disparities in access to educational resources and are more likely to experience underfunded schools. Costs of entrance examinations, examination preparation materials, and applications are additional barriers. Moreover, these students have more limited access to shadowing experiences and mentorship.[12] Combined, these factors contribute to differential attainment in the ability to apply.

During Medical School

Medical school curricula do not adequately address issues related to health equity and perpetuates bias. The concept of race as a biologic construct, rather than a social construct of health, remains entrenched not only within curricula but also embedded

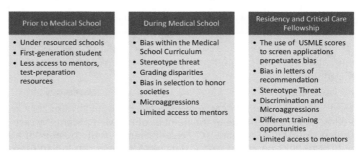

Fig. 3. Disadvantages experienced by UIM trainees across the continuum of training.

in diagnosis and clinical management practices across specialties.[13] Learners experience racialized stereotypes perpetuated through curricular and standardized testing preparation materials.[14] Without curricula about race and racism in medical school, UIM learners are relied upon to teach concepts related to race through their personal experiences.[15] From these such experiences, UIM learners experience social isolation, othering, and stereotype threat.[16]

Research shows grading disparities during medical school that favor White students.[17] Compared with non-UIM, underrepresented in medicine students receive slightly lower clerkship director ratings that subsequently lead to fewer honors grades; these sequential differences in assessments create inequities in future awards that impacts downstream opportunities.[18] Analysis of written evaluations of medical students has demonstrated that words describing competence and knowledge are used more commonly when describing men and non-UIM learners whereas women and UIM learners are described with more muted language related to effort or collaboration.[19] With differential clinical assessments, it has been demonstrated that students with marginalized identities were less likely than peers to be selected to the honor society Alpha Omega Alpha.[20]

Residency and Fellowship Selection

The cascade of inequity resultant from bias in clinical assessments is further amplified by an inappropriate reliance on the United States Medical Licensing Exam (USMLE) for residency and fellowship selection decisions. This examination, designed to assess competency decisions for licensing, does not meet validity criteria to use for postgraduate applicant selection.[21] Performance on the USMLE, while it may correlate with future written examinations, does not predict residency performance competencies or success in practice.[22–24] Furthermore, when scores are used as a screening tool for postgraduate interview invitations, UIM applicants are precluded from being considered for positions.[25] Despite this, threshold scores are used by nearly half of program directors in PCCM to make decisions in who to interview and rank.[26]

Beyond bias in grading and selection to honors societies, research shows that biases in letters of recommendation (LORs) disproportionately affect women and UIM applicants.[27] LORs for men and white candidates are often longer and use different adjectives as compared to letters for women and UIM candidates. Agentic language, descriptions of accomplishments and agency, is more often used for White and male candidates than UIM and female candidates.[28,29] Doubt-raising language and faint praise are more often present in LORs for women and UIM candidates.[29]

Learning Environment Experiences Across the Continuum of Training

The social and learning environments experienced by UIM students and women negatively impact their learning. From matriculation through postgraduate training, women and UIM trainees experience explicit and implicit messages in how they differ from the traditional image of the White male physician. UIM medical students experience less supportive learning environments, discrimination, and microaggressions.[30] Minority students are more likely to assess their race or ethnicity as adversely affecting their medical school training due to experiences of prejudice, feelings of isolation and different cultural expectations. Students with these experiences are more likely to suffer burnout, depressive symptoms, and low mental quality of life scores.[31] In a qualitative study of resident physician's experience of race and ethnicity in the workplace, participants described experiencing a daily barrage of microaggressions, being tasked to serve as race ambassadors and perform and lead diversity efforts, as well as having feelings of social isolation and limited professional mentorship.[32] These exclusions and tokenism contribute to racial trauma experienced.[12]

During residency, gender impacts training opportunities. Gender disparities exist in procedural training with internal medicine women trainees having fewer opportunities to perform intensive care unit procedures and women surgical residents receiving less autonomy within the operative room.[33,34] As women are underrepresented in surgery and subspecialty medicine procedural fields, particularly in PCCM, these differential procedural experiences, whether resultant from bias or stereotype threat, may have downstream impacts on diversity.

THE IMPORTANCE OF EXPANDING DIVERSITY AND ENHANCING EQUITY WITHIN PULMONARY AND CRITICAL CARE

There is value in diversifying the PCCM workforce at the physician, patient, and population levels. Diversity, inclusion, and representation matter to us as individuals, to our patients, and to our society (**Fig. 4**).[35] Diversity among PCCM physicians matters to the patients we serve. Racial concordance between patients and physicians can improve satisfaction, communication, and trust. Patients cared for by physicians who share their race have higher satisfaction.[36] Black patients, when undergoing lung cancer screening, perceive a more accurate risk assessment when advised by a race concordant physician.[37] Patients are more likely to adhere to medication guidelines when they are treated by a clinician of the same race.[38] At the interpersonal level, shared characteristics and shared experiences promote connection and enhance trust and patients' care experiences.

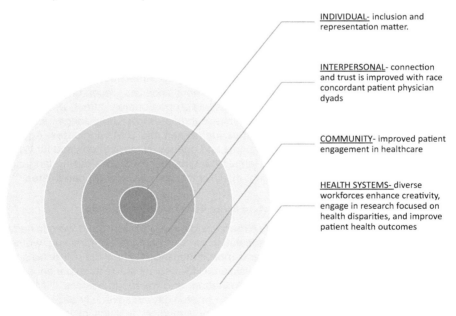

INDIVIDUAL- inclusion and representation matter.

INTERPERSONAL- connection and trust is improved with race concordant patient physician dyads

COMMUNITY- improved patient engagement in healthcare

HEALTH SYSTEMS- diverse workforces enhance creativity, engage in research focused on health disparities, and improve patient health outcomes

Fig. 4. The impacts and importance of expanding diversity within PCCM conceptualized through the socioecological framework. (*From* McLeroy KR, Bibeau D, Steckler A, Glanz K. An ecological perspective on health promotion programs. Health Educ Q. 1988 Winter;15(4):351-77. https://doi.org/10.1177/109019818801500401. PMID: 3068205.)

At the health systems level, a diversified workforce ensures distinct perspectives to innovate and thus paramount to addressing health disparities. UIM physicians are more likely to care for underserved patients from minority backgrounds.[2] UIM faculty are more likely to engage in research focused on health disparities.[39] At a population level, higher Black primary care physician representation levels have been associated with lower all-cause mortality rates among Black individuals.[40] Diverse workforces enhance creativity, increase performance, boost productivity, and improve health outcomes.[41,42] Respiratory health disparities arise from unequal exposure to environmental risk resultant from structural inequities and are aggravated by lack of access to health care, and lack of research in minority populations.[43,44] Therefore, increasing the racial and ethnic diversity within PCCM can address health inequities at multiple levels. Diversity in PCCM is not just a matter of social justice; it has direct implications for patient care, health care outcomes, innovation, and the overall quality of the health care system.

CURRENT THREATS TO EXPANDING DIVERSITY IN PULMONARY AND CRITICAL CARE MEDICINE AND EFFECTIVE STRATEGIES TO ACHIEVE EQUITY AND INCLUSION
Lack of Data and the Need for Reporting Metrics to Track Outcomes

A significant threat to advance diversity, equity, and inclusion (DEI) initiatives within PCCM training programs is the paucity of comprehensive data to inform progress and guide interventions. Existing demographic data pertaining to the number of active pulmonary and critical care physicians and fellowship application and matriculation statistics provide a cursory overview. While these data allow inferences concerning the state of practitioners and prospective fellows, they fall short in providing nuanced insights into academic-affiliated PCCM physicians, the physicians who influence the training of UIM trainees (**Table 1**).

Creating institutional structures and data-reporting measures that promote equity in compensation detail gender and racial distributions as they relate to academic rank, leadership roles, and committee membership are described strategic and effective practices.[45] To increase diversity of fellows and academic PCCM faculty, it is paramount to first gain a thorough understanding of the existing landscape of academic pulmonary faculty. In addition to implementation of transparent data metrics at training centers, opportunities exist to harness data related to gender and racial demographic composition within national PCCM societies; an important step toward equity would begin with an assessment of the current member demographics with the goal to track impacts of changes over time. Transparency and outcomes data would not only serve to evaluate the current environment in which UIM fellows are undergoing training but also would facilitate the establishment of programmatic objectives aimed at diversifying pulmonary and critical care training.

Insufficient Mentorship and Imperative Support for Mentoring

The importance of mentorship for career development is recognized within academic medicine, but UIM trainees often face challenges finding representation within their areas of training. Mentorship can deeply and positively impact a student's choice of residency and career goals.[46] UIM mentors, given their similar background, share similar experiences with UIM students and trainees.[47] This shared background enables UIM mentors to provide guidance that non-UIM mentors might lack, fostering a more relatable and tailored mentorship relationship.[47] Consequently, the low representation of minoritized faculty members in academic PCCM has significant effect of UIM fellows.

Table 1
Threats to expanding diversity in pulmonary and critical care medicine and effective strategies to achieve equity and inclusion

Threats to Diversity	Inclusive and Equitable Practices
• Lack of actionable data to guide and assess diversity efforts	• Transparent data summarizing compensation, academic rank, leadership positions stratified by gender and race
• Limited access to UIM mentors and sponsors	• Visibility of diverse faculty and trainees • Recognition and compensation for diversity work and mentorship • Pathway programs

• Exclusionary recruitment practices
  ○ Meritocracy
  ○ Use of USMLE scores as screening
  ○ Bias in LORs
	• Inclusive and equitable recruitment practices
	  ○ Recognition of differential attainment
	  ○ Bias training
	  ○ Holistic review
	  ○ Standard templates for LORs
	  ○ Behavioral-based and standardized interview questions
	  ○ Implicit Bias Training

• Structural barriers, institutional bias, and inertia	• Evolving to academic climate to promote equity redefining value and devoting resources to DEI work
	  ○ Mitigating bias in the learning environment through diversity training
	  ○ Retention efforts, equitable compensation for UIM fellows and faculty

• Legal and policy constraints: The end of affirmative action	• Multifaceted processes to support institutional missions to enhance diversity, equity and inclusion

To develop UIM mentors requires recognition of their unique barriers experienced. In addition to their scarcity, UIM faculty also face a set of challenges that are not universally experienced by their counterparts. Moreover, they suffer from micro/macroaggressions, unconscious bias, and racism from their peers.[48] In addition, minority faculty are frequently expected to take a disproportionate responsibility of activities that are not viewed as "career-advancing" such as mentoring minority students or trainees, community outreach, and participation within service committees. Collectively, these activities are uncompensated and without similar academic merit levels and hence, collectively known as the "minority tax."[48] Moreover, UIM faculty disproportionately treat patients of lower socioeconomic status with greater social complexity that takes more time and generate less revenue for their organizations facing added pressure from their employers.[49] These challenges unique to UIM faculty necessitate unique support. Collectively, this evidence summarizes the need for restructuring mentorship relationships, ensuring equitable support and recognition of UIM faculty work with strategies to compensate financially or with the provision of protected time.

Exclusionary Recruitment Practices and the Requisite to Prioritize Equity over Meritocracy

The exclusionary nature of the current screening, interviewing, and broader recruitment practices in PCCM widen prevalent disparities to marginalized groups. From the previously stated use of USMLE scores, and medical school grades to biases in LORs, and honor society induction, commonly used metrics fall short in ensuring equity.[50,51] These practices are perpetuated by institutional inertia as many leaders of academic departments belong to dominant groups that fail to recognize the shortcoming of traditional screening methods. Within the academic environment, there is a recurring failure and reliance on meritocracy without acknowledging differential opportunity or considering differential attainment, the assessment of one's "distance traveled" and the acknowledgment of intergenerational mobility.

Historically, meritocracy refers to the assignment of an individual's roles and/or responsibilities based on "objective" evaluations such as tests and grades[52] with the accompanying shortsighted belief that the process of diversifying medicine is a threat to meritocracy. Razack and colleagues posit that "medical practice today requires a reformulation of the notion of merit in medicine."[53] A more sophisticated and accurate approach would be to include a consideration of differential attainment—the unequal outcomes in educational performances among members of different societal groups. The ability to understand and address differential attainment based on opportunities provided is key to achieving equity within educational systems. Markers of resilience, grit and determination, such intergenerational mobility and "distance traveled" are overlooked by traditional screening methods.

Therefore, a shift in the recruitment process is needed. As previously emphasized, conventional metrics such as standardized test scores, research publications and LORs fail to acknowledge the unique disadvantages that UIM applicants face. Factors like lower family income, lower availability of UIM mentors, racism, and other exclusionary practice significantly impact these metrics for UIM applicants.[12] Standardized testing should not be used as a screening metric and, instead, be used for its intended role, to ascertain competency. Consideration should be made to use standardized LORs accompanied by bias training as racial bias in emergency medicine residency applications standardized letters has been described.[54] One previously proposed solution includes holistic review of applications. Holistic review of medical school applications balances an individual's academic performance and achievements with their individual experiences.[55] At the residency level, holistic review has been demonstrated to improve recruitment of UIM applicants.[56] Recently, a single institution study evaluated the implementation of holistic reviews for a PCCM program demonstrating that the implementations were feasible and well received by both fellows and faculty.[57] Moreover, alternative interview methodologies have been studied in PCCM fellowships. Behavioral-based interviewing, a technique in which the job candidate demonstrates their potential for success by providing specific examples of how they handled similar situations in their past experiences, can be practically incorporated within the fellowship recruitment process.[58] Other recommended interventions include the use of standardized questions and interviewer training.[59,60] Using standardized questions aims at reducing gender and racial bias as it utilizes open-ended questions that evaluate the applicant's thought process.[60] Furthermore, unconscious bias training for candidate interviewers is effective as implicit biases can hinder an applicant's success. Implicit racial bias training when used in medical school admissions has been associated with improved diversity among matriculating classes and has been effectively operationalized for graduate medical education.[61,62]

The Academic Climate, Necessary Culture Shifts, and Retention Efforts

It is important to recognize that while bias training is important, there are limitations in its capacity to address organizational biases.[63] In part, this is due to the institutional inertia that exists within academics resultant from homogenous leadership, ingrained biases, and resistance to change. The establishment of a divisional culture that prioritizes diversity is pivotal and requires a cultural shift. "Buy-in" from division heads, senior faculty members, and other staff to challenge traditional recruitment practices is necessary and allocate resources toward implementation of inclusive practices to lead to significant change.

Another shift needed to increase diversity in PCCM is to ensure a safe training environment. It has been previously demonstrated that UIM trainees suffer disproportionately from microaggressions and racism, which have been associated with poorer mental health.[32] UIM trainees often receive disproportionally lower evaluations when compared to their peers. It is not uncommon for UIM trainees to be heavily sought out just to join a training program that is unsafe and perpetuates trauma. Divisions and associated fellowship programs must ensure the proper environment that allows for UIM fellows to thrive. Recommended practices to mitigate bias in the learning environments include periodic diversity needs assessments, diversity training to include identification and mitigation of implicit bias, reporting systems for microaggressions and acts of bias, provision of speakers from diverse backgrounds and the development of programs and activities that highlight different backgrounds to foster inclusivity.[26]

Finally, attention must be devoted to the transition from fellow to faculty as it represents the final step along the training path. Early faculty years bring additional challenges to UIM faculty, one of them being professional isolation. It is imperative that Divisions and Departments offer mentorship to young UIM faculty as to ensure that they have necessary guidance and resources to navigate the intricacies of the promotion process. It is crucial to recognize and compensate UIM faculty's role in mentoring and recruiting other UIM trainees and faculty. This work to foster diversity may require a diversion of time and effort from research productivity or other activities traditionally viewed more favorably in the promotion process. Institutions committed to diversity should redefine academic success to recognize UIM faculty's meaningful contributions for their advancement.

Legal and Policy Constraints, a New Threat

On June 29, 2023, the Supreme Court of the United States (SCOTUS) ruled against affirmative action admission policies in the Students for Fair Admission, Inc (SFFA) v President & Fellows of Harvard College and SFFA v University of North Carolina (UNC) cases. Though the ruling did not completely disallow universities from considering race, as universities can still take race into account if an applicant describes how race has affected their life, it signifies a major shift and change in the landscape for college admissions. Many have pondered the ramifications of this judicial decision on the demographics of students entering colleges and medical schools. It is more than plausible that this ruling will result in a lower proportion of Black, Latinx, and Indigenous students matriculating into colleges and medical schools mirroring what happened in California when affirmative action ended in California's public colleges. In 1996, the affirmative action ban for public universities in California led to a significant drop in diversity, known as Proposition 209.[64] Following its implementation, there was a significant drop in the diversity of matriculants of public universities in California. Prior to the passing of Proposition 209, the demographics of universities such as University of California Los Angeles (UCLA) and UC Berkeley were similar to the demographics of the graduating classes. By 1998, the enrollment of Black and Latinx students had dropped by 40%. The "California case" serves as a cautionary tale that highlights the potential impact of the SCOTUS ruling. It is imperative, if equity is desired, that admissions leadership are proactive in finding innovative ways to preserve and improve current diversifying strategies and academic leaders maintain strategic plans, policies, processes, and practices to diversity efforts in the face of a new legal landscape.

SUMMARY

Although workforce diversity within PCCM has been recognized as critical to reduce and eliminate health disparities, the composition of our workforce has not changed. This is not due to lack of evidence-based practices to expand diversity but instead from insufficient implementation. The growing proportion of diverse applicants that are not matriculating into critical care fellowships indicates the pipeline is not leaking but rather obstructed. Causes of this obstruction include bias across the continuum of training impacting access to mentors, grading, letters of reference, and selection by training programs. In a recent article, authors Lahia Yemane and Emma Omoruyi state, "We must acknowledge that medicine perpetuates the myth of inherent scarcity of qualified UIM applicants rather than identify and address the structures of their exclusion. We should not be pathologizing race but rather the systems and structures that perpetuate racism."[65] It is through systems and structural change to address and mitigate bias that exists across the continuum of learning that we will provide a path toward health care excellence.

CLINICS CARE POINTS

- Implicit and explicit biases within medical education affects the selection of diverse candidates within PCCM. These biases not only impact grading and clinical evaluations, selection to honor societies, LORs, and interview offers but negatively impact their learning environments.

- Effective strategies to mitigate biases must be implemented systematically at both the undergraduate and graduate medical education levels and include inclusive and equitable practices related to both recruitment and retention.

- Inclusive recruitment practices to expand diversity within PCCM include holistic review, recognition of differential attainment, use of standardized templates for LORs, and interview questions and bias training.

- Inclusive practices to retain trainees from diverse backgrounds include deliberate attention to UIM mentorship through recognition and compensation for diversity work and service efforts as well as work to foster an equitable and inclusive academic learning environment.

DISCLOSURE

The authors have nothing to disclose.

REFERENCES

1. Santhosh L, Babik JM. Diversity in the pulmonary and critical care medicine pipeline. Trends in gender, race, and ethnicity among applicants and fellows. ATS Sch 2020;1(2):152–60.
2. Marrast LM, Zallman L, Woolhandler S, et al. Minority physicians' role in the care of underserved patients: diversifying the physician workforce may be key in addressing health disparities. JAMA Intern Med 2014;174(2):289–91.
3. Saha S, Arbelaez JJ, Cooper LA. Patient-physician relationships and racial disparities in the quality of health care. Am J Publ Health 2003;93(10):1713–9.

4. Bureau USC. Census illuminates racial and ethnic composition of the country. 2021. 2020. Available at: https://www.census.gov/library/stories/2021/08/improved-race-ethnicity-measures-reveal-united-states-population-much-more-multiracial.html. [Accessed 30 October 2023].

5. Colleges AoAM. Active physicians who identified as White. 2021. Available at: https://www.aamc.org/data-reports/workforce/data/active-physicians-white-2021. [Accessed 30 October 2023].

6. Colleges AoAM. Active physicians who identified as hispanic (alone or with any race). 2021. Available at: https://www.aamc.org/data-reports/workforce/data/active-physicians-hispanic-alone-or-any-race-2021. [Accessed 30 October 2023].

7. Colleges AoAM. Active physicians who identified as Black or African-American. 2021. Available at: https://www.aamc.org/data-reports/workforce/data/active-physicians-black-african-american-2021. [Accessed 30 October 2023].

8. Colleges AoAM. Historical specialty specific data. 2022. Available at: https://www.aamc.org/data-reports/data/eras-statistics-data. [Accessed 30 October 2023].

9. Colleges AoAM. Number of active MD residents, by race/ethnicity (alone or in combination) and GME specialty. 2022. Available at: https://www.aamc.org/data-reports/students-residents/data/report-residents/2022/table-b5-md-residents-race-ethnicity-and-specialty. [Accessed 30 October 2023].

10. Lett E, Murdock HM, Orji WU, et al. Trends in racial/ethnic representation among US Medical Students. JAMA Netw Open 2019;2(9):e1910490.

11. Solomon SR, Atalay AJ, Osman NY. Diversity is not enough: advancing a framework for antiracism in medical education. Acad Med 2021;96(11):1513–7.

12. Colon Hidalgo D, McElroy I. Racial trauma perpetuated by academic medicine to those in its ranks. Ann Am Thorac Soc 2021;18(11):1773–5.

13. Vyas DA, Eisenstein LG, Jones DS. Hidden in plain sight - reconsidering the use of race correction in clinical algorithms. N Engl J Med 2020;383(9):874–82.

14. Krishnan A, Rabinowitz M, Ziminsky A, et al. Addressing race, culture, and structural inequality in medical education: a guide for revising teaching cases. Acad Med 2019;94(4):550–5.

15. Olsen LD. The conscripted curriculum and the reproduction of racial inequalities in contemporary U.S. medical education. J Health Soc Behav 2019;60(1):55–68.

16. Bullock JL, Lockspeiser T, Del Pino-Jones A, et al. They don't see a lot of people my color: a mixed methods study of racial/ethnic stereotype threat among medical students on core clerkships. Acad Med 2020. S58–s66, 95(11S Association of American Medical Colleges Learn Serve Lead: Proceedings of the 59th Annual Research in Medical Education Presentations).

17. Low D, Pollack SW, Liao ZC, et al. Racial/ethnic disparities in clinical grading in medical school. Teach Learn Med 2019;31(5):487–96.

18. Teherani A, Hauer KE, Fernandez A, et al. How small differences in assessed clinical performance amplify to large differences in grades and awards: a cascade with serious consequences for students underrepresented in medicine. Acad Med 2018;93(9):1286–92.

19. Rojek AE, Khanna R, Yim JWL, et al. Differences in narrative language in evaluations of medical students by gender and under-represented minority status. J Gen Intern Med 2019;34(5):684–91.

20. Hill KA, Desai MM, Chaudhry SI, et al. Association of marginalized identities with alpha omega alpha honor society and gold humanism honor society membership among medical students. JAMA Netw Open 2022;5(9):e2229062.

21. McGaghie WC, Cohen ER, Wayne DB. Are United States Medical Licensing Exam Step 1 and 2 scores valid measures for postgraduate medical residency selection decisions? Acad Med 2011;86(1):48–52.
22. Stohl HE, Hueppchen NA, Bienstock JL. Can medical school performance predict residency performance? Resident selection and predictors of successful performance in obstetrics and gynecology. J Grad Med Educ 2010;2(3):322–6.
23. Sutton E, Richardson JD, Ziegler C, et al. Is USMLE Step 1 score a valid predictor of success in surgical residency? Am J Surg 2014;208(6):1029–34 [discussion 1034].
24. Shirkhodaie C, Avila S, Seidel H, et al. The association between USMLE step 2 clinical knowledge scores and residency performance: a systematic review and meta-analysis. Acad Med 2023;98(2):264–73.
25. Gardner AK, Cavanaugh KJ, Willis RE, et al. Can better selection tools help us achieve our diversity goals in postgraduate medical education? comparing use of USMLE Step 1 scores and situational judgment tests at 7 surgical residencies. Acad Med 2020;95(5):751–7.
26. Tatem GB, Gardner-Gray J, Standifer B, et al. While you don't see color, I see bias: identifying barriers in access to graduate medical education training. ATS Sch 2021;2(4):544–55.
27. Machen JL, Gandhi SM, Moreland CJ, Salib S. Promoting equity in letters of recommendation: recognizing and overcoming bias. Am J Med 2023;136(12): 1216–21.
28. Madera JM, Hebl MR, Martin RC. Gender and letters of recommendation for academia: agentic and communal differences. J Appl Psychol 2009;94(6): 1591–9.
29. Zhang N, Blissett S, Anderson D, et al. Race and gender bias in internal medicine program director letters of recommendation. J Grad Med Educ 2021;13(3): 335–44.
30. Orom H, Semalulu T, Underwood W 3rd. The social and learning environments experienced by underrepresented minority medical students: a narrative review. Acad Med 2013;88(11):1765–77.
31. Dyrbye LN, Thomas MR, Eacker A, et al. Race, ethnicity, and medical student well-being in the United States. Arch Intern Med 2007;167(19):2103–9.
32. Osseo-Asare A, Balasuriya L, Huot SJ, et al. Minority resident physicians' views on the role of race/ethnicity in their training experiences in the workplace. JAMA Netw Open 2018;1(5):e182723.
33. Olson EM, Sanborn DM, Dyster TG, et al. Gender disparities in critical care procedure training of internal medicine residents. ATS Sch 2023;4(2):164–76.
34. Meyerson SL, Sternbach JM, Zwischenberger JB, et al. The effect of gender on resident autonomy in the operating room. J Surg Educ 2017;74(6):e111–8.
35. McLeroy KR, Bibeau D, Steckler A, et al. An ecological perspective on health promotion programs. Health Educ Q 1988;15(4):351–77.
36. Takeshita J, Wang S, Loren AW, et al. Association of racial/ethnic and gender concordance between patients and physicians with patient experience ratings. JAMA Netw Open 2020;3(11):e2024583.
37. Persky S, Kaphingst KA, Allen VC, et al. Effects of patient-provider race concordance and smoking status on lung cancer risk perception accuracy among African-Americans. Ann Behav Med 2013;45(3):308–17.
38. Nguyen AM, Siman N, Barry M, et al. Patient-physician race/ethnicity concordance improves adherence to cardiovascular disease guidelines. Health Serv Res 2020;55(Suppl 1):51.

39. Pololi LH, Evans AT, Gibbs BK, et al. The experience of minority faculty who are underrepresented in medicine, at 26 representative U.S. medical schools. Acad Med 2013;88(9):1308–14.
40. Snyder JE, Upton RD, Hassett TC, et al. Black representation in the primary care physician workforce and its association with population life expectancy and mortality rates in the US. JAMA Netw Open 2023;6(4):e236687.
41. Resar LM, Jaffee EM, Armanios M, et al. Equity and diversity in academic medicine: a perspective from the JCI editors. J Clin Invest 2019;129(10):3974–7.
42. Gomez LE, Bernet P. Diversity improves performance and outcomes. J Natl Med Assoc 2019;111(4):383–92.
43. Celedón JC. Building a diverse workforce in pulmonary, critical care, and sleep medicine. ATS Sch 2021;2(2):145–8.
44. Burchard EG, Oh SS, Foreman MG, et al. Moving toward true inclusion of racial/ethnic minorities in federally funded studies. A key step for achieving respiratory health equality in the United States. Am J Respir Crit Care Med 2015;191(5):514–21.
45. Pino-Jones AD, Cervantes L, Flores S, et al. Advancing diversity, equity, and inclusion in hospital medicine. J Hosp Med 2021;16(4):198–203.
46. Bhatnagar V, Diaz S, Bucur PA. The need for more mentorship in medical school. Cureus 2020;12(5):e7984.
47. Bonifacino E, Ufomata EO, Farkas AH, et al. Mentorship of underrepresented physicians and trainees in academic medicine: a systematic review. J Gen Intern Med 2021;36(4):1023–34.
48. Rodríguez JE, Campbell KM, Pololi LH. Addressing disparities in academic medicine: what of the minority tax? BMC Med Educ 2015;15:6.
49. Richert A, Campbell K, Rodríguez J, et al. ACU workforce column: expanding and supporting the health care workforce. J Health Care Poor Underserved 2013;24(4):1423–31.
50. Pope AJ, Carter K, Ahn J. A renewed call for a more equitable and holistic review of residency applications in the era of COVID-19. AEM Educ Train 2021;5(1):135–8.
51. Ross DA, Boatright D, Nunez-Smith M, et al. Differences in words used to describe racial and gender groups in Medical Student Performance Evaluations. PLoS One 2017;12(8):e0181659.
52. Polastri M, Truisi MC. Meritocracy? Ask yourself. J Intensive Care Soc 2017;18(4):276–8.
53. Razack S, Risør T, Hodges B, et al. Beyond the cultural myth of medical meritocracy. Med Educ 2020;54(1):46–53.
54. Kukulski P, Schwartz A, Hirshfield LE, et al. Racial bias on the emergency medicine standardized letter of evaluation. J Grad Med Educ 2022;14(5):542–8.
55. Grbic D, Morrison E, Sondheimer HM, et al. The association between a holistic review in admissions workshop and the diversity of accepted applicants and students matriculating to medical school. Acad Med 2019;94(3):396–403.
56. Sungar WG, Angerhofer C, McCormick T, et al. Implementation of holistic review into emergency medicine residency application screening to improve recruitment of underrepresented in medicine applicants. AEM Educ Train 2021;5(Suppl 1):S10–s18.
57. Bailey J, Desai B, Wang A, et al. Implementing holistic review practices in a pulmonary and critical care fellowship. ATS Scholar 2023;4(4). ats-scholar. 2022-0108IN.

58. Tatem G, Kokas M, Smith CL, et al. A feasibility assessment of behavioral-based interviewing to improve candidate selection for a pulmonary and critical care medicine fellowship program. Ann Am Thorac Soc 2017;14(4):576–83.
59. Bergelson I, Tracy C, Takacs E. Best practices for reducing bias in the interview process. Curr Urol Rep 2022;23(11):319–25.
60. Dao AT, Garcia MM, Correa R, et al. AAIM recommendations to promote equity and inclusion in the internal medicine residency interview process. Am J Med 2022;135(12):1509–16.e1.
61. Capers Qt. How clinicians and educators can mitigate implicit bias in patient care and candidate selection in medical education. ATS Sch 2020;1(3):211–7.
62. Capers Qt, Clinchot D, McDougle L, et al. Implicit racial bias in medical school admissions. Acad Med 2017;92(3):365–9.
63. National Institutes of Health (US), Office of the Director (OD), Chief Officer for Scientific Workforce Diversity (COSWD). Is Implicit Bias Training Effective? [Internet] National Institutes of Health (NIH); Bethesda, MD, Available a:t https://www.ncbi.nlm.nih.gov/books/NBK603840/. 2021.
64. California Uo. Research and analyses on the impact of proposition 209 in California. 2023. Available at: https://www.ucop.edu/academic-affairs/prop-209/index.html.
65. Yemane L, Omoruyi E. Underrepresented in medicine in graduate medical education: historical trends, bias, and recruitment practices. Curr Probl Pediatr Adolesc Health Care 2021;51(10):101088.

Social Disparities and Critical Illness during the Coronavirus Disease 2019 Pandemic: A Narrative Review

Yhenneko J. Taylor, PhD[a],*, Marc Kowalkowski, PhD[b],
Jessica Palakshappa, MD, MSc[c]

KEYWORDS

- COVID-19 • Social determinants of health • Critical illness • Health disparities
- Patient journey

KEY POINTS

- Structural and social determinants of health influence COVID-19 outcomes at multiple points along the patient journey prior to, during and following hospitalization with critical illness.
- Prior to hospitalization, structural factors contribute to disparities in vaccination rates, access to COVID-19 testing and preventive care, rates of pre-existing chronic conditions and healthcare and other resources at the neighborhood level.
- During hospitalization, structural factors contribute to racial and ethnic differences in clinical presentation, access to treatment and supportive therapies as well as hospital capacity and resource strain.
- Following hospitalization, inequitable access to long term care, skilled nursing and culturally appropriate post-discharge resources contribute to worse outcomes for persons from racial and ethnic minority groups.
- Strategies addressing systemic factors including the distribution of healthcare resources, and standardized care pathways that prioritize equity, shared decision-making are promising approaches for advancing equitable outcomes beyond the COVID-19 pandemic.

[a] Center for Health System Sciences, Atrium Health, 1300 Scott Avenue, Charlotte, NC 28204, USA; [b] Department of Internal Medicine, Center for Health System Sciences, Wake Forest University School of Medicine, 1300 Scott Avenue, Charlotte, NC 28204, USA; [c] Department of Internal Medicine, Wake Forest University School of Medicine, 2 Watlington Hall, 1 Medical Center Boulevard, Winston-Salem, NC 27157, USA
* Corresponding author.
E-mail address: yhenneko.taylor@atriumhealth.org

Crit Care Clin 40 (2024) 805–825
https://doi.org/10.1016/j.ccc.2024.05.010
0749-0704/24/© 2024 Elsevier Inc. All rights are reserved, including those for text and data mining, AI training, and similar technologies.

criticalcare.theclinics.com

INTRODUCTION

When the coronavirus disease 2019 (COVID-19) global health emergency ended on May 5, 2023, over 765 million confirmed cases had been reported globally and nearly 7 million deaths.[1] The 3 year long pandemic devastated families and communities worldwide with significant social and economic consequences. From the earliest reports, inequalities in the impact of the pandemic were clear. Historically marginalized racial/ethnic groups, individuals working in low-wage jobs and with low socioeconomic status, and persons living in crowded housing were getting infected and dying at higher rates than others. In the United States, individuals identifying as Black, Hispanic/Latino, or Native American were getting infected, needing hospitalization, and dying at rates 2 to 4 times higher than the general population.[2] These same groups were overrepresented among bus drivers, grocery store clerks, farmworkers, and other "essential worker" occupations that were required to report to work in person and did not have the option of staying at home to avoid infection.[3] For health equity scholars, these outcomes were inevitable.[4–6] Years of research have described how social and economic factors including structural racism influence health and health care by influencing opportunities for health, like jobs and living conditions, as well as the ability to receive health care and the quality and outcomes of care. Failure to correct these underlying systems and address observed inequities left communities vulnerable to poor outcomes.

The factors contributing to social disparities in COVID-19 outcomes are not new to critical care. Reviews of the critical care literature prior to the pandemic indicate that racial/ethnic, socioeconomic, and sex disparities exist throughout the course of critical illness, with more data on racial/ethnic disparities and specifically differences between Black persons and White persons than other groups.[7–10] For example, incidence of respiratory failure is higher for Black persons, and both incidence and mortality are higher for those with low socioeconomic status and those with male sex.[10] Higher mortality has also been reported among Black persons for sepsis and in-hospital cardiac arrest among other conditions.[8] Limited research examining the causes of these disparities cite structural factors and biases in treatment practices.[11] These studies also highlight a patient trajectory with multiple opportunities to influence inequitable outcomes beginning in the community setting with individual susceptibility to infection to the time of clinical presentation at the hospital, clinical management in the hospital setting, and outcomes of care.[8]

In the context of COVID-19, new considerations arise for social disparities in critical illness. These include hospital capacity and access to personal protective equipment, vaccinations, and virtual care. Critical care also evolved in the context of limited resources to handle issues like the distribution of ventilators, use of newly developed therapies, and family visitation.[12] Understanding how social disparities manifested in this context can provide useful lessons for mitigating health disparities in the future. The goal of this narrative review is to explore evidence about racial/ethnic and socioeconomic differences in critical illness during the COVID-19 pandemic, factors driving those differences, and promising solutions for mitigating inequities. While the root causes of health disparities are common between adults and children, we focus our review on adult studies because of variations in COVID-19 infection in adults and children.

Defining Health Disparities

We begin this review with a definition of health disparities to serve as a foundation for further discussion. Healthy People 2030 defines a health disparity as *a particular type of health difference that is closely linked with social, economic, and/or environmental disadvantage. Health disparities adversely affect groups of people who have systematically experienced greater obstacles to health based on their racial or ethnic group; religion; socioeconomic status; gender; age; mental health; cognitive, sensory, or physical disability; sexual orientation or gender identity; geographic location; or other characteristics historically linked to discrimination or exclusion.*[13]

In this context, health disparities research focuses on inequities in health that are the result of unjust systems, policies and practices, and not individual behavior. When these unjust systems create and perpetuate racial/ethnic inequities, this is described as structural racism.[14] In writing this review, we acknowledge the role of structural racism in perpetuating racial/ethnic health disparities, while examining specific ways in which structural racism contributes to poor health outcomes through access to care, experiences of discrimination and access to resources to prevent and treat disease.

PATIENT JOURNEY FRAMEWORK

This review is organized using a patient journey framework to identify social disparities at various stages before, during, and after patient interactions with critical care services (**Fig. 1**). The use of patient journeys is becoming more common in health care studies.[15] The concept is borrowed from the marketing field where consumer journeys are used to understand user experience with a product or service.[16] Journey mapping is an ethnographic technique that considers the context within which customers/users experience a product or service and how that experience influences their thoughts, actions, and emotions. We apply this framework to critical care during the COVID-19 pandemic and focus on 3 periods: prehospitalization, early hospitalization, and posthospitalization. At each phase, we consider evidence of health disparities and highlight solution-oriented lessons for eliminating disparities in the future.

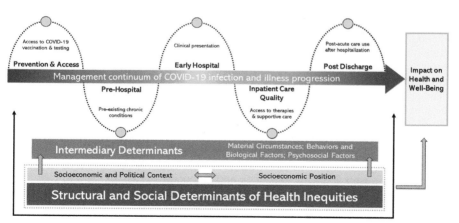

Fig. 1. Impact of structural and social determinants of health on health and well-being along the patient's journey prior to, during, and after hospitalization for critical illness. (*Adapted from* Solar O, Irwin A. A conceptual framework for action on the social determinants of health. Social Determinants of Health Discussion Paper 2.)

PREHOSPITAL DISPARITIES IN CORONAVIRUS DISEASE 2019

Much of the evidence for racial/ethnic and socioeconomic disparities in COVID-19 is reported in the prehospitalization period. A number of reviews have examined associations between race/ethnicity, socioeconomic status, and COVID-19 infection.[17,18] To avoid replicating those narratives, here we focus on associations between those prehospitalization factors, hospitalization, and death. This includes differences in vaccination rates, access to care, prevalence, and control of chronic diseases like hypertension and diabetes and neighborhood and community resources.

Vaccination Rates

COVID-19 vaccination has been shown to be highly effective against severe illness and intensive care unit (ICU) admission. One meta-analysis reported vaccine effectiveness of 97.4% (95% CI: 96.0%–98.8%) based on 4 studies,[19] while another reported 66% lower odds of severe COVID-19 (OR = 0.34; 95% CI: 0.24–0.49) among fully vaccinated individuals.[20] Unfortunately, despite effective vaccines, uptake of vaccinations among people from racial and ethnic minority groups has been hampered by limited access to health care, a lack of resources to schedule a vaccine appointment, misinformation, and health care systems that have not always engendered trust, among other factors. One study reported vaccination coverage among Black and Hispanic persons to be 5% to 8% points lower than that of White persons, with age and socioeconomic factors (income, health insurance, and education) contributing to much of the difference in vaccine receipt and vaccine intention.[21,22] The impact of misinformation on Black and Hispanic communities is thought to be greater owing to lower levels of educational attainment and lower levels of health literacy.[23] For individuals who wanted to get a vaccine, a lack of access to online scheduling platforms and knowledge to navigate complex vaccine scheduling systems were additional barriers. A cross-sectional study of 1342 resource-constrained adults with chronic illness reported that 20% of survey respondents had trouble finding and making vaccine appointments.[24] While this specific study did not find a higher prevalence of appointment barriers for racial/ethnic minorities,[24] other studies have reported that technological barriers to making appointments had a notable impact on Black, Hispanic, and immigrant communities.[25–27]

Racially segregated and socioeconomically disadvantaged communities also experienced slower vaccine uptake because they were not prioritized in early vaccine distribution strategies.[28,29] Low vaccination rates coupled with higher infection rates put people from racial and ethnic minority groups at an increased risk of severe illness. Data from 382,979 hospitalizations in the COVID-19–Associated Hospitalization Surveillance Network from March 2020 to August 2022 showed that while racial/ethnic disparities in hospitalization and ICU admission persisted over the period, the magnitude of difference was reduced during the period when vaccines were available.[30] Thus, strategies designed to improve equitable vaccine uptake have the potential to directly impact disparities in incidence of critical illness and subsequent patient outcomes as shown in a North Carolina case study.[31] Successful models include those that have addressed financial, logistical, and language access barriers to COVID-19 vaccination (e.g., mobile clinics with no insurance requirements) and leveraged trusted community relationships.[25,27,32,33]

Access to Coronavirus Disease 2019 Testing and Preventive Care

Timely access to COVID-19 testing and preventive care have both been associated with COVID-19 outcomes. Across the pandemic, persons from minoritized racial/

ethnic groups and those with lower socioeconomic status were less likely to get tested, but had higher positivity rates once tested. In Pennsylvania, for example, Hispanic persons had 4.2 times greater odds of testing positive compared to White persons and 1.8 times greater odds of hospitalization.[34] The same study found that high neighborhood social vulnerability was associated with 2.4 times greater odds of testing positive and 1.3 times greater odds of hospitalization compared to low social vulnerability, with increasing magnitude of racial/ethnic differences in more vulnerable neighborhoods. Myriad barriers to timely testing for COVID-19 have been reported and include structural disparities like access to testing sites, allocation of funding, and ability to take time off work to seek care.[35] When tested, Black patients were more likely to get care at an emergency department than in an outpatient setting,[36] a potential result of lower rates of established primary care relationships. Analysis by Walls and colleagues of cohort data from 1604 patients hospitalized with COVID-19 found that patients with a primary care provider had 27% lower odds of 30 day ICU admission and 41% lower odds of 30 day all-cause mortality.[37] Patients who were uninsured had 28% higher odds of 30 day all-cause mortality, while odds were 2 times as high for Medicaid beneficiaries. In their analysis, both Black and Hispanic patients had higher odds of ICU admission and death compared to Whites and differences were not explained by clinical and socioeconomic characteristics alone.[37] Notably, having a primary care provider remained strongly associated with lower odds of all-cause mortality in stratified models for Black patients.

Preexisting Chronic Conditions

Reports of the higher rates of COVID-19 hospitalizations and deaths among Black persons and other minoritized racial ethnic groups commonly cite the higher rates of comorbid conditions as a contributing factor.[38–40] Indeed, chronic conditions that increase the risk of severe COVID-19 including diabetes, hypertension, and obesity are more prevalent among Black persons and other people from racial and ethnic minority groups than among non-Hispanic White persons. Excess rates of comorbid conditions have been tied to structural factors including residential segregation and intergenerational wealth, which in turn influence access to healthy foods and safe spaces to exercise, stress, and other factors that influence incidence and management of chronic health conditions.[41–43]

Findings regarding the association between pre-existing chronic conditions and disparities in critical illness vary with some studies finding no racial/ethnic differences after adjusting for comorbidities, and others showing that differences persist. Marmarchi and colleagues[44] reported on 288 ICU hospitalized patients in the early phase of the pandemic and found no difference in in-hospital mortality between African American patients and other patients despite higher rates of comorbidities like hypertension (80% vs 59%) and diabetes (49% vs 34%). A cohort study including 1047 hospitalized patients in a large New York City hospital reported lower odds of critical illness for Black patients versus White patients after adjusting for comorbidities and neighborhood characteristics, while there was no significant difference for Hispanic patients.[45] The Study of the Treatment and Outcomes in Critically Ill Patients with COVID-19 including ICU data from 67 US hospitals found higher rates of 28 day mortality for Hispanic patients versus non-Hispanic Whites (odds ratio: 1.44, 95% CI: 1.12–1.84) after adjustment for clinical characteristics despite younger age and fewer comorbidities.[46] In contrast, a large national cohort of 124,780 Black and White patients with COVID-19 found that having a comorbidity attenuated the risk of ICU admission but did not eliminate racial differences in ICU admission, which was higher for Black patients than White patients and increased with age.[47]

Lopez and colleagues analyzed data from 2125 COVID-19-positive adult patients requiring ICU admission at the Cleveland Clinic Health System and found no differences in mortality by race or ethnicity after adjusting for chronic conditions including chronic kidney disease and malignant neoplasms, and disease severity (as measured by the Acute Physiologic Assessment and Chronic Health Evaluation score), which were all significantly associated with death.[48] The authors proposed that standardized care pathways, limited resource strain, and equitable distribution of resources as likely factors contributing to this finding. The study by Marmarchi and colleagues also cited a lack of resource strain as a potential contributing factor influencing the lack of significant differences in in-hospital mortality between Black patients and other patients in their dataset.[44]

Neighborhood and Community Setting

The association between place of residence and health outcomes is well established.[49,50] Social determinants of health are defined as the conditions in which individuals live, work, and play. During the pandemic, morbidity and mortality were highest in communities with higher poverty rates, lower levels of education, higher populations from minoritized racial/ethnic groups, and greater levels of crowding.[51] ICU data from 70 US hospitals showed that the socioeconomic status of the community surrounding a hospital contributed at least 12% of the mortality risk for hospitalized patients, of whom 30% identified as Black and 38% as White.[52] Analysis of New York City data showed that boroughs with higher percent of Hispanic and Black residents also had higher poverty levels and lower per capita ICU beds.[53]

Health outcomes during the pandemic were also impacted by access to broadband Internet, which was essential for accessing primary care for chronic disease management.[54] Broadband Internet access varies across community settings, and reports suggest that the pandemic widened the existing digital divide for Black and Hispanic persons and individuals with lower incomes who have lower rates of access to reliable broadband services.[55] Limited access to virtual care during the pandemic likely exacerbated existing lower rates of disease control for chronic conditions like hypertension and diabetes, which influence COVID-19 severity.

EARLY HOSPITALIZATION

Once hospitalized with COVID-19, disparities exist in both the risk of developing severe or critical illness as well as access to therapies and critical care resources. Many of the social factors at play in the prehospitalization period continue to influence health care and outcomes during early hospitalization. Minoritized racial/ethnic groups including Black, Latino, and Indigenous persons are more likely to be hospitalized with COVID-19 than White persons, a finding that has been consistent across different health settings globally.[56–58] These same groups are significantly more likely to require ICU care. In a longitudinal analysis during the first year of the COVID-19 pandemic, compared with White patients, Asian or Pacific Islander and Latino patients had significantly higher percentages of invasive mechanical ventilation and vasopressor use and Black patients had significantly higher rates of renal replacement therapy.[2] Contributing factors include differences in clinical presentation, access to therapies during hospitalization, and hospital capacity and resource strain.

Differences in Clinical Presentation

Many of the chronic health conditions that impact the susceptibility to critical illness disproportionally impact minoritized racial/ethnic groups.[8,59] Black persons and persons from other minoritized racial/ethnic groups with COVID-19 are more likely to have one or more comorbid conditions compared to White patients with COVID-19.[60,61] Chronic kidney disease, diabetes, human immunodeficiency virus, and obesity all disproportionately affect Black persons and persons from other minoritized racial/ethnic groups and have been found to be consistent risk factors for a severe outcome from COVID-19.[62–67] In addition to differences in prevalence, rates of disease control for conditions like hypertension and diabetes are lower among some minoritized racial/ethnic groups owing to less access to primary care. These differences were likely exacerbated during the pandemic as people from racial and ethnic minority groups were more likely to delay medical care for chronic conditions.[68,69] Timing of seeking care may also influence observed disparities in critical illness. Studies have shown that Black and Latino persons were more likely to have treatment and testing delays for COVID-19 because of factors including lack of paid time off to seek medical care, access to treatment and testing facilities, misinformation about COVID-19, and prior discriminatory experiences with the health care system.[70]

Access to Therapies and Supportive Care

Evidence suggests differences between racial and ethnic groups in receipt of supportive care and therapeutics while hospitalized for COVID-19. In a national cohort of veterans, Black race was associated with lower odds of receiving evidence-based treatment of COVID-19, including dexamethasone, remdesivir, and immunomodulatory medications.[71] Oxygen saturation thresholds have been particularly important in guiding decisions about eligibility for COVID-19 treatments. Pulse oximetry systematically overestimates arterial oxygen saturation among patients from racial and ethnic minority groups,[72,73] and was associated with higher likelihood of occult hypoxemia in patients from racial and ethnic minority groups hospitalized with COVID-19.[74] This overestimation resulted in a delay in recognizing eligibility for COVID-19 therapeutics among Black and Hispanic patients, with implications for population-level disparities seen in COVID-19 outcomes.[75] Implicit biases among health care providers may also have contributed to disparities observed in treatment for severe COVID-19 and access to limited therapeutic options, as have been found with clinician-patient interactions across diverse care settings.[76,77]

Hospital Capacity and Resource Strain

During the pandemic, hospital capacity and resources influenced both treatment decisions and care delivery processes that impact outcomes of care. Kanter and colleagues found that 49% of the lowest income communities had no ICU beds in their communities compared to only 3% of the highest income communities.[78] The gap was most pronounced in rural areas but income disparities were still present in dense, urban areas. Striking disparities were reported in New York City where majority White zip code tabulation areas (ZCTAs) had on average 69.5 to 75.5 licensed beds at various timepoints compared to 8.0 to 10.1 beds in majority Black and Hispanic ZCTAs.[79] Even in areas with access to ICU beds, disparities persist. Patients admitted to hospitals with fewer ICU beds had a higher mortality from COVID-19.[80] This finding replicates a prepandemic finding that patients with respiratory failure have better outcomes if cared for in hospitals with a high case volume of mechanical ventilation.[81] In our current health care system, patients with COVID-19 most likely to be cared for at strained and underresourced hospital systems are more often Medicaid recipients, uninsured, and from a minoritized racial and ethnic group.[82] This differential access to well-resourced hospitals significantly contributed to wide variations in mortality in critically ill adults with COVID-19.[52]

Triage and Allocation Policies

The strain on limited health care resources during the pandemic led to the development of new and revised triage scores and policies to manage critical care resources (eg, intensive care unit beds and mechanical ventilators) across states, health care systems, and individual hospitals. A systematic review of ventilator allocation guidelines in the United States found that only 26 states had publicly available guidelines as of May 2020, with considerable variation across states.[83] A similar mixed-methods analysis of ventilator triage policies at 67 hospitals in the United States found that 53.7% did not have a policy as of March 2020 and that there was substantial heterogeneity in triage criteria and a lack of guidance on fair and equitable implementation among those with policies.[84] Most triage policies (including those in the majority of states with allocation guidelines) apply the utilitarian approach of directing resources to those most likely to benefit and use severity of illness scores such as the Sequential Organ Failure Assessment (SOFA) score to allocate resources to those sick enough, but not too sick to benefit.[83] However, such policies create structural disadvantage for people from racial and ethnic minority groups. For example, a cohort study of COVID-19-positive patients in the Yale-New Haven Health System concluded that the use of SOFA scores for ventilator triage would exacerbate racial disparities because although Black patients had higher SOFA scores compared to patients of other races indicating higher acuity, this did not translate into higher in-hospital mortality or ICU admission.[85] Similar studies demonstrate an overestimation of mortality risk for Black patients compared to White patients using SOFA,[86,87] thus systematically deprioritizing Black patients for care. While no clear solutions to equitable ventilator allocation emerged during the pandemic, simulation studies[88–90] highlight the limitations of widely used approaches like SOFA in the context of COVID-19 and the opportunity to consider health disparities and save more lives using alternative strategies. Additional reviews of triage and allocation guidelines during the pandemic call for a focus on justice and the inclusion of race/ethnicity and other social factors in the development and evaluation of the criteria to improve equity.[91–93]

POSTHOSPITAL DISCHARGE

A growing number of studies have examined care delivery and outcomes that occur after index hospitalization for COVID-19. However, current evidence regarding disparities that persist into the recovery period is limited, and few data exist on differences between racial, ethnic, and socioeconomic groups after critical illness with COVID-19. Emerging areas of interest include access to and utilization of postdischarge health care services, incidence of symptoms and sequelae consistent with postintensive care syndrome and postacute COVID-19 syndrome (ie, "Long COVID," multiorgan system effects of COVID-19 and its treatment), and hospital readmission and mortality outcomes.

Access to Postdischarge Services

COVID-19 hospitalization can be lengthy and complex and thus requires careful attention to prospective rehabilitation needs, particularly for severely ill patients who received organ support during hospitalization. In our current health care system, postacute health care services can address medical needs and provide timely response to potential complications that develop during transitions of care.[94] Yet, access to these services was restricted early in the COVID-19 pandemic,[95] and existing data indicate the majority of adults who survived hospitalization for COVID-19 were discharged to home without additional supportive services. One large Centers for Disease Control and Prevention study of 126,137 patients hospitalized with COVID-19 found that 60% of 106,543 patients discharged alive went home, while 10% received home health assistance, and 15% went to a skilled nursing facility.[96] Similar findings have been observed in multiple other cohorts.

Although few studies have examined subgroup differences in the provision of these transitional rehabilitation services, examples demonstrate decreased use of postdischarge services among traditionally marginalized populations. Among 6248 patients hospitalized at an academic health system in the midwestern United States,[97] patients identifying as Black, Asian, and Hispanic were less likely than White patients to be discharged to postacute care (ie, skilled nursing, inpatient rehabilitation, or long-term acute care; relative risk ratio, Black: 0.64, 0.47–0.88; Asian: 0.48, 0.34–0.67, Hispanic: 0.59, 0.35–0.98). Additionally, in a separate chart review study of patients discharged from a single academic medical center in the United States,[98] , Hispanic ethnicity was shown to be associated with more frequent discharge home without additional health care services (adjusted odds ratio: 2.52, 95% CI: 1.50 to 4.25; compared to patients with non-Hispanic ethnicity). Patients admitted to the ICU during their hospitalization were more frequently discharged to nonhome settings. In one multicenter, international observational study of ICU survivors,[99] 47% were discharged home without assistance, while 24% were discharged home with health assistance, and 29% were discharged to a facility outside the home (eg, 11% long-term acute care, 8% skilled nursing, and 2% hospice). In this study, nonhome discharge was more prevalent among non-Hispanic White persons, reinforcing the observed limitations persons from minoritized racial/ethnic groups experienced in accessing potentially beneficial postacute services—even when illness severity was high. Together, these findings are consistent with literature from before the COVID-19 pandemic demonstrating racial/ethnic disparities with people from racial and ethnic minority groups traditionally having poorer access to postacute care services and worse recovery outcomes.

Differences in Post-coronavirus Disease 2019-related Symptoms and Sequelae Following Hospitalization

Approximately 70% of patients hospitalized with COVID-19 experience prolonged symptoms for at least 2 months after the acute illness, known as postacute sequelae of severe acute respiratory syndrome coronavirus 2 infection (PASC), including physical weakness, fatigue, dyspnea, cognitive dysfunction (eg, memory and concentration problems), and psychological distress.[100,101] There is ongoing epidemiologic, mechanistic, and clinical research seeking to better understand recovery following acute COVID-19 hospitalization.[102,103] In one large electronic health record-based study from 5 health systems in New York City in the Researching COVID to Enhance Recovery (RECOVER) Program,[104] there were significant racial and ethnic differences in symptoms identified by International Classification of Diseases, Tenth Revision (ICD-10) diagnosis codes at health care encounters up to 180 days after index hospitalization. Higher adjusted incidences of dyspnea, headache, chest pain, abdominal pain, and joint pain were observed among Black and Hispanic versus White individuals, while lower adjusted incidences of sleep disorders, hair loss, pressure ulcers, and malnutrition were observed between the same comparison groups.[104] When grouped by condition type, any respiratory, circulatory, endocrine, and general conditions were all observed to be more frequent among Black and Hispanic persons versus White persons. Another study identified PASC symptom clusters with differential proportions of racial groups represented across subtypes.[105] These findings highlight persistent disparities beyond the acute illness, along with potentially unique needs to be addressed in diverse patient groups. Early in the pandemic, there were calls to extend ICU recovery programs to individuals hospitalized with COVID-19; however, one qualitative study found that health systems were not prepared to address the needs of historically marginalized populations who are more likely to be uninsured or underinsured and have limited access to technology or poor digital literacy.[106] These gaps suggest other recovery care models[107] along with additional integration of community-based support may be useful to more comprehensively address the multifaceted needs observed in diverse populations.[108,109]

Differences in Readmission and Mortality Outcomes Following Hospitalization

Despite the established high burden of disease associated with COVID-19-related hospitalization and subsequent sequelae, hospital readmission rates have been observed to be relatively low—with less than 10% of hospitalized patients readmitted within 30 days in most existing reports,[110,111] including reports of ICU survivors.[112] In a large retrospective analysis of 965,231 adults hospitalized with COVID-19 in the United States,[113] 30,651 (3.2%) were readmitted within 30 days. Higher rates of readmission were observed among persons with lower median income (adjusted hazard ratio: 1.20, 95% CI: 1.14–1.28; <US$49,999 vs >US$86,000), Medicaid payor status (adjusted hazard ratio: 1.60, 95% CI: 1.50–1.70; vs private insurance), along with illness severity on index hospitalization (adjusted hazard ratio, mechanical ventilation: 1.22, 95% CI: 1.16–1.30). Similarly, a study of 883,394 Medicare beneficiaries found higher risk of hospital readmission at 30, 90, and 180 days among dual Medicaid-Medicare eligible versus nondual eligible patients (36% vs 29% at 180 days) and for Black versus White patients (35% vs 30% at 180 days).[114] Conversely, one study of 106,543 adults discharged from hospitals in the United States found non-Hispanic White persons had higher adjusted odds of same-hospital readmission within 60 days than those of other racial and ethnic groups.[96] In another report of readmission and mortality outcomes within 60 days of hospital discharge among patients discharged from the nationwide Veterans Affairs health care system, 19% of patients were readmitted and 9% of patients died; there were no nonage-related associations identified between patient characteristics and outcomes of interest.[115] In England, one study of 47,780 adults discharged from National Health Service (NHS) hospitals found the rate ratio of posthospital discharge mortality, comparing individuals with COVID-19 and matched controls, was greater among people from racial and ethnic minority groups than in White individuals.[116] The relatively limited data and conflicting evidence highlight the need for additional research on observed disparities in posthospital outcomes after COVID-19.

SEPARATE AND UNEQUAL

The story of the Martin Luther King, Jr. (MLK) Community Hospital, a safety-net hospital in South Los Angeles, California, is a striking example of the impact of structural racism and social determinants of health on critical care outcomes during the pandemic.[117] South Los Angeles was at the epicenter of the pandemic with nearly twice as many COVID-19 cases per capita compared to Los Angeles County, which led the United States in number of COVID-19 cases and deaths.[118] The community has evolved over time and is considered a product of racial residential segregation, employment discrimination, and disinvestment.[119] Once consisting of a majority Black population, the community includes residents who are 79% Hispanic/Latino and 18% Black, with 42% of adults employed in industries with high COVID-19 infection risk (manufacturing, retail, transportation, and warehousing).[118] Multiple indicators of elevated risk of COVID-19 infection including high social vulnerability, crowding, preexisting medical conditions, and barriers to accessing health care are concentrated within the community.[120]

Against this backdrop, the MLK Community Hospital sought to carry out its mission "to provide compassionate, collaborative, quality care."[121] At one point, 66% of their hospitalized patients had COVID-19 and their emergency department with 29 beds had 70 patients.[122] MLK Community Hospital staff converted spaces like their meditation room and gift shop into patient care rooms and converted medical units into critical care units to expand capacity. While they were able to save some lives, many others succumbed to COVID-19. According to one report, 86% of patients with COVID-19 who were intubated at MLK hospital died.[123] As before the pandemic, they had limited success transferring their patients who were predominantly Medicaid beneficiaries to larger, well-resourced hospitals that may have been able to offer more life-saving treatment options.[117,122,123] Elaine Batchlor, chief executive officer of MLK Hospital offers that while some characterize the experience of her hospital during the pandemic as overwhelming, it reflects effects of structural racism including underfunding of health care in racial and ethnic minority and low-income communities.[117] The acute challenges that MLK Hospital faced were addressed by receiving help from the National Guard, yet the need for comprehensive reform of a health care system that doles out unequal opportunity for health to racial and ethnic minority groups and persons with low incomes remained.

LEARNING FROM CORONAVIRUS DISEASE 2019 TO IMPROVE FUTURE OUTCOMES

Three key lessons emerge from this review regarding how we can learn from the pandemic to advance equitable critical care in the future (**Box 1**). The first is that improving disparities in critical care outcomes begins outside of the hospital. In this review, we focused on access to preventive care and chronic disease management, vaccines, and neighborhood and community resources as prehospital factors that influence the development of severe COVID-19 disease and subsequent outcomes. As new strains of COVID-19 emerge, vaccines remain a valuable tool for disease

---

Box 1
Three lessons from the coronavirus disease 2019 pandemic to advance equitable critical care in the future

1. Improving disparities in critical care outcomes begins outside of the hospital.
   - Access to preventive care and chronic disease management
   - Equitable access to vaccines
   - Neighborhood and community resources, poverty rates, and access to broadband Internet
   - Sociopolitical context including societal values and policies that guide allocation of critical care resources to mitigate effects of critical illness on historically marginalized populations

2. Implementing equitable care pathways may reduce disparate outcomes.
   - Standardized care pathways ensure that all patients receive evidence-based care that matches their local context
   - More research is needed to quantify the impact of care pathways on racial/ethnic and socioeconomic disparities

3. Offer person-centered care that prioritizes shared decision-making and respect for cultural values.
   - Prioritize patient-centered and family-centered care
   - Train providers to recognize and address implicit and explicit biases and their impact on patient care and outcomes

prevention. Yet, Black and Hispanic people have lower rates of vaccination against new COVID-19 strains compared to other racial and ethnic minority groups and White people.[124] Vaccination rates are also lower in communities with high social vulnerability, which often have a higher proportion of persons from racial and ethnic minority groups.[124] Equitable vaccination strategies built on trust and understanding in partnership with the impacted communities are needed to overcome gaps in vaccination for those who need it most.

In addition to these immediate prehospital factors, the World Health Organization framework for social determinants of health highlights the important role of sociopolitical context including societal values and policies on health and well-being.[50] The framework suggests that policies can be implemented at multiple levels to reduce: (1) effects of social stratification (eg, policies about health care available to individuals with low incomes on public insurance); (2) exposures to factors to lead to poor health (eg, policies about availability of personal protective equipment for essential workers); (3) vulnerabilities of people who are disadvantaged (eg, policies about access to healthy food, green spaces, and chronic disease care to prevent disease and reduce poor health outcomes); and (4) unequal consequences of ill health (eg, policies about loss of income due to illness and about access to treatment of illnesses). For example, the Crisis Standards of Care, one of the guidelines used for allocating scarce critical care resources during the pandemic, does not consistently account for equity in distribution of resources to people who are disadvantaged.[125] Policies that require equitable approaches to resource distribution could mitigate future gaps in outcomes of care for persons from historically marginalized groups. In the critical care context, policies to promote equitable care distribution of ventilators and other life-saving therapies should be developed in collaboration with community members prior to the next health emergency.

A second lesson is that implementing equitable care pathways may reduce disparate outcomes. Care pathways involve a standardized approach to care that ensures patients meeting certain clinical criteria receive evidence-based care to achieve the best outcome in their local context. Lopez and colleagues[48] reported that the Cleveland Clinic, which implemented standardized COVID-19 critical care protocols adapted from the World Health Organization, observed limited differences in ICU therapies and no difference in mortality by race or ethnicity. The use of standardized care pathways for COVID-19,[126] cancer care,[127] heart failure,[128] and venous thromboembolism[129] is a promising approach for improving health care outcomes. However, more research is needed to quantify the direct impact of implementation of care pathways on racial/ethnic and socioeconomic disparities to guide future practice.

A third lesson is that health systems should aim to offer person-centered care that prioritizes shared decision-making and respect for cultural values. We found that people from racial and ethnic minority groups were more likely to experience treatment biases during hospitalization and less likely to receive postdischarge care that was designed to meet their needs and cultural values. Providing ICU care that is patient-centered and family-centered is essential to health care quality and beneficial to the experience of patients, families, and clinicians.[130] Implicit and explicit biases are a key barrier to receipt of person-centered care for people from racial and ethnic minority groups. Provider education about biases and developing a culture of equitable care are potential strategies to overcome these barriers.

SUMMARY

The COVID-19 pandemic exacerbated existing racial/ethnic and socioeconomic disparities in critical illness through its disproportionate impact on already marginalized communities including Black, Hispanic/Latino, and American Indian/Alaska Native persons. These groups had increased vulnerability to COVID-19 exposure and infection, higher rates of preexisting chronic health conditions, less access to vaccines, and lived in communities with fewer critical care resources. Moreover, in the critical care setting, individuals from marginalized groups were more likely to present with severe disease, be treated in facilities with fewer resources, and experience discrimination. Structural and social determinants of health continue to influence posthospitalization outcomes including access to long-term care and culturally appropriate recovery programs for PASC. Strategies addressing systemic factors including the distribution of health care resources, universal access to preventive care, and standardized care pathways that prioritize equity, shared decision-making, and respect for cultural values are promising approaches for advancing equitable outcomes beyond the COVID-19 pandemic.

CLINICS CARE POINTS

- Social disparities in critical care originate from systemic inequities that influence health behavior and outcomes.
- The COVID-19 pandemic exacerbated existing racial/ethnic and socioeconomic disparities in access to health care and control of chronic health conditions resulting in higher disease severity among already marginalized populations.
- Risk of critical illness from COVID-19 infection was higher for Black and Hispanic persons and persons from other minority racial and ethnic groups compared to White persons, while risk of death did not differ by race and ethnicity in most settings.
- Multiple factors at the point of care including ICU capacity of individual hospitals, triage protocols and treatment biases worked together to either mitigate or exacerbate disparities.
- Community factors including variable availability of postdischarge resources, long-term care facilities, and nursing homes further influence COVID-19 recovery; however, further research is needed to quantify their impact on posthospital outcomes.
- Critical care units implementing standardized care protocols and those operating outside of capacity constraints in better resourced communities achieved more equitable outcomes across racial/ethnic categories.

DISCLOSURE

The authors have no conflicts of interest to disclose.

FUNDING

No funding for this article. Dr Kowalkowski reports receiving grant support from the National Institutes of Health (R01NR018434, R01HL169533), Agency for Healthcare Research and Quality (R01HS029656, R21HS027248), and Duke Endowment (7056-SP, 6993-SP) outside of the submitted work. Dr Palakshappa is supported by the National Institute of Aging (K23 AG073529).

REFERENCES

1. WHO chief declares end to COVID-19 as a global health emergency press release. 2023. Available at: https://news.un.org/en/story/2023/05/1136367.

2. Acosta AM, Garg S, Pham H, et al. Racial and ethnic disparities in rates of COVID-19-associated hospitalization, intensive care unit admission, and in-hospital death in the United States from March 2020 to february 2021. JAMA Netw Open 2021;4(10):e2130479.

3. Rogers TN, Rogers CR, VanSant-Webb E, et al. Racial disparities in COVID-19 mortality among essential workers in the United States. World Med Health Pol 2020;12(3):311–27.

4. Baptiste DL, Commodore-Mensah Y, Alexander KA, et al. COVID-19: shedding light on racial and health inequities in the USA. J Clin Nurs 2020;29(15–16): 2734–6.

5. Krishnan L, Ogunwole SM, Cooper LA. Historical insights on coronavirus disease 2019 (COVID-19), the 1918 influenza pandemic, and racial disparities: illuminating a path forward. Ann Intern Med 2020;173(6):474–81.

6. Williams DR, Cooper LA. COVID-19 and health equity-A new kind of "herd immunity". JAMA 2020;323(24):2478–80.

7. Foreman MG, Willsie SK. Health care disparities in critical illness. Clin Chest Med 2006;27(3):473–86, vii.

8. Soto GJ, Martin GS, Gong MN. Healthcare disparities in critical illness. Crit Care Med 2013;41(12):2784–93.

9. Mitchell HK, Reddy A, Perry MA, et al. Racial, ethnic, and socioeconomic disparities in paediatric critical care in the USA. Lancet Child & adolescent health 2021;5(10):739–50.

10. Blank JA, Armstrong-Hough M, Valley TS. Disparities among patients with respiratory failure. Curr Opin Crit Care 2023;29(5):493–504.

11. Hilton EJ, Goff KL, Sreedharan R, et al. The flaw of medicine: addressing racial and gender disparities in critical care. Anesthesiol Clin 2020;38(2):357–68.

12. Hensley MK, Prescott HC. Caring for the critically ill patient with COVID-19. Clin Chest Med 2022;43(3):441–56.

13. Office of Disease Prevention and Health Promotion. Health Equity in Healthy People 2030. Available at: https://health.gov/healthypeople/priority-areas/health-equity-healthy-people-2030. [Accessed 1 November 2023].

14. Neely AN, Ivey AS, Duarte C, et al. Building the transdisciplinary resistance collective for research and policy: implications for dismantling structural racism as a determinant of health inequity. Ethn Dis 2020;30(3):381–8.

15. Davies EL, Bulto LN, Walsh A, et al. Reporting and conducting patient journey mapping research in healthcare: a scoping review. J Adv Nurs 2023;79(1): 83–100.

16. Crosier A, Handford A. Customer journey mapping as an advocacy tool for disabled people:A case study. Soc Market Q 2012;18(1):67–76.

17. Duong KNC, Le LM, Veettil SK, et al. Disparities in COVID-19 related outcomes in the United States by race and ethnicity pre-vaccination era: an umbrella review of meta-analyses. Front Public Health 2023;11:1206988.

18. Khanijahani A, Iezadi S, Gholipour K, et al. A systematic review of racial/ethnic and socioeconomic disparities in COVID-19. Int J Equity Health 2021;20(1):248.

19. Zheng C, Shao W, Chen X, et al. Real-world effectiveness of COVID-19 vaccines: a literature review and meta-analysis. Int J Infect Dis 2022;114:252–60.

20. Flacco ME, Acuti Martellucci C, Baccolini V, et al. COVID-19 vaccines reduce the risk of SARS-CoV-2 reinfection and hospitalization: meta-analysis. Front Med 2022;9:1023507.

21. Williams AM, Clayton HB, Singleton JA. Racial and ethnic disparities in COVID-19 vaccination coverage: the contribution of socioeconomic and demographic factors. Am J Prev Med 2022;62(4):473–82.

22. Kim D. Associations of race/ethnicity and socioeconomic factors with vaccination among US adults during the COVID-19 pandemic, January to March 2021. Preventive medicine reports 2023;31:102021.

23. Arigbede OM, Aladeniyi OB, Buxbaum SG, et al. The use of five public health themes in understanding the roles of misinformation and education toward disparities in racial and ethnic distribution of COVID-19. Cureus 2022;14(10): e30008.

24. Spees LP, Biddell CB, Angove RSM, et al. Barriers to COVID-19 vaccine uptake among resource-limited adults diagnosed with chronic illness. Front Public Health 2023;11:1046515.

25. Tay ET, Fernbach M, Chen H, et al. A community-based volunteer service to reduce COVID-19 vaccination inequities in New York City. Journal of Public Health 2023.

26. Moore R, Rojo MO, Purvis RS, et al. Overcoming barriers and enhancing facilitators to COVID-19 vaccination in the Hispanic community. BMC Publ Health 2022;22(1):2393.

27. Nawaz S, Moon KJ, Anagbonu F, et al. Evaluation of the COVID-19 Vaccination Campaign ¡Ándale! ¿Qué Esperas? in Latinx Communities in California, June 2021-May 2022. Public Health Rep. 2023:333549231204043. doi: 10.1177/00333549231204043.

28. Medcalfe SK, Slade CP. Racial residential segregation and COVID-19 vaccine uptake: an analysis of Georgia USA county-level data. BMC Publ Health 2023;23(1):1392.

29. DiRago NV, Li M, Tom T, et al. COVID-19 vaccine rollouts and the reproduction of urban spatial inequality: disparities within large US cities in March and april 2021 by racial/ethnic and socioeconomic composition. J Urban Health 2022; 99(2):191–207.

30. Ko JY, Pham H, Anglin O, et al. Vaccination status and trends in adult coronavirus disease 2019-associated hospitalizations by race and ethnicity: March 2020-august 2022. Clin Infect Dis 2023;77(6):827–38.

31. Wong CA, Dowler S, Moore AF, et al. COVID-19 vaccine administration, by race and ethnicity - North Carolina, december 14, 2020-april 6, 2021. MMWR Morb Mortal Wkly Rep 2021;70(28):991–6.

32. Mayfield CA, Priem JS, Inman M, et al. An equity-focused approach to improving access to COVID-19 vaccination using mobile health clinics. Healthc (Amst) 2023; 11(2):100690.

33. Wu TY, Yang X, Lally S, et al. Using community engagement and geographic information systems to address COVID-19 vaccination disparities. Tropical medicine and infectious disease 2022;7(8).

34. Bilal U, Jemmott JB, Schnake-Mahl A, et al. Racial/ethnic and neighbourhood social vulnerability disparities in COVID-19 testing positivity, hospitalization, and in-hospital mortality in a large hospital system in Pennsylvania: a prospective study of electronic health records. Lancet regional health Americas 2022;10: 100220.

35. Mody A, Pfeifauf K, Geng EH. Using lorenz curves to measure racial inequities in COVID-19 testing. JAMA Netw Open 2021;4(1):e2032696.

36. Sparling A, Walls M, Mayfield CA, et al. Racial/ethnic disparities in health care setting choice for adults seeking severe acute respiratory syndrome coronavirus 2 testing. Med Care 2022;60(1):3–12.
37. Walls M, Priem JS, Mayfield CA, et al. Disparities in level of care and outcomes among patients with COVID-19: associations between race/ethnicity, social determinants of health and virtual hospitalization, inpatient hospitalization, intensive care, and mortality. Journal of racial and ethnic health disparities 2023; 10(2):859–69.
38. Saini G, Swahn MH, Aneja R. Disentangling the coronavirus disease 2019 health disparities in african Americans: biological, environmental, and social factors. Open Forum Infect Dis 2021;8(3):ofab064.
39. Gupta R, Agrawal R, Bukhari Z, et al. Higher comorbidities and early death in hospitalized African-American patients with Covid-19. BMC Infect Dis 2021; 21(1):78.
40. Alcendor DJ. Racial disparities-associated COVID-19 mortality among minority populations in the US. J Clin Med 2020;9(8).
41. Rodgers GP, Gibbons GH. Obesity and hypertension in the time of COVID-19. JAMA 2020;324(12):1163–5.
42. Bleich SN, Ard JD. COVID-19, obesity, and structural racism: understanding the past and identifying solutions for the future. Cell Metabol 2021;33(2):234–41.
43. Gravlee CC. Systemic racism, chronic health inequities, and COVID-19: a syndemic in the making? Am J Hum Biol 2020;32(5):e23482.
44. Marmarchi F, Liu M, Rangaraju S, et al. Clinical outcomes of critically Ill patients with COVID-19 by race. Journal of racial and ethnic health disparities 2022;9(2): 385–9.
45. Ogedegbe G, Ravenell J, Adhikari S, et al. Assessment of racial/ethnic disparities in hospitalization and mortality in patients with COVID-19 in New York city. JAMA Netw Open 2020;3(12):e2026881.
46. Ricardo AC, Chen J, Toth-Manikowski SM, et al. Hispanic ethnicity and mortality among critically ill patients with COVID-19. PLoS One 2022;17(5):e0268022.
47. Poulson M, Geary A, Annesi C, et al. National disparities in COVID-19 outcomes between Black and white Americans. J Natl Med Assoc 2021;113(2):125–32.
48. Lopez DC, Whelan G, Kojima L, et al. Critical care among disadvantaged minority groups made equitable: trends throughout the COVID-19 pandemic. Journal of racial and ethnic health disparities 2023;10(2):660–70.
49. Swope CB, Hernández D, Cushing LJ. The relationship of historical redlining with present-day neighborhood environmental and health outcomes: a scoping review and conceptual model. J Urban Health 2022;99(6):959–83.
50. Solar O, Irwin A. A conceptual framework for action on the social determinants of health. Geneva: World Health Organization; 2010.
51. Pan W, Miyazaki Y, Tsumura H, et al. Identification of county-level health factors associated with COVID-19 mortality in the United States. Journal of biomedical research 2020;34(6):437–45.
52. Churpek MM, Gupta S, Spicer AB, et al. Hospital-level variation in death for critically ill patients with COVID-19. Am J Respir Crit Care Med 2021;204(403–411): 403–11.
53. Arasteh K. Prevalence of comorbidities and risks associated with COVID-19 among Black and hispanic populations in New York city: an examination of the 2018 New York city community health survey. Journal of racial and ethnic health disparities 2021;8(4):863–9.

54. Jain V, Al Rifai M, Lee MT, et al. Racial and geographic disparities in internet use in the U.S. Among patients with hypertension or diabetes: implications for telehealth in the era of COVID-19. Diabetes Care 2021;44(1):e15–7.

55. Early J, Hernandez A. Digital disenfranchisement and COVID-19: broadband internet access as a social determinant of health. Health Promot Pract 2021; 22(5):605–10.

56. Irizar P, Pan D, Kapadia D, et al. Ethnic inequalities in COVID-19 infection, hospitalisation, intensive care admission, and death: a global systematic review and meta-analysis of over 200 million study participants. EClinicalMedicine 2023;57: 101877.

57. Mirajkar A, Oswald A, Rivera M, et al. Racial disparities in patients hospitalized for COVID-19. J Natl Med Assoc 2023;115(4):436–40.

58. Gold JAW, Wong KK, Szablewski CM, et al. Characteristics and clinical outcomes of adult patients hospitalized with COVID-19 - Georgia, March 2020. MMWR Morb Mortal Wkly Rep 2020;69(18):545–50.

59. Esper AM, Moss M, Lewis CA, et al. The role of infection and comorbidity: factors that influence disparities in sepsis. Crit Care Med 2006;34(10):2576–82.

60. Webb Hooper M, Nápoles AM, Pérez-Stable EJ. COVID-19 and racial/ethnic disparities. JAMA 2020;323(24):2466–7.

61. Hsu HE, Ashe EM, Silverstein M, et al. Race/ethnicity, underlying medical conditions, homelessness, and hospitalization status of adult patients with COVID-19 at an urban safety-net medical center - Boston, Massachusetts, 2020. MMWR Morb Mortal Wkly Rep 2020;69(27):864–9.

62. Khan MMA, Khan MN, Mustagir MG, et al. Effects of underlying morbidities on the occurrence of deaths in COVID-19 patients: a systematic review and meta-analysis. J Glob Health 2020;10(2):020503.

63. McClellan W, Warnock DG, McClure L, et al. Racial differences in the prevalence of chronic kidney disease among participants in the reasons for geographic and racial differences in stroke (REGARDS) cohort study. J Am Soc Nephrol 2006; 17(6):1710–5.

64. Fadini GP, Morieri ML, Longato E, et al. Prevalence and impact of diabetes among people infected with SARS-CoV-2. J Endocrinol Invest 2020;43(6): 867–9.

65. Ssentongo P, Heilbrunn ES, Ssentongo AE, et al. Epidemiology and outcomes of COVID-19 in HIV-infected individuals: a systematic review and meta-analysis. Sci Rep 2021;11(1):6283.

66. Hales CM, Carroll MD, Fryar CD, et al. Prevalence of obesity and severe obesity among adults: United States, 2017-2018. NCHS Data Brief 2020;360:1–8.

67. Zhou Y, Yang Q, Chi J, et al. Comorbidities and the risk of severe or fatal outcomes associated with coronavirus disease 2019: a systematic review and meta-analysis. Int J Infect Dis 2020;99:47–56.

68. Gertz AH, Pollack CC, Schultheiss MD, et al. Delayed medical care and underlying health in the United States during the COVID-19 pandemic: a cross-sectional study. Preventive medicine reports 2022;28:101882.

69. Ahmed A, Song Y, Wadhera RK. Racial/ethnic disparities in delaying or not receiving medical care during the COVID-19 pandemic. J Gen Intern Med 2022;37(5):1341–3.

70. Buikema AR, Buzinec P, Paudel ML, et al. Racial and ethnic disparity in clinical outcomes among patients with confirmed COVID-19 infection in a large US electronic health record database. EClinicalMedicine 2021;39:101075.

71. Castro AD, Mayr FB, Talisa VB, et al. Variation in clinical treatment and outcomes by race among US veterans hospitalized with COVID-19. JAMA Netw Open 2022;5(10):e2238507.

72. Sjoding MW, Dickson RP, Iwashyna TJ, et al. Racial bias in pulse oximetry measurement. N Engl J Med 2020;383(25):2477–8.

73. Wong AI, Charpignon M, Kim H, et al. Analysis of discrepancies between pulse oximetry and arterial oxygen saturation measurements by race and ethnicity and association with organ dysfunction and mortality. JAMA Netw Open 2021; 4(11):e2131674.

74. Fawzy A, Wu TD, Wang K, et al. Racial and Ethnic Discrepancy in Pulse Oximetry and Delayed Identification of Treatment Eligibility Among Patients With COVID-19. JAMA Intern Med 2022;182(7):730–8.

75. Fawzy A, Wu TD, Wang K, et al. Clinical outcomes associated with overestimation of oxygen saturation by pulse oximetry in patients hospitalized with COVID-19. JAMA Netw Open 2023;6(8):e2330856.

76. FitzGerald C, Hurst S. Implicit bias in healthcare professionals: a systematic review. BMC Med Ethics 2017;18(1):19.

77. White DB, Lo B. Mitigating Inequities and Saving Lives with ICU Triage during the COVID-19 Pandemic. Am J Respir Crit Care Med 2021;203(3):287–95.

78. Kanter GP, Segal AG, Groeneveld PW. Income disparities in access to critical care services. Health Aff 2020;39(8):1362–7.

79. Douglas JA, Subica AM. COVID-19 treatment resource disparities and social disadvantage in New York City. Prev Med 2020;141:106282.

80. Gupta S, Hayek SS, Wang W, et al. Factors associated with death in critically ill patients with coronavirus disease 2019 in the US. JAMA Intern Med 2020; 180(11):1436–47.

81. Kahn JM, Goss CH, Heagerty PJ, et al. Hospital volume and the outcomes of mechanical ventilation. N Engl J Med 2006;355(1):41–50.

82. Kelly C., Parker W.F., Pollack H.A., Low-income COVID-19 patients die needlessly because they are stuck in the wrong hospitals—while the right hospitals too often shut them out. Health Affairs Blog. Available at: https://www.healthaffairs.org/content/forefront/low-income-covid-19-patients-die-needlessly-because-they-stuck-wrong-hospitals-while.

83. Piscitello GM, Kapania EM, Miller WD, et al. Variation in ventilator allocation guidelines by us state during the coronavirus disease 2019 pandemic: a systematic review. JAMA Netw Open 2020;3(6):e2012606.

84. Antommaria AHM, Gibb TS, McGuire AL, et al. Ventilator triage policies during the COVID-19 pandemic at U.S. Hospitals associated with members of the association of bioethics program directors. Ann Intern Med 2020;173(3):188–94.

85. Roy S, Showstark M, Tolchin B, et al. The potential impact of triage protocols on racial disparities in clinical outcomes among COVID-positive patients in a large academic healthcare system. PLoS One 2021;16(9):e0256763.

86. Miller WD, Han X, Peek ME, et al. Accuracy of the sequential organ failure assessment score for in-hospital mortality by race and relevance to crisis standards of care. JAMA Netw Open 2021;4(6):e2113891.

87. Ashana DC, Anesi GL, Liu VX, et al. Equitably allocating resources during crises: racial differences in mortality prediction models. Am J Respir Crit Care Med 2021;204(2):178–86.

88. Bhavani SV, Luo Y, Miller WD, et al. Simulation of ventilator allocation in critically ill patients with COVID-19. Am J Respir Crit Care Med 2021;204(10):1224–7.

89. Chuang E, Grand-Clement J, Chen JT, et al. Quantifying utilitarian outcomes to inform triage ethics: simulated performance of a ventilator triage protocol under sars-CoV-2 pandemic surge conditions. AJOB empirical bioethics 2022;13(3): 196–204.

90. Walsh BC, Zhu J, Feng Y, et al. Simulation of New York city's ventilator allocation guideline during the spring 2020 COVID-19 surge. JAMA Netw Open 2023; 6(10):e2336736.

91. Stone JR. Social justice, triage, and COVID-19: ignore life-years saved. Med Care 2020;58(7):579–81.

92. Long R, Cleveland Manchanda EC, Dekker AM, et al. Community engagement via restorative justice to build equity-oriented crisis standards of care. J Natl Med Assoc 2022;114(4):377–89.

93. Clarification of triage scoring criteria. JAMA Netw Open 2021;4(2):e212183.

94. Werner RM, Coe NB, Qi M, et al. Patient outcomes after hospital discharge to home with home health care vs to a skilled nursing facility. JAMA Intern Med 2019;179(5):617–23.

95. Grabowski DC, Mor V. Nursing home care in crisis in the wake of COVID-19. JAMA 2020;324(1):23–4.

96. Lavery AM, Preston LE, Ko JY, et al. Characteristics of hospitalized COVID-19 patients discharged and experiencing same-hospital readmission - United States, march-august 2020. MMWR Morb Mortal Wkly Rep 2020;69(45):1695–9.

97. Ikramuddin F, Melnik T, Ingraham NE, et al. Predictors of discharge disposition and mortality following hospitalization with SARS-CoV-2 infection. PLoS One 2023;18(4):e0283326.

98. Patel S, Truong GT, Rajan A, et al. Discharge disposition and clinical outcomes of patients hospitalized with COVID-19. Int J Infect Dis 2023;130:1–5.

99. Siddiqui S, Kelly L, Bosch N, et al. Discharge disposition and loss of independence among survivors of COVID-19 admitted to intensive care: results from the SCCM discovery viral infection and respiratory illness universal study (VIRUS). J Intensive Care Med 2023;38(10):931–8.

100. Thaweethai T, Jolley SE, Karlson EW, et al. Development of a definition of post-acute sequelae of SARS-CoV-2 infection. JAMA 2023;329(22):1934–46.

101. Nalbandian A, Sehgal K, Gupta A, et al. Post-acute COVID-19 syndrome. Nat Med 2021;27(4):601–15.

102. Horwitz LI, Thaweethai T, Brosnahan SB, et al. Researching COVID to Enhance Recovery (RECOVER) adult study protocol: rationale, objectives, and design. PLoS One 2023;18(6):e0286297.

103. RECOVER COVID initiative. 2023. Available at: https://recovercovid.org/. [Accessed 1 November 2023].

104. Khullar D, Zhang Y, Zang C, et al. Racial/ethnic disparities in post-acute sequelae of SARS-CoV-2 infection in New York: an EHR-based cohort study from the RECOVER program. J Gen Intern Med 2023;38(5):1127–36.

105. Reese JT, Blau H, Casiraghi E, et al. Generalisable long COVID subtypes: findings from the NIH N3C and RECOVER programmes. EBioMedicine 2023;87: 104413.

106. Eaton TL, Sevin CM, Hope AA, et al. Evolution in care delivery within critical illness recovery programs during the COVID-19 pandemic: a qualitative study. Annals of the American Thoracic Society 2022;19(11):1900–6.

107. Danesh V, Boehm LM, Eaton TL, et al. Characteristics of post-ICU and post-COVID recovery clinics in 29 U.S. Health systems. Critical care explorations 2022;4(3):e0658.

108. Johnson KA, Quest T, Curseen K. Will you hear me? Have you heard me? Do you see me? Adding cultural humility to resource allocation and priority setting discussions in the care of african American patients with COVID-19. J Pain Symptom Manag 2020;60(5):e11–4.

109. Johnson SF, Tiako MJN, Flash MJE, et al. Disparities in the recovery from critical illness due to COVID-19. Lancet Psychiatr 2020;7(8):e54–5.

110. Akbari A, Fathabadi A, Razmi M, et al. Characteristics, risk factors, and outcomes associated with readmission in COVID-19 patients: a systematic review and meta-analysis. Am J Emerg Med 2022;52:166–73.

111. Atalla E, Kalligeros M, Giampaolo G, et al. Readmissions among patients with COVID-19. Int J Clin Pract 2021;75(3):e13700.

112. Anesi GL, Jablonski J, Harhay MO, et al. Characteristics, outcomes, and trends of patients with COVID-19-related critical illness at a learning health system in the United States. Ann Intern Med 2021;174(5):613–21.

113. Muzammil TS, Gangu K, Nasrullah A, et al. Thirty-Day readmissions among COVID-19 patients hospitalized during the early pandemic in the United States: insights from the Nationwide Readmissions Database. Heart Lung 2023;62:16–21.

114. Oseran AS, Song Y, Xu J, et al. Long term risk of death and readmission after hospital admission with covid-19 among older adults: retrospective cohort study. BMJ 2023;382:e076222.

115. Donnelly JP, Wang XQ, Iwashyna TJ, et al. Readmission and death after initial hospital discharge among patients with COVID-19 in a large multihospital system. JAMA 2021;325(3):304–6.

116. Ayoubkhani D, Khunti K, Nafilyan V, et al. Post-covid syndrome in individuals admitted to hospital with covid-19: retrospective cohort study. BMJ 2021;372:n693.

117. Batchlor E., Were COVID-19 patients in the wrong hospital—or the wrong community? What really drove COVID-19 outcomes in South Los Angeles. Health Affairs Blog. Vol 20232021. Available at: https://www.healthaffairs.org/content/forefront/were-covid-19-patients-wrong-hospital-wrong-community-really-drove-covid-19-outcomes.

118. Schoen E, Hulburd K, Yap C, et al. Resilience & rebuilding: recommendations for an equitable recovery from COVID-19 in South Los Angeles. Sol price center for social innovation. San Diego, CA: University of Southern California; 2021.

119. Comandon A, Ong P. South Los Angeles Since the 1960s: race, place, and class. Rev Black Polit Econ 2020;47(1):50–74.

120. Ong P. Los Angeles neighborhoods and COVID-19 medical vulnerability indicators: a local data model for equity in public health decision-making. UCLA: Center for Neighborhood Knowledge 2020.

121. MLK Community Healthcare. About MLK community healthcare. 2023. Available at: https://www.mlkch.org/about. [Accessed 1 November 2023].

122. Fadel L. All things considered [internet]: NPR; 2021 january 21, 2021 [cited 11/1/2023]. Podcast. Available at: https://www.npr.org/2021/01/21/959091838/the-separate-and-unequal-health-system-highlighted-by-covid-19.

123. Fink S. Dying of covid in a 'separate and unequal' L.A. Hospital. New York, NY: New York Times; 2021.

124. Centers for Disease Control and Prevention. COVID data tracker. 2023. Available at: https://covid.cdc.gov/covid-data-tracker. [Accessed 1 November 2023].

125. Cleveland Manchanda EC, Sanky C, Appel JM. Crisis standards of care in the USA: a systematic review and implications for equity amidst COVID-19. Journal of racial and ethnic health disparities 2021;8(4):824–36.

126. Sangal RB, Liu RB, Cole KO, et al. Implementation of an electronic health record integrated clinical pathway improves adherence to COVID-19 hospital care guidelines. Am J Med Qual 2022;37(4):335–41.
127. Jobling IT, Waddington C, Lee D, et al. Piloting a novel cancer care pathway: socioeconomic background as a barrier to access. Clin Med (Lond) 2022; 22(3):241–5.
128. González-Juanatey JR, Comín-Colet J, Pascual Figal D, et al. Optimization of patient pathway in heart failure with reduced ejection fraction and worsening heart failure. Role of vericiguat. Patient Prefer Adherence 2023;17:839–49.
129. Misky GJ, Carlson T, Thompson E, et al. Implementation of an acute venous thromboembolism clinical pathway reduces healthcare utilization and mitigates health disparities. J Hosp Med 2014;9(7):430–5.
130. Secunda KE, Kruser JM. Patient-centered and family-centered care in the intensive care unit. Clin Chest Med 2022;43(3):539–50.

A Clinician's Guide to Understanding Bias in Critical Clinical Prediction Models

João Matos, MSc[a,b,c], Jack Gallifant, MBBS, MSc[c,d],
Anand Chowdhury, MD, MMCi[e],
Nicoleta Economou-Zavlanos, PhD[f],
Marie-Laure Charpignon, MS[g], Judy Gichoya, MD[h],
Leo Anthony Celi, MD, MS, MPH[c,i,j], Lama Nazer, PharmD[k],
Heather King, PhD[l,m,n], An-Kwok Ian Wong, MD, PhD[e,o,*]

KEYWORDS

- Bias • Prediction models • Artificial intelligence • AI • Machine learning

KEY POINTS

- This narrative review focuses on the role of clinical prediction models in supporting informed clinical decision-making in critical care, emphasizing their 2 forms: traditional scores and artificial intelligence-based models.
- Clinicians should evaluate these prediction models for their validity in ways similar to how ICU clinicians assess validity of pulse pressure variation.
- The assessment of pulse pressure variation is one of the many tasks critical care practitioners perform daily.
- Clinical prediction models play a crucial role in handling complex data to support clinicians to make more informed and timely decisions.

[a] University of Porto (FEUP), Porto, Portugal; [b] Institute for Systems and Computer Engineering, Technology and Science (INESC TEC), Porto, Portugal; [c] Laboratory for Computational Physiology, Institute for Medical Engineering and Science, Massachusetts Institute of Technology, Cambridge, MA, USA; [d] Department of Critical Care, Guy's and St Thomas' NHS Trust, London, UK; [e] Division of Pulmonary, Allergy, and Critical Care Medicine, Department of Medicine, Duke University, Durham, NC, USA; [f] Duke Health, AI Health, Durham, NC, USA; [g] Institute for Data Systems and Society, Massachusetts Institute of Technology, Cambridge, MA, USA; [h] Department of Radiology, Emory University, Atlanta, GA, USA; [i] Department of Biostatistics, Harvard T.H. Chan School of Public Health, Boston, MA, USA; [j] Department of Medicine, Beth Israel Deaconess Medical Center, Boston, MA, USA; [k] Department of Pharmacy, King Hussein Cancer Center, Amman, Jordan; [l] Durham VA Health Care System, Health Services Research and Development, Center of Innovation to Accelerate Discovery and Practice Transformation (ADAPT), Durham, NC, USA; [m] Department of Population Health Sciences, Duke University, Durham, NC, USA; [n] Division of General Internal Medicine, Duke University, Duke University School of Medicine, Durham, NC, USA; [o] Department of Biostatistics and Bioinformatics, Duke University, Division of Translational Biomedical Informatics, Durham, NC, USA
* Corresponding author. Duke University, 2 Genome Court, Box 103000 Durham, NC 27710.
E-mail address: med@aiwong.com

Crit Care Clin 40 (2024) 827–857
https://doi.org/10.1016/j.ccc.2024.05.011
0749-0704/24/© 2024 Elsevier Inc. All rights reserved, including those for text and data mining, AI training, and similar technologies.

criticalcare.theclinics.com

INTRODUCTION

With the rapid deployment of medical sensors, devices, and software systems in hospitals, the practice of critical care medicine has evolved and now relies extensively on the use of scoring tools and models to better monitor or predict clinical endpoints. For example, the assessment of volume status is critical to determine whether a hypotensive patient requires either more fluid or the initiation of vasopressors. To address this need, models such as pulse pressure variation (PPV) were created to predict volume responsiveness.[1,2] In clinical medicine, we are taught that PPV is predictive of fluid responsiveness but that certain conditions must be met to ensure its validity.[1,2] For example, initial studies required 2 criteria: positive pressure ventilation of 8 to 12 cc/kg and a regularly regular heart rate (ie, not in atrial fibrillation). Outside of these conditions, the accuracy of PPV is debatable; therefore, using this surrogate metric to guide clinical decision-making may not result in the intended effects.[1,2]

The assessment of PPV is one of the many tasks critical care practitioners perform daily. While this tool and other scoring systems (eg, Sequential Organ Failure Assessment [SOFA], Pneumonia Patient Outcomes Research Team [PORT] cohort study, and pneumonia severity index [PSI]) were studied in great detail during clinical training and subsequently put into practice, a large number of the prediction models embedded into the workflow involve recent advances in artificial intelligence and machine learning (AI/ML) approaches (eg, epic sepsis model [ESM][3] and Glucommander[4]). Further, although clinical teams are familiar with physiology-based measures such as PPV, they may not be equally versed in model-based tools. Given the speed at which new model architectures emerge in computer science, continued education is needed not only to familiarize with the content and methods underlying clinical prediction models but also to become aware of the associated risk of bias and inaccuracy.[3,5]

Given the unprecedented complexity, and potential for widespread impact, many governments are taking steps to regulate AI that may impact the daily lives of their citizens. The EU AI Act, approved by the European Parliament in June 2023, establishes obligations for providers and users depending on the level of risk from AI.[6] Just recently, in October 2023, the Biden–Harris Administration issued an executive order on safe, secure, and trustworthy AI,[7] reflecting the global concern over the potential implications of unregulated AI advancement.

As the field advances, it is critical for clinicians to understand the applicability and limitations of the many prediction models used in the intensive care unit (ICU), especially those based on AI/ML. In this narrative review, we take the perspective of critical care clinicians evaluating the practical aspects of a clinical prediction model that is available for use in the ICU. Through case studies and a listing of existing educational materials, our objective is to raise awareness and encourage the clinical end-user to be more inquisitive when apprehending a new prediction model.

CHALLENGES INHERENT TO THE INTENSIVE CARE UNIT

Clinical prediction tools, encompassing various scoring systems and models, play an indispensable role in the field of critical care.[8] In the ICU, clinicians face challenges akin to analyzing "big data," due to their quantity, sampling frequency, multimodality, and varying resolution and quality.[9] Health care practitioners in the critical care setting must incorporate information from multiple data sources, ranging from patient interviews to physical examinations, laboratory results, imaging, consultant reports, physiologic sensors, and scientific evidence. The complexities arising from this wide array of data are further compounded by patient heterogeneity, ranging from clinical features such as comorbidities and surgical histories to vital signs[10] and, to a lesser extent in critical care, social determinants of health.[11]

Furthermore, observational studies of physician decision-making over time and in cognitively demanding clinical settings have suggested that repeated engagement in cognitively intense thinking can lead to a degradation in the quality of decisions.[12] In the demanding milieu of critical care, clinicians are burdened with multifaceted goals. Balancing patient safety, optimizing postillness outcomes, employing resources judiciously, and tailoring care through personalized medicine necessitate processing this vast amount of information. The criticality of each decision is heightened by the inherent ambiguity and challenge of establishing causal connections between treatment and outcomes.[13]

To navigate the challenges posed by big data and mitigate the impact of cognitive limitations, clinicians turn to clinical prediction tools. These tools assist in identifying the salient aspects of the data that are most critical for a particular decision.[14] Similar to applying a filter to a database search, clinical prediction models seek to clarify which data elements contain the most information pertinent to a particular problem and isolate these essential data into easy-to-interpret scales, such as categories or percentage risks. This summarization process involves strategically discarding nonessential information, ensuring that what remains is of utmost importance for the intended decision.

CLINICAL PREDICTION MODELS IN THE INTENSIVE CARE UNIT

Clinical prediction models have the potential to enhance the quality of care delivery and contribute to improved patient outcomes within the dynamic and demanding environment of critical care.[15]

Traditionally, these models are score-based, meaning they consist of a set of operations that consider various clinical variables, ultimately yielding a numerical score. By assessing the scale and distribution of data, thresholds can be established to facilitate informed decision-making. These models can aid in critical decisions involving risks versus benefits of specific treatments (eg, MELD,[16] congestive heart failure, hypertension, age $\geq$75 [doubled], diabetes, stroke [doubled], vascular disease, age 65 to 74 and sex category [female] [CHADS$_2$-VASC], and Hypertension, Abnormal Renal/Liver Function, Stroke, Bleeding History or Predisposition, Labile INR, Elderly, Drugs/Alcohol Concomitantly [HAS-BLED][17]), detection of early or atypical disease presentations (eg, the laboratory risk indicator for necrotizing fasciitis [LRINEC] score for necrotizing soft tissue infection,[18] or Hscore for hemophagocytic lymphohistiocytosis[19]), test selection and interpretation (eg, Wells score for PE prediction), prognosis assessment (eg, Acute Physiology and Chronic Health Evaluation [APACHE] IV[20] and Oxford Acute Severity of Illness Score (OASIS)[21] for mortality risk assessment), and risk adjustment for benchmarking and comparison (eg, Medicare Severity Diagnosis Related Group [MS-DRG],[22] Charlson comorbidity,[23] and Elixhauser scores[24]). At times, these models have been used to inform decisions related to resource allocation, even when not originally designed for such purposes (eg, SOFA for extracorporeal cardiopulmonary resuscitation [eCPR][25] and extracorporeal membrane oxygenation [ECMO][26]).

As AI/ML technologies become the foundation of these prediction models, some of the more recent developments have shifted toward leveraging advanced computational algorithms to handle complex, high-dimensional data and to extract intricate patterns that might not be discernible through conventional statistical methods.[8] AI-based models, distinguished from their traditional score-based counterparts, can tackle a wider range of tasks, adapt to evolving clinical environments, and refine their predictive accuracy over time. Examples of predictive models of this nature include monitoring, early diagnosis (eg, sepsis), treatment decision support systems (eg, onset of mechanical ventilation), and outcome and prognosis assessment (eg, in-hospital mortality).[27]

These AI-based models can incorporate sophisticated modeling approaches such as deep learning architectures[28] or reinforcement learning techniques,[29] enabling a more dynamic and adaptive approach to data analysis and decision-making within critical care settings. AI-based models can also integrate multimodal input,[30] real-time data streams, and offer personalized predictions, thereby contributing to a more precise and tailored approach to patient care, treatment optimization, and resource allocation.[31]

In this section, we explore both "traditional score-based" and "AI-based" prediction models, which reveal distinct approaches and capabilities (**Table 1**). Traditional score-based models are typically limited in their scope, addressing specific problems such as mortality prediction, illness severity, and early warning scores (EWS).[37] These models rely on prespecified patient characteristics and are relatively simple, often summarized as a sequence of operations and easily computed using tools like MDCalc.[32] On the other hand, AI-based models have a much broader range of tasks, including monitoring, diagnosis, treatment, and outcome prediction.[27] However, their complexity lies in their often opaque, "black-box" structures, which require significant computational resources for both training and inference.[33]

Although traditional models generally do not consider fairness during development,[38] AI-based models are starting to incorporate fairness metrics from their initial design, even though there is still progress to be made in this area.[34] In terms of longevity and generalization, traditional score-based models are commonly used across various geographic and clinical settings, often remaining relevant for decades, even when not designed with that objective.[23,25,26] In contrast, AI-based models are more customized and designed to be adaptable, often tailored to specific populations, hospitals, or units and intended for iterative improvement.[35] Finally, while traditional models heavily emphasize clinical expertise, the development of AI-based models necessitates collaboration between individuals with clinical expertise and those possessing data science skills.[36]

Traditional Scores as Clinical Prediction Models

Clinical prediction models in the form of traditional scores have long served as vital tools for informing clinical decision-making. These scores often serve the purpose of either providing valuable information or aiding in specific decision-making processes, such as treatment assignment and resource allocation within a defined time frame. However, there are instances where these models, initially developed for specific purposes, may be repurposed or applied in different clinical contexts. An example of this is the utilization of the SOFA score for patient triage, highlighting the versatility of these tools beyond their original intended scope. In this section, we review some common score-based prediction models in the ICU, highlighting some of their limitations and factors to consider when using them in clinical practice.

Ashana and colleagues' investigation of the SOFA score's predictive capabilities for in-hospital mortality risks unearths marked racial disparities.[39] Their findings show that the risk of mortality is frequently underestimated among White patients but overestimated among Black patients. In scenarios where crisis standards of care (CSCs) apportion resources based on predicted mortality risks, this bias could inadvertently skew resource allocation. This is particularly evident among patients with projected mortality rates under 30%—the demographic arguably benefiting most from intensive care.[39] This bias persisted after adjustment for age, sex, and comorbidities, hinting at

Table 1
Comparison of "traditional" with "artificial intelligence-based" clinical prediction models

	"Traditional Score-based" Prediction Models	"AI-based" Prediction Models
Range of addressed problems	Limited range: eg, mortality prediction, illness severity, or EWS	Wide range of tasks, encompassing monitoring, diagnosis, treatment, and outcomes
Underlying patient characteristics	Often prespecified	May not always be specified
Complexity and interpretability	Simple, usually summarized as a sequence of operations and easily computed with tools like MDCalc[32]	Often resemble "black-box" models,[33] with complex structures and higher computational times both for training and inference
Fairness	Generally not considered during development; mostly evaluated post hoc and after the scores have been deployed	Although fairness metrics have a long way to go,[34] it is beginning to be considered from the initial design
Longevity and generalization	Used across diverse geographic and clinical settings. Use often grows stale and lasts for decades	More customized, "disposable," often limited to certain populations, hospitals, or units. Designed to be reiterated[35]
Talent and teams	Emphasis on clinical expertise	Collaboration between clinical expertise and data science skills for development, and implementation scientists for deployment[36]

Abbreviation: AI, artificial intelligence.

systemic factors like structural racism influencing mortality differentials. Ashana and colleagues' study demonstrates the pernicious consequences of this miscalibration on resource allocation, highlighting the pitfalls of using a model outside of its intended scope, and arguing for a reassessment of the SOFA score's place within CSCs.[40]

Model predictions can be skewed by information unrelated to the patient's clinical condition, such as the rate at which data are sampled. A case in point is the utilization of the APACHE II and simplified acute physiology score (SAPS) II severity scores in intensive care contexts.[37] Suistomaa and colleagues' exploration at a university hospital's ICU involved varying the sampling rates of laboratory and hemodynamic data and observing the consequential effects on severity scores.[37] Three distinct scoring paradigms were assessed: traditional scores (manual hemodynamic data paired with sporadic laboratory values), clinical information management system (CIMS) scores (2 minute median hemodynamic data with laboratory values based on clinical needs), and high rate scores (2 minute median hemodynamic data with 2 hourly laboratory assessments). The results revealed that increasing the sampling rate for hemodynamic monitoring and laboratory testing amplified the APACHE II and SAPS II scores considerably, leading to heightened predicted probabilities of hospital deaths. Notably, these increased scores did not correspond to heightened mortality rates, suggesting that predictive overestimations can distort clinical judgments. Additionally, the APACHE II score, despite its widespread use, harbors intrinsic limitations: operational complexity (its intricate nature poses operational challenges to routine use), predictive limitations (not a reliable prognostic tool, especially within the first 24 hours postadmission), and generalizability issues (initial validation was tailored for ICU-admitted patients, thereby reducing its efficacy for patients transferred from other wards or institutions). Suistomaa and colleagues' findings, juxtaposed with the inherent limitations of APACHE II, underscore the necessity for methodological rigor when interpreting the predictions from this model in the context of delivering care to individual patients.

EWS, like the United Kingdom's National Early Warning Score 2 (NEWS2), have become indispensable for identifying early decompensation in a complicated clinical milieu. The instrumentality of oxygen saturation by pulse oximetry (SpO$_2$), a core component, accentuates its utility in assessing respiratory functions. Nonetheless, recent studies spotlight biases in pulse oximetry, especially pertinent during the coronavirus disease 2019 (COVID-19) pandemic.[41] A retrospective analysis of 7126 patients with COVID-19 revealed a concerning racial bias in oxyhemoglobin measurement by pulse oximeters, with the device disproportionately overestimating arterial oxygen saturation for Asian, Black, and Hispanic patients vis-à-vis White patients.[41] These miscalibrations led to a substantial number of Black and Hispanic patients being overlooked for COVID-19-specific treatments. An exhaustive cross-sectional study further substantiated these discrepancies and highlighted the "hidden hypoxemia" phenomenon, which portends dire clinical ramifications.[42] These findings underscore the necessity for continuous re-evaluation of scores like NEWS2, with special emphasis on rectifying inherent biases to ensure clinical equity. In summation, it is paramount for clinicians to continuously scrutinize and understand the intricacies, correct application, and potential biases of traditional clinical prediction models. Doing so ensures that these tools maintain their efficacy and reliability, ultimately safeguarding the quality and equity of patient care.

Artificial Intelligence-based Clinical Prediction Models

In recent years, the landscape of clinical risk prediction models in critical care has witnessed a significant shift toward AI-based solutions. This precedent—including successes and failures in design and/or implementation—can inform the training and deployment of new models, especially in situations where traditional scores might come short and alternatives are urgently needed.[8,43] Unlike traditional scores that can be easily computed,[32] AI-based models often necessitate integration within the health care system infrastructure, making them less readily available for scrutiny or interpretation by individual clinicians. This trend toward AI-based models also raises concerns about the purchase of newly developed and commercialized medical software and devices by health care institutions. Specifically, the selection of commercial products for use in the ICU may not be by end-user clinicians, although they should be part of the decision-making process.[44] Assessing the risks associated with these models becomes a critical consideration in this context, especially given the increased complexity of the algorithms, as well as the varying expertise of the teams developing them, which may differ significantly from traditional medical expertise.[36]

In this section, we explore the realm of clinical prediction models, emphasizing the role of AI in shaping their evolution. **Table 2** outlines the main categories for the tasks where AI/ML is being leveraged, similar to the taxonomy proposed by Hong and colleagues.[27] The 4 categories outlined can be grouped into 2 broader classifications. The first category is related to a "current assessment," involving (1) *real-time monitoring*, which evaluates the progression of patients' physiologic variables (22), or the settings of an ongoing treatment like mechanical ventilation.[46,48] The reviewed studies often utilized simpler modeling approaches. On the other hand, the second broad category focuses on predicting the "future" state of the patient and encompasses (2) *early diagnosis*, (3) *treatment decision support systems*, and (4) *outcome assessment*. These have recently garnered significant attention in research, leveraging state-of-the-art technologies in the realm of AI/ML.

Examples of prediction models for early diagnosis include acute kidney injury,[49] sepsis,[85] and respiratory disease,[56,57] all of which are associated with increased mortality in the ICU, and abnormal blood glucose levels.[86] As for treatment decision support systems, our review describes prediction models related to therapies that have a decisive impact on the management and outcomes of critically ill patients, including mechanical ventilation,[60–62,87] antibiotics dosing,[63] intravenous fluids and vasopressor administration,[64,65] heparin dosing,[66] morphine dosing,[67] and insulin dosing.[68,70] Regarding outcome prediction, prevalent tasks identified in the literature include predicting ICU and in-hospital mortality (20), ICU length of stay,[78–80] ICU readmission,[82,83] and long-term survival and quality of life.[84]

These prediction models can potentially improve patient outcomes, the salience of information, and, thus, the quality of decisions taken by the clinical teams and enhance bed management, aiding in resource allocation. Yet, the current reality remains that the algorithms prominently featured in research literature are largely impractical for direct implementation at the forefront of clinical practice.[44,88,89] Implementation may often be significantly harder than development on retrospective data; data management, model development, and clinical workflow implementation are 3 common hurdles that must all be passed.[88] In the following section, we explore the current limitations, challenges, and suggestions for clinicians to mitigate the risk of bias associated with such prediction tools in the ICU.[45,47,50–55,58,59,69,71–77,81,89]

RISK OF BIAS: RECOMMENDATIONS FOR A CLINICIAN USING AN ARTIFICIAL INTELLIGENCE TOOL IN THE INTENSIVE CARE UNIT

In this section, we apply the taxonomy proposed by Nazer and colleagues[90] on the bias in the AI/ML development pipeline, with a focus on an example application of

Table 2
Nonexhaustive description of categories of intensive care unit artificial intelligence-based clinical prediction models in literature

Category	Specific Task	Examples in Research Literature
1. Real-time monitoring	Physiologic indicators	Zhang and Szolovits[45] proposed patient-specific, bedside, real-time alarm algorithms based on neural network learning for adaptive monitoring in the ICU
	Mechanical ventilation settings	Kwok et al.[46] used a linear regression model and a nonlinear adaptive neuro-fuzzy inference system to estimate Fio$_2$; Rehm et al.[47] and Gholami et al.[48] created an ML classifier to detect patient-ventilator asynchrony
2. Early diagnosis	Acute kidney injury (AKI)	Sun et al.[49] proposed the use of clinical notes and deep learning for an early detection of AKI onset; Sanchez-Pinto and Khemani[50] delved into AKI prediction among critically ill children, using multivariable logistic regression
	Sepsis and infection	Desautels et al.[51] presented "InSight," a gradient-boost ML model to predict sepsis using a minimal set of EHR variables. Calvert et al.[52] studied the same model among an alcohol use disorder patient population. Mao et al.[53] from the same company, validated the same model across different centers in the United States. Ghosh et al.[54] explored coupled hidden Markov models to predict septic shock in the ICU. Bedoya et al.[55] developed a multioutput Gaussian process and recurrent neural network to predict sepsis upon emergency department admission. Wong et al.[3] attempted to externally validate the ESM, a proprietary early warning system for sepsis that has shown poor discrimination and calibration in predicting sepsis
	Respiratory disease	Le et al.[56] proposed gradient-boosted tree models for early prediction of acute respiratory distress syndrome (ARDS) in the ICU. Sauthier et al.[57] used random forest models to predict prolonged acute hypoxemic respiratory failure in influenza-infected critically ill children
	Abnormal glucose	Tang et al.[58] used deep neural networks to predict blood glucose concentrations after short-acting insulin injections
3. Treatment decision support system	Mechanical ventilation timing, duration, weaning, reinitiation	Miu et al.[59] created a multivariable logistic regression model to predict the need for reintubation in the ICU. Ghazal et al.[60] trained bagged complex trees to predict SpO2 value after a ventilator setting change. Yu et al.[61] 2020 proposed a supervised-actor-critic reinforcement learning modeling approach to aid in the decision-making problems of ventilation and sedative dosing in the ICU. Sayed et al.[62] used gradient-boosted tree models to predict invasive mechanical ventilation duration after ARDS onset

Antibiotics dosing	Janssen et al.[63] proposed a framework for informed precision dosing, requiring accurate pharmacokinetic or ML
Intravenous (IV) fluid and vasopressor administration	Komorowski et al.[64] developed a reinforcement learning agent to achieve optimal administration of IV fluids and vasopressors. Srinivasan and Doshi-Velez[65] developed a novel interpretable batch variant of Adversarial Inverse Reinforcement Learning algorithm to optimize vasopressor and IV fluid administration in the ICU
Heparin dosing	Nemati et al.[66] developed a deep reinforcement learning model to learn an optimal heparin dosing policy in the ICU
Morphine dosing	Lopez-Martinez et al.[67] proposed a decision-making framework for opioid dosing based on reinforcement learning
Insulin dosing	DeJournett et al.[68] proposed an AI-based closed-loop glucose controller for an ICU setting using an adaptive modeling approach proposed by Van Herpe et al.[69] Nguyen et al.[70] proposed an ensemble model to predict patients requiring more than 6 units of total daily insulin dose
4. Outcome Assessment — In-hospital and ICU mortality/survival	Hsieh et al.[71] created a Fuzzy Hyper-Rectangular Composite Neural Network to predict the survival of ICU patients in a Taiwanese center. Johnson and Mark[72] developed a gradient-boosting model to predict mortality among ICU patients in MIMIC-III.[73] Monteiro et al.[74] proposed the use of a linear support-vector machine model coupled with a multivariate feature selection process to predict ICU mortality using the 3 datasets of the PhysioNet/Computing in Cardiology Challenge.[75] Iwase et al.[76] created random forest models to predict ICU mortality and length of stay in a Japanese center. Choi et al.[77] trained, among others, light gradient-boosted machine models to predict ICU mortality in 2 university hospitals in South Korea
ICU length of stay (LoS)	Abd-Elrazek et al.[78] employed fuzzy logic to predict LoS in the ICU using general admission features
	Alghatani et al.[79] created a binary model to predict whether the ICU stay is short or long, using MIMIC-III
	Hempel et al.[80] found random forest models to attain the highest performance for ICU LoS prediction using MIMIC-IV[81]
ICU readmission	Rojas et al.[82] proposed a gradient-boosted machine model to predict ICU readmission using MIMIC-III. Lin et al.[83] used recurrent neural networks with long short-term memory to predict unplanned readmission using MIMIC-III
Long-term survival and quality of life	Oyeen et al.[84] developed a prediction model for quality of life 1 y after ICU discharge based upon data available at the first ICU day using Lasso regression

Abbreviations: AKI, acute kidney injury; ARDS, acute respiratory distress syndrome; ESM, epic sepsis model; HMM, hidden Markov models; ICU, intensive care unit; LoS, length of stay; MIMIC-III, medical information mart for intensive care-III.
Taxonomy based on Hong and colleagues.[27]

this framework in the ICU. We emphasize how to effectively utilize these tools while maintaining a critical stance that addresses the potential risks of bias. *The premise is that a new AI tool has just been deployed in an ICU.* Prior to deployment, it has presumably been carefully analyzed by the hospital administration, who reviewed the framing of the problem and model, ensured that the modeling overarching approach is well-suited to solve the problem at hand; the team of developers was well suited for the task; and the methodology was sound and well executed. It is imperative for the clinicians to be well-versed in their institution's governance process, as it plays a pivotal role in querying developers and vendors. Following this initial step, we analyze the different steps of the ML development pipeline in the context of critical care, as defined by Nazer and colleagues.[90] For each step, we provide specific ICU examples; recommendations for bias risk assessment; and highlight how these can be put into practice in the context of the well-known overhaul and withdrawal of the epic sepsis prediction model.[3,91]

Guidelines for the ethical and equitable development, implementation, utilization, and governance of AI/ML models in the health care sector as a whole have attracted considerable attention in scholarly studies in recent times. Wiens and colleagues[92] presented guidelines on the translation of ML-based interventions into health care. Faes and colleagues[93] focused on promoting clinicians' critical appraisal studies of clinical applications of ML. Van de Sande and colleagues[94] summarized current guidelines, challenges, regulatory documents, and good practices that are needed to develop and safely implement AI in medicine. Nazer and colleagues[90] highlighted sources of bias within the process of developing AI algorithms in health care. Hassan and colleagues[95] provided a road map to develop predictive models that can be used in clinical practice.

With the increasing recognition of the importance of prioritizing fairness and uncovering biases among AI/ML developers,[96] reviews similar to the one performed by Nazer and colleagues[90] have been extensively performed across medical specialties. Arbet and colleagues[97] outlined common misconceptions about ML studies using electronic health record (EHR) data. Similarly, Sauer and colleagues[98] elaborated on potential pitfalls to be avoided when dealing with leveraging EHR data. Roberts and colleagues[99] conducted a systematic review that showed that all examined models intended to detect COVID-19 presented methodological flaws that hampered their utility. Delgado and colleagues[100] reviewed biases of AI algorithms developed for contact tracing and medical triage for COVID-19. Drukker and colleagues[101] delved into the different sources of bias in medical imaging-based ML methods. Gichoya and colleagues[102] reviewed pitfalls framed in the larger AI lifecycle for radiology applications. Nakayama and colleagues[103] listed the biases that can lurk in the AI lifecycle in ophthalmology. This abundance of studies suggests that the field is cognizant of the need for more structure; however, consensus is still needed for a set of common operating principles.[104–114]

Table 3 outlines the main sources of bias for an ML-based critical clinical prediction model. In the context of critical care, we explored: *data sources*, which include limitations related to selection bias,[104,111] unequally performing medical devices (80), and label bias; *data preprocessing*, where missingness handling (82, 83) and outlier removal can drive harmful spurious correlations; *model development*, which encompasses understanding the input features and their potential to leak information that compromises the utility of the model in real clinical practice (84); and *model validation* and *implementation*, which are associated with the performance of the algorithms, external validation, and postdeployment monitoring.[3,35,114]

Table 3

A checklist for intensive care unit clinicians to evaluate artificial intelligence-based clinical prediction models

ML Step	Risk of Bias/Challenge	What to do about it as a Clinician in the ICU	Case Study: ESM[3,91]
Data sources	Selection bias A mismatch between the training set and the real-world target; it can occur due to data and clinician drifts,[104] population shift,[105] and others	• Understand the population and datathon model was trained on • Compare the ICU typical composition with the cohorts behind the algorithms • Does the task at hand require any exclusion that I should be aware of?	Underlying patient characteristics are not reported (typically done in "**Table 1**"[106,107]) "*This model was developed and validated by Epic Systems Corporation based on data from 405,000 patient encounters across 3 health systems from 2013 to 2015.*" We are unable to assess potential selection bias, which would require looking at the inclusion/exclusion criteria of the cohort and represented demographics
	Biased medical devices Pulse oximeters, ECG, EEG, temporal thermometers, and sphygmometers are ubiquitously used in the ICU but have been shown to yield inaccuracies among certain subpopulations[108]	• Are these device limitations taken into account in the model? • Is the model's incorporation of these limitations enough to produce biased results? • Which groups of patients should I be especially worried about?	There is limited information on the input data due to the proprietary nature of ESM "*Data elements included vital signs, medication orders, lab values, comorbidities, and demographic information.*" The inclusion of vital signs could raise concerns as, for example, pulse oximetry readings are likely to be biased against Black and Hispanic patients[42]
	Label bias The label (or ground-truth) may be missing or inaccurate, thus leading to assumptions or limitations.	• Is the ground-truth a good ground-truth? • Is there any problem with the way we document the label that the model uses? • Is there anything I can do to increase the accuracy of the way possible labels are reported in the future?	"*(...) sepsis was defined as any encounter associated with an International Classification of Diseases (ICD-9) code indicating diagnosis of sepsis. Time of sepsis onset was defined as 6 h prior to clinical intervention (...)*" The label seems to be derived from billing information and based on ICD-9, which

(continued on next page)

Table 3
(continued)

ML Step	Risk of Bias/Challenge	What to do about it as a Clinician in the ICU	Case Study: ESM[3,91]
			may mean the model was not trained on patients with sepsis documented differently. This could raise questions about mismatches with actual practice
Data preprocessing	Handling missingness Some variables may not be missing at random, driving spurious correlations[109,110]; eg, the measurement of arterial blood gas in the ICU seems to be less likely among certain subpopulations[42] Outlier removal In the ICU, extreme values often take place (eg, blood pressure, glycemia)	• How does the model handle missingness? • Does it mirror my practice? • Does it embed any biases? • Is it consistent across subgroups? • Should I change anything in the way I report or not readings/measurements? • Does the outlier handling remove data points that I should be aware of? • Can I trust the model for such edge cases? • Can I recognize such edge cases and know when to fully ignore the model?	Data preprocessing is not mentioned by the vendors. *"This limited information is of concern because proprietary models are difficult to assess owing to their opaque nature and have been shown to decline in performance over time."* We recommend not to accept a model with such opaqueness and requesting these details from the development team
Model development	Diagnostic suspicion bias[111] An uneven diagnostic procedure in the target population, where some of the variables used to train the model (eg, timing and results of a test order) already convey information about the outcome, which constitutes a subtle yet common example of data leakage and limiting performance in patients where staff are not already suspicious Included variables The input data must contain relevant predictors that avoid leakages and go in line with clinical causal intuition	• Does the model require any variables that depend on my suspicion? • Is there any variable that reflects my bias and can be further confirmed or reinforced by the model's output? • Is there any reinforcement loop that I can or should avoid? • Do the included features follow a causal rationale that makes sense according to my clinical intuition? • Understand that variable importance tools (eg, SHAP[112]) are not causal	The only information on the modeling is: *"The ESM is a penalized logistic regression model (...)"* As the input features are not disclosed, assessing the soundness of this step is very challenging, posing a significant concern for this model. The study conducted by Wong et al.[3] suggested that one input variable to the model was antibiotic orders by a provider—a classic example of diagnostic suspicion bias since the suspicion of the clinical team would be necessary for the model to work. Further, we are unable to assess whether the possible relations between the features and the output have a causal rationale behind them

Model validation	Model performance The model will never work for 100% of the patients. External validation can help assess the utility of a model,[3] but it does not represent a definitive answer[35,113]	• What was the reported performance of the model? • Does the evaluation look sound? • Was it equally effective across groups? • To what extent can I trust this model?	In the final ESM, "(...) AUC ranged between 0.76–0.83.", which seems to be fairly calibrated. However, the external validation performed by Wong et al.[3] showed a significant deterioration, with poor discrimination in predicting the onset of sepsis—AUC of 0.63—and a large burden of alert fatigue. Critically appraising these metrics is fundamental to gaining trust
Implementation	Postdeployment monitoring Models are prone to drifts of different kinds over time[114]	• Is the model being updated? • Is it adaptable to possible changes? • Can I trust it in the long term? • Are there plans for real world monitoring?	This model bypassed peer review and regulatory oversight. The postdeployment monitoring seems to have been poorly conducted, considering the drop in performance verified by Wong et al.[3]

Abbreviations: AUC, area under the curve; ECG, electrocardiogram; EEG, electroencephalogram; ESM, epic sepsis model; ICD, International Classification Of Diseases; ICU, intensive care unit.
Taxonomy of ML steps based on Nazer and colleagues.[90]

As a case study, we delved into the ESM, which has been withdrawn following a publication from Wong and colleagues.[3] It presents various risk factors, biases, and, more importantly, uncertainties that raise significant structural concerns for its use in the ICU setting. First, the lack of transparency on the sources for the model's training data hampers our ability to assess the introduction of bias.[115] Additionally, the model's reliance on medical devices that were later shown to introduce racial bias, such as pulse oximeters, poses a risk since such medical devices may yield biased readings for certain patient groups as described earlier.[108] The use of billing data for label generation could also raise questions about the accuracy of the ground-truth, and the lack of information on missingness handling and outlier removal complicates the model's reliability.[103] The model's dependence on diagnostic suspicion poses a serious limitation to its real-world applicability and may perpetuate biases inherent in clinical decision-making.[3] The absence of information on model variables and causal rationale further challenges its clinical applicability. Furthermore, the discrepancy between vendor-reported and externally validated performance metrics, along with the apparent lack of postdeployment monitoring and transparency, diminishes trust in the model's long-term reliability.[3]

Despite all these concerns, the ESM was implemented in hundreds of US hospitals, bypassing peer review and regulatory oversight.[3] In light of the concerns and potential risks associated with the ESM, our recommendations for a clinician utilizing a similar model emphasize 3 core principles: curiosity, questioning, and skepticism. It is imperative for clinicians to actively engage with the model's documentation, approaching the model's reported training processes and underlying architecture with a critical and inquisitive mindset. This involves probing the model's data sources, underlying assumptions, and algorithms, as well as seeking transparency and detailed information from the developers regarding data preprocessing, feature selection, model development, and validation. Clinicians should continuously question the model's accuracy, especially in the context of their specific ICU patient population and remain vigilant for any potential biases or limitations.

HOW TO LEARN ABOUT CLINICAL PREDICTION MODELS AND SOURCES OF BIAS?

AI in health care is a field that is developing and expanding rapidly, and therefore, clinicians should be constantly updated on the most recent advances in this field, as well as understand the various sources of bias and potential strategies to mitigate them. This has traditionally been taught in the framework of scientific articles.[116] Historically, continued education and professional development used to be limited to individuals and institutions that can cover the cost of training and educational resources; however, over the past several years, the increased availability of open-access resources and virtual conferences/webinars has facilitated upskilling in data science for health care for practitioners and institutions within various resource settings. **Table 4** outlines major resources that clinicians may utilize to advance their skills and knowledge in the field of AI and the potential sources of bias. These include dedicated textbooks and journals as well as more modern resources such as datathons and workshops, which allow interactions around real-time, hands-on case studies. The launch of the first SCCM datathon in August 2023 illustrates the importance of the venue in fostering collegial information sharing and learning about the development, implementation, and evaluation of clinical prediction models in critical care.

Textbooks have traditionally been considered as the primary source of knowledge; however, as with all textbooks, the information quickly becomes outdated.[120] Though

Table 4
Resources available for clinicians to learn more about artificial intelligence in critical care and potential biases[a]

Source	Examples
Books	Chayakrit Krittanawong. Artificial intelligence in clinical practice. 1st Edition, 2023[117] MIT Critical Data. Secondary Analysis of Electronic Health Records.[118] Asselbergs FW. Clinical Applications of Artificial Intelligence in Real-World Data. 1st Edition, 2023
Journals[b]	Journal of American Medical Informatics Association Lancet Digital Health PLOS Digital Health BMC Digital Health BMJ Health & Care Informatics
Preprint servers	arXiv medRxiv
News Web sites	Stat News Guardian Technology MIT Technology Review Stanford HAI News ProPublica Technology Wired Science
Social media (Linkedin, X (Twitter), others)	SCCM ESICM YouTube—for interest-oriented learning. Keywords relevant to these topics include "AI Bias," "ML Fairness," "Health Equity"
Societies/professional groups	SCCM Discovery Data Science ESICM Data Science Section BrainX WiDS
Others	Datathons—eg, MIT Critical Datathon 2023, focused on Pulse Oximetry Bias; and SCCM Discovery Datathon 2023, which included Patient Safety and Health Equity tracks Conferences Coursera—eg, Emma Pierson's "Practical Steps for Building Fair AI Algorithms" course[119] Udemy

Abbreviations: ESICM, European Society of Intensive Care Medicine; SCCM, Society of Critical Care Medicine.
[a] This is a nonexhaustive list of common sources.
[b] All critical care journals have been publishing articles related to AI and ML in critical care.

most textbooks may be expensive to purchase, there are a few AI textbooks that are freely available, such as *Secondary Analysis of Electronic Health Records*.[118] Journals are another major resource that clinicians constantly rely on to stay up to date on recent science. In general, most critical care journals publish in the field of AI, but there are also journals that specialize in digital health and AI, such as the Journal of the American Medical Informatics Association, Lancet Digital Health, PLoS Digital Health, and BMC Digital Health. However, not all of these journals are open access. Preprint servers, such as arXiv or medRix, serve as valuable platforms for researchers to rapidly disseminate their findings to the scientific community before formal peer review, fostering early communication and collaboration. However, while enabling swift knowledge sharing, preprint servers may present challenges in terms of quality control and the potential spread of unvalidated or misleading information.[121]

News Web sites also play an interesting role in scientific dissemination by simplifying complex technical articles and making them accessible to diverse audiences. News Web sites offer curated information sources, facilitating access to complex technical and conceptual material for those who may find it challenging to navigate on their own; as an example in the scope of technology and critical care, technical computer science articles tailored to the comprehension of a medical audience can often be found within these resources. Additionally, news Web sites serve as a means for the early distribution of preprints and diverse viewpoints, contributing to the rapid flow of information within the scientific community. Although institutions usually have partnerships with these Web sites, hefty subscription fees may pose an obstacle to accessibility. Examples include *Stat News*,[122] *MIT Technology Review*,[123] *Stanford HAI News*,[124] *Guardian Technology*,[125] and *ProPublica Technology*.[126] Social media is becoming a major educational source for health care practitioners as it provides an update on what has been recently published in science, as well as creates a platform for discussing various aspects. The diversity of members on social media in terms of their backgrounds and settings creates an enriching platform to understand limitations and bias within various fields, including AI. Most critical care societies and journals post on social media platforms, mainly LinkedIn and X/Twitter, and to a lesser extent on Facebook and Instagram. However, though there is significant value to learning through social media, one should keep in mind that the content does not undergo any form of peer review and, therefore, should be carefully assessed for its validity.

Societies are also an important venue for various educational programs. There are data science groups within societies that conduct various educational activities during their annual conferences as well as webinars and other educational sessions. For example, the Society of Critical Care Medicine (SCCM) has a Data Science Campaign through their Discovery Research Section,[127] and the European Society of Intensive Care Medicine (ESICM) has a Data Science section.[128] However, activities through such societies and sections are limited to those who have membership. There are also other societies that are more specialized in AI and big data, such as the BrainX Community[129] and Women in Data Science (WiDS),[130] both of which offer free membership. In addition, they both provide various educational programs, many of which require no registration fees.

Datathons are a helpful way to build capacity and collaborations.[131–133] Conceived in 2016, it places clinical staff and data scientists/informaticists in direct contact. As opposed to a clinician who blindly relies on a black box/"magical" thinking, codevelopment and working together breaks down silos and provides firsthand experience with the process of model development. In-person datathons create fellow student and researcher teams so that data scientists and clinicians can combine their skills when addressing a problem. This unique opportunity to bring clinicians and data scientists together allows for the creation of an interface layer.[131] Not all academic centers have both in sufficient concentrations or naturally encounter each other. Working together on a project through a datathon can be a time-efficient manner to increase effective learning.[134] Datathon organizers include institutions (eg, Massachusetts Institute of Technology) and clinical societies (eg, ESICM and SCCM).[135] Datathons have been conducted in-person and virtually and have been received positively.[117,119,136] They have also generated diverse groups of research teams that continue to work together after the datathons. However, such datathons are restricted to a small group of participants, given that most of them require financial support for the travel of the participants to the site of the event or the travel of instructors. While some virtual data-thons have been organized, their impact remains to be assessed and compared with that of in-person events.

DISCUSSION
Modeling Limitations

Despite rapid progress in ML for health in the last decade, estimating the causal effects of interventions taking place in ICU settings remains challenging. Indeed, ICU patients often present multiple comorbidities upon admission, and their status may further complicate during their stay, resulting in a large number of time-varying confounders of any treatment-outcome relationships of interest. Moreover, ICU clinicians often prescribe several treatments concurrently (eg, antibiotics, anticoagulants, and antiarrhythmics).[137] The complexity of ICU pharmacotherapy thus makes isolating the effect of a single drug difficult and preventing harmful drug–drug interactions complicated.[138–140]

Beyond the presence of measurement errors emanating from numerous medical devices used in ICU settings (eg, pulse oximeters and sphygmomanometers),[141,142] observational studies conducted in critical care are also more prone to immortal time bias[143] than in other fields of medicine due to a high mortality rate in the first 24 hours following ICU admission. Indeed, a recent retrospective cohort study performed in Alberta, Canada, found that patients who die within 1 day comprise one-third of ICU deaths.[144] Therefore, if we were interested in evaluating the effect of an intervention only made available after the first day on ICU length-of-stay, patients who survived to their first ICU day would have a period of unexposed immortal time before receiving the intervention, an easily missed sampling bias. In 2009, Shintani and colleagues[145] had already warned about the prevalent but misleading use of standard Cox regression models in ICU survival analyses, showcasing the extent of bias when using time-fixed covariates to analyze the effect of a time-varying exposure on ICU length of stay. In a newly published perspective,[146] Vail and colleagues have again called for increased attention to immortal time bias in critical care, illustrating their argumentation with flawed observational studies of exposure to hydrocortisone, ascorbic acid, and thiamine therapy among patients with sepsis and septic shock—all published between 2017 and now. The authors took a step forward by providing a checklist for clinicians to more easily evaluate the characteristics of study design and analysis that may result in immortal time bias or detect a lack of sufficient reporting to rule out its absence. Two simple recommendations emanate from the studies of Shintani and colleagues and Vail and colleagues: first, carefully checking the methods section of any clinical article to ensure that time-varying analytical techniques were used appropriately, and second, ensuring that follow-up begins after the intervention eligibility period ends and at a time that is aligned across all patients.

For practitioners who are also greatly involved in research, the detailed specification of a "target trial" is advisable when retrospectively analyzing routinely collected patient data, that is, following the same procedure as when writing the detailed protocol of a randomized controlled trial. Practices such as listing inclusion/exclusion criteria, describing the static or dynamic treatment strategies under investigation, defining the follow-up period, and eliciting the causal estimands of interest all contribute to improving the transparency of statistical inferences. For instance, by considering more realistic treatment eligibility criteria and strategies, Wanis and colleagues[147] have shown that ICU patients captured in the medical information mart for intensive care (MIMIC)-IV database who were intubated earlier versus later during their stay had similar 30 day mortality rates. Their findings contrast with prior studies, which often used infeasible treatment strategies, and highlight the sensitivity of treatment effect estimates to critical but often neglected study design decisions.

The challenges faced in the ICU, including those related to the complexity of establishing causality within a context of multiple concurrent treatments, biases from medical devices, and the presence of immortal time bias, have the potential to generate misleading and harmful spurious correlations. Spurious correlations are noncausal relationships between the input and the outcome, which may shift in deployment.[105] These spurious correlations are particularly concerning, especially when they arise from systemic social discrimination, as seen in the case of bias in critical care medical devices.[108] Allowing the embedding of these errors, biases, and limitations in subsequent AI models could perpetuate and exacerbate existing disparities.[148,149] Therefore, modeling efforts in the realm of critical care must be approached with caution,[150] and a careful inspection of such sources of bias must be conducted a priori.[151]

Geographic Variability

Another challenge to the body of knowledge of clinical prediction models in the ICU is the significant variability observed across different ICU units, hospitals, and geographic locations. Numerous factors contribute to this variation, encompassing aspects such as differential patient illness severity, clinical outcomes, hospital type (eg, academic, community), size, number of beds, occupancy, staffing coverage, weekend coverage, demographics of the served population, reasons for ICU admission, or types of ICU units within the hospital.[152] For instance, comparing the health care systems in the United Kingdom and the United States reveals substantial dissimilarities.[153,154] The United States has 7 times as many ICU beds per capita as the United Kingdom.[153] In the United Kingdom, hospital stays before ICU admission are longer and the severity of illnesses is heightened.[153] This diversity in health care settings presents significant challenges in developing clinical prediction models that aim to effectively function across different contexts. An illustrative example is the NEWS2 in the United Kingdom, which, despite probably not being equally performant for all the different settings and populations,[41] is used nationwide as a guideline. As a result, it is imperative for clinicians to evaluate the architecture of their clinical prediction models critically. The multitude of reasons why a model may not be effective in a new setting underscores the need for a nuanced understanding of the local dynamics. Therefore, any model must be conscious of these challenges, be grounded in its local context, and aim to accommodate the intricacies of geographic variability from design. Similarly, the methodologies and recommendations suggested herein may not universally apply to all settings.

Challenges Related to Explainability, Generalizability, and External Validation

Explainability methodologies are argued to build trust among health care professionals, offering transparency in AI/ML decision-making, and potentially reducing bias.[155] In fact, recent Food and Drug Administration guidance recommends incorporating explanations into clinical decision support software so that clinicians are informed about the foundations of recommendations.[156] Nevertheless, the added value of such explanations remains debatable. In fact, a recent randomized clinical survey conducted by Jabbour and colleagues[157] showed that AI model explanations did not aid clinicians in identifying systematically biased models. In the absence of suitable explainability techniques, it is argued that the emphasis should be on careful internal and external validation of clinical models.[158]

Generalizability, that is, the ability of AI/ML models to extrapolate their knowledge to unobserved data, has also attracted considerable attention from researchers. Futoma and colleagues[113] highlighted that generalizability is not a binary concept but a multi-faceted one, involving not only temporal considerations like prospective application within the original center but also external validation across new centers and time-frames. However, neglecting such limitations in generalizability could lead to missed opportunities for leveraging AI/ML models in situations with potential clinical utility. Instead, narrow, "overfit," local models that work under certain circumstances and for certain subpopulations may actually be acceptable and yield value in real-world ICU practice.[35]

This has been confirmed in subsequent studies such as Youssef and colleagues[35] that argue that external validation of a clinical prediction model does not necessarily imply that it is useful in real-world settings. To ensure the practical usefulness of AI-based clinical models, we recommend complementing offline internal and external validations by the implementation of prospective impact studies; these can subsequently be used to timely determine the need to retrain the model locally. Wide adoption of the proposed recurring and local validation framework should allow for addressing distribution shifts in treatment, outcome, or both. In addition, if a change in health insurance contracts affects the mix of patients coming to the ICU, if critical care protocols are updated (eg, following the modification to sepsis recommendation guidelines), or if a hospital deploys a new EHR system, a timely update to the model using local patient cohorts would incorporate these new operational inputs.

Hence, as clinicians critically appraises a clinical prediction model, despite extensive external validation, it is crucial to approach any prediction model with caution and skepticism, as success in various centers and environments does not guarantee optimal performance within a specific ICU setting.

Postdeployment Detection and Mitigation of Disparities

Detecting and mitigating disparities after model deployment involves a multistep process, from data collection to data analysis, model correction development, dashboard creation, and near real-time monitoring of the revised models once implemented. While existing models may take at most a week to get updated and released on Hugging Face (Brooklyn, New York, NY), methods to evaluate the extent of their biases have not been standardized, and there is no platform where investigators can similarly post the results of model investigations or stress tests.

Disparity Dashboards

Despite the limited offer, a few initiatives have recently emerged. For example, Yi and colleagues[159] have described the steps needed to design and develop a digital equity dashboard for the emergency department of UC San Francisco hospitals. The use of disparity dashboards in clinical care delivery is growing. To sustain such efforts, Gallifant and colleagues[160] have recommended the setup of incentive systems to accelerate health data collection and reporting and of rewards that acknowledge successful mitigation of health disparities. Nonetheless, certain biases are more subtle and may remain undetected.[161] For instance, cognitive biases may affect the way clinicians handle conversations regarding end-of-life care with a patient's family.

Frameworks and Guidance Initiatives

High-level frameworks, recommendations, and guidance initiatives are also being designed to address these issues. Specifically, initiatives like STANDINGTogether[162] have the objective of ensuring the comprehensive representation of diverse populations in health datasets for the development of AI systems, which could solve part of the problem. The primary focus lies in offering guidance on the collection and reporting of crucial demographic details, including but not limited to gender, race, ethnicity, and others. Emphasizing transparency, the recommendations advocate for clear disclosure of any limitations within the dataset. This transparency facilitates informed decision-making by developers when selecting datasets for their AI models or tools. Furthermore, the STANDINGTogether guidelines provide insights into identifying potential harm to specific groups when employing medical AI systems, thereby contributing to the responsible and ethical use of such technologies. Other initiatives, such as the Coalition for Healthcare AI, are addressing this by convening experts from health care systems experts from multiple institutions representing health care systems, academia, government, and industry to identify problems and propose solutions to enable trustworthy AI in health care.[163] By developing a framework for an assurance standard and releasing a blueprint as a first step to building consensus on the execution, they attempt to develop an executable path toward assurance laboratories for continued assessment and monitoring of deployed and implemented systems.

The Potential of Artificial Intelligence/Machine Learning Models to Help Level the Playing Field

Chen and colleagues[164] have also argued that AI can help address health disparities, including by identifying and mitigating well-documented societal bias. A foundational study by Obermeyer and colleagues[165] estimated the calibration bias of an algorithm used to predict the health needs of insured patients 1 year ahead and showed significant differences based on race. Practically, a Black patient with the same algorithmic risk score as a White patient would on average have worse outcomes than their counterpart a year later. This retrospective analysis suggests that the insurer's model was underestimating the health needs of Black patients. Because they also had access to yearly health care costs per patient, the authors were able to identify the source of this bias, namely the use of individual-level health costs as a misleading proxy for health needs.

When the mechanisms underlying existing disparities can be interrogated and the sources of bias can be identified even partially, the development of correction models is facilitated. For example, underrepresentation of women and minority groups in clinical trials for cardiovascular diseases is known to affect the fairness of risk prediction models for atherosclerotic cardiovascular disease; yet, explicit adjustment in new models can alleviate the repercussions of a lack of inclusion in past trials.[166] Using the Southern Community Cohort Study, Zink and colleagues[167] identified differences in data quality as another source of bias in colorectal cancer risk prediction models.

Detecting or addressing disparities or biased practices sometimes involves stratifying or adjusting for race, ethnicity, and other social determinants of health. However, the decision of using race and ethnicity as input variables in risk prediction models remains highly contentious[168] and should be made on a case-by-case basis, with desired health outcome targets and fairness metrics clearly stated. Indeed, while the push[169,170] to remove such variables from risk scoring systems is legitimate, simply omitting race and ethnicity could yield worse prediction accuracy for racially minority groups,[171,172] as recently demonstrated by Khor and colleagues[173] in the context of a risk prediction model for colorectal cancer recurrence. Similarly, Zink and colleagues showed that implementing race-based corrections into colorectal cancer risk prediction models can counterbalance differences in data collection (eg, missingness, quality) by race.

In Pursuit of Fair, Performant, Sustainable, and Transparent Models

What do we ultimately seek from critical clinical prediction models? The answer, we posit, is 4 fold: fairness, performance, sustainability, and transparency. Fairness is essential to prevent the perpetuation and exacerbation of harmful societal biases within our models. Performance is crucial for ensuring the reliability and accuracy of these prediction models. Sustainability is pivotal to enable the necessary continual, automated updates of the models. Finally, transparency will democratize the ability to examine the underlying cohorts, methodologies, and architectures, which will ultimately foster fairness, performance, and sustainability.

While implementation poses challenges, it is imperative to enhance the hospital's capacity to accommodate the demands of these ever-evolving, lifelong learning AI/ML models. This requires not only building and improving data infrastructures within our hospitals but also providing comprehensive training to clinicians, specifically intensivists in the context of this review, to enable them to critically analyze the risk of bias, and effectively utilize the new generation of ICU tools.

SUMMARY

Clinical prediction models play a crucial role in handling complex data to support clinicians to make more informed and timely decisions. These models come in 2 forms: traditional scores and AI-based, each addressing a different range of tasks, with varying levels of complexity, interpretability and generalizability; these differences are typically inherent to the differences of expertise between the development teams of each type of model. Bias is not limited to either traditional or AI-based models, as both types have been found to potentially perpetuate harmful societal biases. Mitigating bias in AI models requires collaboration among diverse teams well-versed in understanding the underlying datasets and AI methodologies, as well as the critical appraisal of these tools by both hospital leadership and clinicians, particularly in the ICU. As bias can emerge at every stage of the AI lifecycle, from data sources to model deployment, we outline 6 steps, accompanied by examples that serve as a scaffold to design strategies to manage the risk of bias. In a more holistic view, bias mitigation will require ensuring the sustainability of clinical data pipelines within hospitals, prioritizing transparency and fairness in model development, and providing a more interdisciplinary training to clinicians. For clinicians interested in expanding their understanding of bias, resources like books, journals, social media platforms, professional societies, and events like datathons can be valuable sources of information.

CLINICS CARE POINTS

- Critical clinical prediction models enable clinicians to distill complex data into actionable insights, facilitating well-informed and timely decisions. These algorithms can be "traditional score-based" and "AI-based," yielding different properties regarding their range of addressed problems, underlying patient characteristics, generalization capabilities, development teams, fairness assessment, and complexity and interpretability.

- Biases can be present in traditional clinical prediction models (eg, SOFA, NEWS), as well as in AI-based models (eg, ESM), and both models have demonstrated the risk to perpetuate harmful societal biases.

- Effectively mitigating bias and reducing potential harm in AI-based models necessitates the collaboration of diverse teams possessing expertise in understanding both underlying datasets and AI methodologies. Equally important is the critical evaluation of these tools in the ICU by hospital leadership and clinicians. Biases, spanning the entire AI lifecycle, originate from data sources, preprocessing, model development, evaluation, and deployment stages.

- Clinicians seeking to expand their knowledge on bias can explore resources such as books, journals, social media platforms, societies and professional groups, and other decentralized events like datathons.
- Enhancing transparency and fairness in the development of predictive models, ensuring sustainability in hospitals' clinical data pipelines, and providing comprehensive training to clinicians are fundamental steps to identify and mitigate biases in critical clinical prediction models.

DISCLOSURE

A.I. Wong holds equity and management roles in Ataia Medical. A.I. Wong is supported by the Duke CTSI by the National Center for Advancing Translational Sciences, United States (NCATS) of the National Institutes of Health, United States under UL1TR002553 and REACH Equity under the National Institute on Minority Health and Health Disparities, United States (NIMHD) of the National Institutes of Health under U54MD012530. All other authors have no conflicts to disclose.

REFERENCES

1. Myatra SN, Prabu NR, Divatia JV, et al. The changes in pulse pressure variation or stroke volume variation after a "tidal volume challenge". Reliably predict fluid responsiveness during low tidal volume ventilation 2017. https://doi.org/10.1097/CCM.0000000000002183.
2. De Backer D, Heenen S, Piagnerelli M, et al. Pulse pressure variations to predict fluid responsiveness: influence of tidal volume. Intensive Care Med 2005;31(4):517–23.
3. Wong A, Otles E, Donnelly JP, et al. External validation of a widely implemented proprietary sepsis prediction model in hospitalized patients. JAMA Intern Med 2021;181(8):1065–70.
4. Davidson PC, Steed RD, Bode BW. Glucommander: a computer-directed intravenous insulin system shown to be safe, simple, and effective in 120,618 h of operation. Diabetes Care 2005;28(10):2418–23.
5. Obermeyer Z, Powers B, Vogeli C, et al. Dissecting racial bias in an algorithm used to manage the health of populations. Science 2019;366(6464). https://doi.org/10.1126/science.aax2342.
6. EU AI Act: first regulation on artificial intelligence. Available at: https://www.europarl.europa.eu/news/en/headlines/society/20230601STO93804/eu-ai-act-first-regulation-on-artificial-intelligence. [Accessed 1 November 2023].
7. The White House. President biden issues executive order on safe, secure, and trustworthy artificial intelligence. Available at: https://www.whitehouse.gov/briefing-room/statements-releases/2023/10/30/fact-sheet-president-biden-issues-executive-order-on-safe-secure-and-trustworthy-artificial-intelligence/. [Accessed 1 November 2023].
8. Johnson AEW, Ghassemi MM, Nemati S, et al. Machine learning and decision support in critical care. Proc IEEE Inst Electr Electron Eng 2016;104(2):444–66.
9. Celi LA, Mark RG, Stone DJ, et al. "Big data" in the intensive care unit. Closing the data loop. Am J Respir Crit Care Med 2013;187(11):1157–60.

10. Balogh EP, Miller BT, Ball JR, et al. The diagnostic process. (US): National Academies Press; 2015.
11. Katz A, Chateau D, Enns JE, et al. Association of the social determinants of health with quality of primary care. Ann Fam Med 2018;16(3):217–24.
12. Zheng B, Kwok E, Taljaard M, et al. Decision fatigue in the Emergency Department: how does emergency physician decision making change over an eight-hour shift? Am J Emerg Med 2020;38(12):2506–10.
13. Han PKJ, Klein WMP, Arora NK. Varieties of uncertainty in health care: a conceptual taxonomy. Med Decis Making 2011;31(6):828–38.
14. Delétang G, Ruoss A, Duquenne P-A, et al. Language modeling is compression. arXiv [csLG] 2023.
15. Meissen H, Gong MN, Wong A-KI, et al. The future of critical care: optimizing technologies and a learning healthcare system to potentiate a more humanistic approach to critical care. Crit Care Explor 2022;4(3):e0659.
16. Kamath PS, Wiesner RH, Malinchoc M, et al. A model to predict survival in patients with end-stage liver disease. Hepatology 2001;33(2):464–70.
17. Pisters R, Lane DA, Nieuwlaat R, et al. A novel user-friendly score (HAS-BLED) to assess 1-year risk of major bleeding in patients with atrial fibrillation: the Euro Heart Survey. Chest 2010;138(5):1093–100.
18. Tarricone A, Mata KDL, Gee A, et al. A systematic review and meta-analysis of the effectiveness of LRINEC score for predicting upper and lower extremity necrotizing fasciitis. J Foot Ankle Surg 2022;61(2):384–9.
19. Knaak C, Nyvlt P, Schuster FS, et al. Hemophagocytic lymphohistiocytosis in critically ill patients: diagnostic reliability of HLH-2004 criteria and HScore. Crit Care 2020;24(1):244.
20. Zimmerman JE, Kramer AA, McNair DS, et al. Acute Physiology and Chronic Health Evaluation (Apache) IV: hospital mortality assessment for today's critically ill patients. Crit Care Med 2006;34(5):1297–310.
21. Johnson AEW, Kramer AA, Clifford GD. A new severity of illness scale using a subset of Acute Physiology and Chronic Health Evaluation data elements shows comparable predictive accuracy. Crit Care Med 2013;41(7):1711–8.
22. Goldfield N. The evolution of diagnosis-related groups (DRGs): from its beginnings in case-mix and resource use theory, to its implementation for payment and now for its current utilization for quality within and outside the hospital. Qual Manag Health Care 2010;19(1):3–16.
23. Charlson ME, Pompei P, Ales KL, et al. A new method of classifying prognostic comorbidity in longitudinal studies: development and validation. J Chronic Dis 1987;40(5):373–83.
24. Elixhauser A, Steiner C, Harris DR, et al. Comorbidity measures for use with administrative data. Med Care 1998;36(1):8–27.
25. Staudacher D, Supady A, Schroth F, et al. Performance of SOFA, SAVE, and SAPS2 score in venoarterial extracorporeal membrane oxygenation (VA-ECMO) for cardiogenic shock and extracorporeal cardiopulmonary resuscitation (eCPR). Resuscitation 2018;130:e5–6.
26. Hick JL, Rubinson L, O'Laughlin DT, et al. Clinical review: allocating ventilators during large-scale disasters–problems, planning, and process. Crit Care 2007; 11(3):217.
27. Hong N, Liu C, Gao J, et al. State of the art of machine learning-enabled clinical decision support in intensive care units: literature review. JMIR Med Inform 2022;10(3):e28781.
28. LeCun Y, Bengio Y, Hinton G. Deep learning. Nature 2015;521(7553):436–44.

29. Sutton RS, Barto AG. Reinforcement learning. MIT press. Available at: https://mitpress.mit.edu/9780262193986/reinforcement-learning/. [Accessed 21 October 2023].

30. Acosta JN, Falcone GJ, Rajpurkar P, et al. Multimodal biomedical AI. Nat Med 2022;28(9):1773–84.

31. Johnson KB, Wei W-Q, Weeraratne D, et al. Precision medicine, AI, and the future of personalized health care. Clin Transl Sci 2021;14(1):86–93.

32. Elovic A, Pourmand A. MDCalc medical calculator app review. J Digit Imaging 2019;32(5):682–4.

33. Rudin C. Stop explaining black box machine learning models for high stakes decisions and use interpretable models instead. Nat Mach Intell 2019;1(5):206–15.

34. Mbakwe AB, Lourentzou I, Celi LA, et al. Fairness metrics for health AI: we have a long way to go. EBioMedicine 2023;90. https://doi.org/10.1016/j.ebiom.2023.104525.

35. Youssef A, Pencina M, Thakur A, et al. External validation of AI models in health should be replaced with recurring local validation. Nat Med 2023;1–2.

36. Quinn TP, Senadeera M, Jacobs S, et al. Trust and medical AI: the challenges we face and the expertise needed to overcome them. J Am Med Inf Assoc 2021;28(4):890–4.

37. Suistomaa M, Kari A, Ruokonen E, et al. Sampling rate causes bias in Apache II and SAPS II scores. Intensive Care Med 2000;26(12):1773–8.

38. Paulus JK, Kent DM. Predictably unequal: understanding and addressing concerns that algorithmic clinical prediction may increase health disparities. NPJ Digit Med 2020;3:99.

39. Ashana DC, Anesi GL, Liu VX, et al. Equitably allocating resources during crises: racial differences in mortality prediction models. Am J Respir Crit Care Med 2021;204(2):178–86.

40. Miller WD, Han X, Peek ME, et al. Accuracy of the sequential organ failure assessment score for in-hospital mortality by race and relevance to Crisis standards of care. JAMA Netw Open 2021;4(6):e2113891.

41. Fawzy A, Wu TD, Wang K, et al. Racial and ethnic discrepancy in pulse oximetry and delayed identification of treatment eligibility among patients with COVID-19. JAMA Intern Med 2022;182(7):730–8.

42. Wong A-KI, Charpignon M, Kim H, et al. Analysis of discrepancies between pulse oximetry and arterial oxygen saturation measurements by race and ethnicity and association with organ dysfunction and mortality. JAMA Netw Open 2021;4(11):e2131674.

43. Eini-Porat B, Amir O, Eytan D, et al. Tell me something interesting: clinical utility of machine learning prediction models in the ICU. J Biomed Inform 2022;132:104107.

44. Kellogg KC, Sendak M, Balu S. AI on the front lines. MIT Sloan Manag Rev 2022;63(4):44–50. Cambridge.

45. Zhang Y, Szolovits P. Patient-specific learning in real time for adaptive monitoring in critical care. J Biomed Inform 2008;41(3):452–60.

46. Kwok HF, Linkens DA, Mahfouf M, et al. Adaptive ventilator FiO2 advisor: use of non-invasive estimations of shunt. Artif Intell Med 2004;32(3):157–69.

47. Gholami B, Phan TS, Haddad WM, et al. Replicating human expertise of mechanical ventilation waveform analysis in detecting patient-ventilator cycling asynchrony using machine learning. Comput Biol Med 2018;97:137–44.

48. Rehm GB, Han J, Kuhn BT, et al. Creation of a robust and generalizable machine learning classifier for patient ventilator asynchrony. Methods Inf Med 2018;57(4): 208–19.

49. Sun M, Baron J, Dighe A, et al. Early prediction of acute kidney injury in critical care setting using clinical notes and structured multivariate physiological measurements. Stud Health Technol Inform 2019;264:368–72.

50. Sanchez-Pinto LN, Khemani RG. Development of a prediction model of early acute kidney injury in critically ill children using electronic health record data. Pediatr Crit Care Med 2016;17(6):508–15.

51. Desautels T, Calvert J, Hoffman J, et al. Prediction of sepsis in the intensive care unit with minimal electronic health record data: a machine learning approach. JMIR Med Inform 2016;4(3):e28.

52. Calvert J, Desautels T, Chettipally U, et al. High-performance detection and early prediction of septic shock for alcohol-use disorder patients. Ann Med Surg (Lond) 2016;8:50–5.

53. Mao Q, Jay M, Hoffman JL, et al. Multicentre validation of a sepsis prediction algorithm using only vital sign data in the emergency department, general ward and ICU. BMJ Open 2018;8(1):e017833.

54. Ghosh S, Li J, Cao L, et al. Septic shock prediction for ICU patients via coupled HMM walking on sequential contrast patterns. J Biomed Inform 2017;66:19–31.

55. Bedoya AD, Futoma J, Clement ME, et al. Machine learning for early detection of sepsis: an internal and temporal validation study. JAMIA Open 2020;3(2): 252–60.

56. Le S, Pellegrini E, Green-Saxena A, et al. Supervised machine learning for the early prediction of acute respiratory distress syndrome (ARDS). J Crit Care 2020;60:96–102.

57. Sauthier MS, Jouvet PA, Newhams MM, et al. Machine learning predicts prolonged acute hypoxemic respiratory failure in pediatric severe influenza. Crit Care Explor 2020;2(8):e0175.

58. Tang B, Yuan Y, Yang J, et al. Predicting blood glucose concentration after short-acting insulin injection using discontinuous injection records. Sensors 2022;22(21). https://doi.org/10.3390/s22218454.

59. Frandes M, Timar B, Lungeanu D. A risk based neural network approach for predictive modeling of blood glucose dynamics. Stud Health Technol Inform 2016; 228:577–81.

60. Ghazal S, Sauthier M, Brossier D, et al. Using machine learning models to predict oxygen saturation following ventilator support adjustment in critically ill children: a single center pilot study. PLoS One 2019;14(2):e0198921.

61. Yu C, Ren G, Dong Y. Supervised-actor-critic reinforcement learning for intelligent mechanical ventilation and sedative dosing in intensive care units. BMC Med Inform Decis Mak 2020;20(Suppl 3):124.

62. Sayed M, Riaño D, Villar J. Predicting duration of mechanical ventilation in acute respiratory distress syndrome using supervised machine learning. J Clin Med Res 2021;10(17). https://doi.org/10.3390/jcm10173824.

63. Janssen A, De Waele JJ, Elbers PWG. Towards adequate and automated antibiotic dosing. Intensive Care Med 2023;49(7):853–6.

64. Komorowski M, Celi LA, Badawi O, et al. The Artificial Intelligence Clinician learns optimal treatment strategies for sepsis in intensive care. Nat Med 2018; 24(11):1716–20.

65. Srinivasan S, Doshi-Velez F. Interpretable batch IRL to extract clinician goals in ICU hypotension management. AMIA Jt Summits Transl Sci Proc 2020;2020: 636–45.

66. Nemati S, Ghassemi MM, Clifford GD. Optimal medication dosing from suboptimal clinical examples: a deep reinforcement learning approach. Conf Proc IEEE Eng Med Biol Soc 2016;2016:2978–81.

67. Lopez-Martinez D, Eschenfeldt P, Ostvar S, et al. Deep reinforcement learning for optimal critical care pain management with morphine using dueling double-deep Q networks. Conf Proc IEEE Eng Med Biol Soc 2019;2019:3960–3.

68. DeJournett L, DeJournett J. In silico testing of an artificial-intelligence-based artificial pancreas designed for use in the intensive care unit setting. J Diabetes Sci Technol 2016;10(6):1360–71.

69. Van Herpe T, Espinoza M, Haverbeke N, et al. Glycemia prediction in critically ill patients using an adaptive modeling approach. J Diabetes Sci Technol 2007; 1(3):348–56.

70. Nguyen M, Jankovic I, Kalesinskas L, et al. Machine learning for initial insulin estimation in hospitalized patients. J Am Med Inf Assoc 2021;28(10):2212–9.

71. Hsieh Y-Z, Su M-C, Wang C-H, et al. Prediction of survival of ICU patients using computational intelligence. Comput Biol Med 2014;47:13–9.

72. Johnson AEW, Mark RG. Real-time mortality prediction in the intensive care unit. AMIA Annu Symp Proc 2017;2017:994–1003.

73. Johnson AEW, Pollard TJ, Shen L, et al. MIMIC-III, a freely accessible critical care database. Sci Data 2016;3:160035.

74. Monteiro F, Meloni F, Baranauskas JA, et al. Prediction of mortality in Intensive Care Units: a multivariate feature selection. J Biomed Inform 2020;107:103456.

75. Silva I, Moody G, Scott DJ, et al. Predicting in-hospital mortality of ICU patients: the PhysioNet/computing in cardiology challenge 2012. Comput Cardiol 2012; 39:245–8.

76. Iwase S, Nakada T-A, Shimada T, et al. Prediction algorithm for ICU mortality and length of stay using machine learning. Sci Rep 2022;12(1):1–9.

77. Choi MH, Kim D, Choi EJ, et al. Mortality prediction of patients in intensive care units using machine learning algorithms based on electronic health records. Sci Rep 2022;12(1):1–11.

78. Abd-Elrazek MA, Eltahawi AA, Abd Elaziz MH, et al. Predicting length of stay in hospitals intensive care unit using general admission features. Ain Shams Eng J 2021;12(4):3691–702.

79. Alghatani K, Ammar N, Rezgui A, et al. Predicting intensive care unit length of stay and mortality using patient vital signs: machine learning model development and validation. JMIR Med Inform 2021;9(5):e21347.

80. Hempel L, Sadeghi S, Kirsten T. Prediction of intensive care unit length of stay in the MIMIC-IV dataset. NATO Adv Sci Inst Ser E Appl Sci 2023;13(12):6930.

81. Johnson AEW, Bulgarelli L, Shen L, et al. MIMIC-IV, a freely accessible electronic health record dataset. Sci Data 2023;10(1):1.

82. Rojas JC, Carey KA, Edelson DP, et al. Predicting intensive care unit readmission with machine learning using electronic health record data. Ann Am Thorac Soc 2018;15(7):846–53.

83. Lin Y-W, Zhou Y, Faghri F, et al. Analysis and prediction of unplanned intensive care unit readmission using recurrent neural networks with long short-term memory. PLoS One 2019;14(7):e0218942.

84. Oeyen S, Vermeulen K, Benoit D, et al. Development of a prediction model for long-term quality of life in critically ill patients. J Crit Care 2018;43:133–8.

85. Moor M, Rieck B, Horn M, et al. Early prediction of sepsis in the ICU using machine learning: a systematic review. Front Med 2021;8:607952.
86. Zale A, Mathioudakis N. Machine learning models for inpatient glucose prediction. Curr Diab Rep 2022;22(8):353–64.
87. Miu T, Joffe AM, Yanez ND, et al. Predictors of reintubation in critically ill patients. Respir Care 2014;59(2):178–85.
88. van de Sande D, van Genderen ME, Huiskens J, et al. Moving from bytes to bedside: a systematic review on the use of artificial intelligence in the intensive care unit. Intensive Care Med 2021;47(7):750–60.
89. Johnson A.E.W., Pollard T.J., Mark R.G., Reproducibility in critical care: a mortality prediction case study, Machine learning for healthcare conference, 18–19 Aug 2017;68:361–376.
90. Nazer LH, Zatarah R, Waldrip S, et al. Bias in artificial intelligence algorithms and recommendations for mitigation. PLOS Digit Health 2023;2(6):e0000278.
91. Habib AR, Lin AL, Grant RW. The epic sepsis model falls short—the importance of external validation. JAMA Intern Med 2021;181(8):1040–1.
92. Wiens J, Saria S, Sendak M, et al. Do no harm: a roadmap for responsible machine learning for health care. Nat Med 2019;25(9):1337–40.
93. Faes L, Liu X, Wagner SK, et al. A clinician's guide to artificial intelligence: how to critically appraise machine learning studies. Transl Vis Sci Technol 2020; 9(2):7.
94. van de Sande D, Van Genderen ME, Smit JM, et al. Developing, implementing and governing artificial intelligence in medicine: a step-by-step approach to prevent an artificial intelligence winter. BMJ Health Care Inform 2022;29(1). https://doi.org/10.1136/bmjhci-2021-100495.
95. Hassan N, Slight R, Morgan G, et al. Road map for clinicians to develop and evaluate AI predictive models to inform clinical decision-making. BMJ Health Care Inform 2023;30(1):e100784.
96. Ferryman K, Mackintosh M, Ghassemi M. Considering biased data as informative artifacts in AI-assisted health care. N Engl J Med 2023;389(9):833–8.
97. Arbet J, Brokamp C, Meinzen-Derr J, et al. Lessons and tips for designing a machine learning study using EHR data. J Clin Transl Sci 2020;5(1):e21.
98. Sauer CM, Chen L-C, Hyland SL, et al. Leveraging electronic health records for data science: common pitfalls and how to avoid them. The Lancet Digital Health 2022;4(12):e893–8.
99. Roberts M, Driggs D, Thorpe M, et al. Common pitfalls and recommendations for using machine learning to detect and prognosticate for COVID-19 using chest radiographs and CT scans. Nat Mach Intell 2021;3(3):199–217.
100. Delgado J, de Manuel A, Parra I, et al. Bias in algorithms of AI systems developed for COVID-19: a scoping review. J bioeth Inq 2022;407–19. https://doi.org/10.1007/s11673-022-10200-z.
101. Drukker K, Chen W, Gichoya J, et al. Toward fairness in artificial intelligence for medical image analysis: identification and mitigation of potential biases in the roadmap from data collection to model deployment. J Med Imaging (Bellingham) 2023;10(6):061104.
102. Gichoya JW, Thomas K, Celi LA, et al. AI pitfalls and what not to do: mitigating bias in AI. Br J Radiol 2023;96(1150):20230023.
103. Nakayama LF, Matos J, Quion J, et al. Unmasking biases and navigating pitfalls in the ophthalmic artificial intelligence lifecycle: a review. arXiv [csCY] 2023.
104. Hegedus EJ, Moody J. Clinimetrics corner: the many faces of selection bias. J Man Manip Ther 2010;18(2):69–73.

105. Yang Y, Zhang H, Katabi D, et al. Change is hard: a closer look at subpopulation shift. arXiv 2023.

106. Yoshida K., Bohn J. Tableone: create "table 1" to describe baseline characteristics. R Package Version n.d.

107. Pollard TJ, Johnson AEW, Raffa JD, et al. tableone: an open source Python package for producing summary statistics for research papers. JAMIA Open 2018;1(1):26–31.

108. Charpignon M-L, Byers J, Cabral S, et al. Critical bias in critical care devices. Crit Care Clin 2023;39(4):795–813.

109. Nijman S, Leeuwenberg AM, Beekers I, et al. Missing data is poorly handled and reported in prediction model studies using machine learning: a literature review. J Clin Epidemiol 2022;142:218–29.

110. Greenland S, Mansournia MA, Altman DG. Sparse data bias: a problem hiding in plain sight. BMJ 2016;352:i1981.

111. Delgado-Rodríguez M, Llorca J. Bias. J Epidemiol Community 2004;58(8): 635–41.

112. Lundberg S, Lee S-I. A unified approach to interpreting model predictions. arXiv 2017.

113. Futoma J, Simons M, Panch T, et al. The myth of generalisability in clinical research and machine learning in health care. Lancet Digit Health 2020;2(9): e489–92.

114. Finlayson SG, Subbaswamy A, Singh K, et al. The clinician and dataset shift in artificial intelligence. N Engl J Med 2021;385(3):283.

115. Daneshjou R, Smith MP, Sun MD, et al. Lack of transparency and potential bias in artificial intelligence data sets and algorithms: a scoping review. JAMA Dermatol 2021;157(11):1362–9.

116. Young JM, Solomon MJ. How to critically appraise an article. Nat Clin Pract Gastroenterol Hepatol 2009;6(2):82–91.

117. Krittanawong C, editor. *Artificial Intelligence in Clinical Practice: How AI Technologies Impact Medical Research and Clinics*. Amsterdam, Netherlands: Elsevier; 2023.

118. MIT Critical Data. *Secondary analysis of electronic health records*. Berlin, Germany: Springer Nature; 2016. p. 427.

119. Practical steps for building fair AI algorithms. Coursera. Available at: https://www.coursera.org/learn/algorithmic-fairness. [Accessed 6 January 2024].

120. Greene P. Bill gates says the textbook is dying. Is He right? Forbes Magazine 2019.

121. Nabavi Nouri S, Cohen YA, Madhavan MV, et al. Preprint manuscripts and servers in the era of coronavirus disease 2019. J Eval Clin Pract 2021;27(1): 16–21.

122. Facher L, Garde D, Silverman E, et al. Stat. Stat. Available at: https://www.statnews.com/. [Accessed 3 November 2023].

123. Magazine series, MIT Technology Review.

124. News. Stanford Institute for human-centered artificial intelligence. Available at: https://hai.stanford.edu/news. [Accessed 3 November 2023].

125. Magazine series, Guardian Technology.

126. Technology. ProPublica. Available at: https://www.propublica.org/topics/technology. [Accessed 3 November 2023].

127. SCCM. Society of critical care medicine (SCCM). Available at: https://sccm.org/Research/Discovery-Research-Network/datascience. [Accessed 3 November 2023].

128. Data science. ESICM. Available at: https://www.esicm.org/groups/data-science/. [Accessed 3 November 2023].

129. Home. BrainX community. Available at: https://brainxai.org/. [Accessed 3 November 2023].

130. WiDS Worldwide. WiDS worldwide. Available at: https://www.widsworldwide.org/. [Accessed 3 November 2023].

131. Sobel J, Almog R, Celi L, et al. How to organise a datathon for bridging between data science and healthcare? Insights from the Technion-Rambam machine learning in healthcare datathon event. BMJ Health Care Inform 2023;30(1). https://doi.org/10.1136/bmjhci-2023-100736.

132. Aboab J, Celi LA, Charlton P, et al. A "datathon" model to support cross-disciplinary collaboration. Sci Transl Med 2016;8(333):333ps8.

133. Luo EM, Newman S, Amat M, et al. MIT COVID-19 Datathon: data without boundaries. BMJ Innov 2021;7(1):231–4.

134. Piza FM, Celi LA, Deliberato RO, et al. Assessing team effectiveness and affective learning in a datathon. Int J Med Inf 2018;112:40–4.

135. Datathon. Society of critical care medicine (SCCM). Available at: https://sccm.org/Research/Discovery-Research-Network/datascience/Datathon. [Accessed 3 November 2023].

136. Lyndon MP, Pathanasethpong A, Henning MA, et al. Measuring the learning outcomes of datathons. BMJ Innovations 2022;8(2). https://doi.org/10.1136/bmjinnov-2021-000747.

137. Zhou S, Skaar DJ, Jacobson PA, et al. Pharmacogenomics of medications commonly used in the intensive care unit. Front Pharmacol 2018;9:1436.

138. Bakker T, Abu-Hanna A, Dongelmans DA, et al. Clinically relevant potential drug-drug interactions in intensive care patients: a large retrospective observational multicenter study. J Crit Care 2021;62:124–30.

139. Moore P, Burkhart K. Adverse drug reactions in the intensive care unit. Critical Care Toxicol 2017;693–739.

140. Wang H, Shi H, Wang N, et al. Prevalence of potential drug - drug interactions in the cardiothoracic intensive care unit patients in a Chinese tertiary care teaching hospital. BMC Pharmacol Toxicol 2022;23(1):39.

141. Charpignon M-L, Carrel A, Jiang Y, et al. Going beyond the means: exploring the role of bias from digital determinants of health in technologies. PLOS Digit Health 2023;2(10):e0000244.

142. Liu J, Li Y, Li J, et al. Sources of automatic office blood pressure measurement error: a systematic review. Physiol Meas 2022;43(9). https://doi.org/10.1088/1361-6579/ac890e.

143. Yadav K, Lewis RJ. Immortal time bias in observational studies. JAMA 2021;325(7):686–7.

144. Andersen SK, Montgomery CL, Bagshaw SM. Early mortality in critical illness - a descriptive analysis of patients who died within 24 hours of ICU admission. J Crit Care 2020;60:279–84.

145. Shintani AK, Girard TD, Eden SK, et al. Immortal time bias in critical care research: application of time-varying Cox regression for observational cohort studies. Crit Care Med 2009;37(11):2939–45.

146. Vail EA, Gershengorn HB, Wunsch H, et al. Attention to immortal time bias in critical care research. Am J Respir Crit Care Med 2021;203(10):1222–9.

147. Wanis KN, Madenci AL, Hao S, et al. Emulating target trials comparing early and delayed intubation strategies. Chest 2023;164(4):885–91.

148. Angwin J, Larson J, Kirchner L, et al. Machine bias. Available at: https://www. propublica.org/article/machine-bias-risk-assessments-in-criminal-sentencing. [Accessed 22 October 2023].

149. Panch T, Mattie H, Atun R. Artificial intelligence and algorithmic bias: implications for health systems. J Glob Health 2019;9(2):010318.

150. Iqbal U, Celi LA, Hsu Y-HE, et al. Healthcare artificial intelligence: the road to hell is paved with good intentions. BMJ Health Care Inform 2022;29(1). https://doi. org/10.1136/bmjhci-2022-100650.

151. Teotia K, Jia Y, Woite NL, et al. Variation in monitoring: glucose measurement in the ICU as a case study to preempt spurious correlations. bioRxiv 2023. https:// doi.org/10.1101/2023.10.12.23296568.

152. Critical Care Statistics. Society of critical care medicine (SCCM). Available at: https://www.sccm.org/Communications/Critical-Care-Statistics. [Accessed 24 October 2023].

153. Wunsch H, Angus DC, Harrison DA, et al. Comparison of medical admissions to intensive care units in the United States and United Kingdom. Am J Respir Crit Care Med 2011;183(12):1666–73.

154. Angus DC, Shorr AF, White A, et al. Critical care delivery in the United States: distribution of services and compliance with Leapfrog recommendations. Crit Care Med 2006;1016–24.

155. Amann J, Blasimme A, Vayena E, et al. Explainability for artificial intelligence in healthcare: a multidisciplinary perspective. BMC Med Inform Decis Mak 2020; 20(1):310.

156. Center for Devices. Radiological Health. Clinical decision support software - guidance. U.S. Food and Drug Administration. Available at: https://www.fda. gov/regulatory-information/search-fda-guidance-documents/clinical-decision-support-software. [Accessed 6 January 2024].

157. Jabbour S, Fouhey D, Shepard S, et al. Measuring the impact of AI in the diagnosis of hospitalized patients: a randomized clinical vignette survey study. JAMA 2023;330(23):2275–84.

158. Ghassemi M, Oakden-Rayner L, Beam AL. The false hope of current approaches to explainable artificial intelligence in health care. Lancet Digit Health 2021;3(11):e745–50.

159. Yi S, Burke C, Reilly A, et al. Designing and developing a digital equity dashboard for the emergency department. J Am Coll Emerg Physicians Open 2023;4(4):e12997.

160. Gallifant J, Kistler EA, Nakayama LF, et al. Disparity dashboards: an evaluation of the literature and framework for health equity improvement. Lancet Digit Health 2023;5(11):e831–9.

161. Harleen Kaur Johal CD. Challenging cognitive biases in the intensive care unit. BMJ | Journal of Medical Ethics 2020. Available at: https://blogs.bmj.com/ medical-ethics/2020/07/14/challenging-cognitive-biases-in-the-intensive-care-unit/. [Accessed 6 January 2024].

162. Ganapathi S, Palmer J, Alderman JE, et al. Tackling bias in AI health datasets through the STANDING Together initiative. Nat Med 2022;28(11):2232–3.

163. Chai. Available at: https://www.coalitionforhealthai.org/. [Accessed 7 January 2024].

164. Chen IY, Joshi S, Ghassemi M. Treating health disparities with artificial intelligence. Nat Med 2020;26(1):16–7.

165. Obermeyer Z, Powers B, Vogeli C, et al. Dissecting racial bias in an algorithm used to manage the health of populations. Science 2019;447–53. https://doi. org/10.1126/science.aax2342.
166. Pfohl S, Marafino B, Coulet A, et al. Creating fair models of atherosclerotic cardiovascular disease risk, . Proceedings of the 2019 AAAI/ACM conference on AI, ethics, and society. New York, NY, USA: Association for Computing Machinery; 2019. p. 271–8.
167. Zink A, Obermeyer Z, Pierson E. Race corrections in clinical algorithms can help correct for racial disparities in data quality. bioRxiv 2023. https://doi.org/10. 1101/2023.03.31.23287926.
168. Manski CF, Mullahy J, Venkataramani AS. Using measures of race to make clinical predictions: decision making, patient health, and fairness. Proc Natl Acad Sci U S A 2023;120(35):e2303370120.
169. Vyas DA, Eisenstein LG, Jones DS. Hidden in plain sight - reconsidering the use of race correction in clinical algorithms. N Engl J Med 2020;383(9):874–82.
170. Diao JA, Inker LA, Levey AS, et al. In search of a better equation - performance and equity in estimates of kidney function. N Engl J Med 2021;384(5):396–9.
171. Stevens ER, Caverly T, Butler JM, et al. Considerations for using predictive models that include race as an input variable: the case study of lung cancer screening. J Biomed Inform 2023;147:104525.
172. Hammond G, Johnston K, Huang K, et al. Social determinants of health improve predictive accuracy of clinical risk models for cardiovascular hospitalization, annual cost, and death. Circ Cardiovasc Qual Outcomes 2020;13(6):e006752.
173. Khor S, Haupt EC, Hahn EE, et al. Racial and ethnic bias in risk prediction models for colorectal cancer recurrence when race and ethnicity are omitted as predictors. JAMA Netw Open 2023;6(6):e2318495.